Allergy and Clinical Immunology

Allergy and Clinical Immunology

Edited by Fabian Kent

hayle medical

New York

Hayle Medical,
750 Third Avenue, 9ᵗʰ Floor,
New York, NY 10017, USA

Visit us on the World Wide Web at:
www.haylemedical.com

ISBN: 978-1-63241-645-2

Cataloging-in-Publication Data

Allergy and clinical immunology / edited by Fabian Kent.
    p. cm.
Includes bibliographical references and index.
ISBN 978-1-63241-645-2
1. Allergy. 2. Clinical immunology. 3. Immunologic diseases. I. Kent, Fabian.
QR188 .A455 2019
616.97--dc23

Table of Contents

              venom immunotherapy** 167
              Marcello Albanesi, Andrea Nico, Alessandro Sinisi, Lucia Giliberti, Maria Pia Rossi,
              Margherita Rossini, Georgios Kourtis, Anna Simona Rucco, Filomena Loconte,
              Loredana Muolo, Marco Zurlo, Danilo Di Bona, Maria Filomena Caiaffa
              and Luigi Macchia

Chapter 22   **High frequency of IgE sensitization towards kiwi seed storage proteins among
              peanut allergic individuals also reporting allergy to kiwi** 178
              Jenny van Odijk, Sigrid Sjölander, Peter Brostedt, Magnus P. Borres
              and Hillevi Englund

Chapter 23   **The control of allergic rhinitis in real life**... 186
              Federica Gani, Carlo Lombardi, Laura Barrocu, Massimo Landi, Erminia Ridolo,
              Massimo Bugiani, Giovanni Rolla, Gianenrico Senna and Giovanni Passalacqua

Chapter 24   **Amelioration of patients with chronic spontaneous urticaria in treatment with
              vitamin D supplement** 192
              Nazila Ariaee, Shima Zarei, Mojgan Mohamadi and Farahzad Jabbari

Chapter 25   **Role of genetic variations of *chitinase 3-like 1* in bronchial asthmatic patients** 197
              Kazuyuki Abe, Yutaka Nakamura, Kohei Yamauchi and Makoto Maemondo

              Permissions

              List of Contributors

              Index

Preface

This book has been an outcome of determined endeavour from a group of educationists in the field. The primary objective was to involve a broad spectrum of professionals from diverse cultural background involved in the field for developing new researches. The book not only targets students but also scholars pursuing higher research for further enhancement of the theoretical and practical applications of the subject.

The hypersensitivity of the immune system in response to harmless substances in the environment is referred to as an allergy. Allergies are common in society, with a significant percentage of the population affected by atopic dermatitis, allergic rhinitis, food allergies, asthma, anaphylaxis, etc. A wide range of foods cause allergic reactions, such as eggs, soy, cow's milk, peanuts, etc. Insect stings can also generate allergic responses. An allergic response to a trigger starts when the immunoglobulin E antibodies bind to the allergen and then to a receptor on mast cells where it triggers the release of histamine and other inflammatory chemicals. The management of allergies is under the scope of clinical immunology. The professionals specialized in this field are known as clinical immunologists. This book traces the progress of clinical immunology and highlights some of its concepts and principles. Also included in this book is a detailed explanation of the mechanisms and manifestations of diverse kinds of allergies. A number of latest researches have been included to keep the readers up-to-date with the global concepts in these areas of study.

It was an honour to edit such a profound book and also a challenging task to compile and examine all the relevant data for accuracy and originality. I wish to acknowledge the efforts of the contributors for submitting such brilliant and diverse chapters in the field and for endlessly working for the completion of the book. Last, but not the least; I thank my family for being a constant source of support in all my research endeavours.

Editor

Sublingual grass allergen specific immunotherapy: a retrospective study of clinical outcome and discontinuation

Christer Janson[1]*, Fredrik Sundbom[1], Peter Arvidsson[2] and Mary Kämpe[1]

Abstract

Background: Sublingual immunotherapy (SLIT) is effective, tolerable, and convenient for many allergic patients. Still, real-world evidence is scarce and the aim of this study is to assess the patient reported outcome of treatment with SLIT against grass pollen allergy in a consecutive patient population.

Methods: Patients (n = 329) who were confirmed to be allergic to timothy grass and had been prescribed SLIT were consecutively enrolled in the study and completed a questionnaire online or in hard copy.

Results: 207 (62.9%) patients responded to the questionnaire. The female/male ratio was 105/102 with a mean age of 39 ± 11 years (range 19–70 years). 113 (55%) patients reported they had completed the full 3-year treatment period, 49 (24%) were still on treatment, and 45 (22%) had discontinued treatment prematurely. Respondents who had completed the full treatment period reported that their allergy symptoms in the most recent grass pollen season had improved to a larger extent than subjects still on treatment or discontinuing the treatment prematurely. Improvement of asthma was twice as common among patients who completed compared to discontinued treatment (42 vs. 20%). Younger age (37 ± 12 vs. 41 ± 11 years, p < 0.001) and a higher prevalence of reported oral and/or gastrointestinal side effects (49 vs. 24%, p = 0.02) characterised the group that terminated SLIT. Forgetfulness was the most commonly reported specific reason.

Conclusion: Treatment perseverance resulted in improved patient reported outcome. Forgetfulness was the most frequently reported reason for discontinuing SLIT treatment against grass pollen allergy.

Keywords: Grass pollen allergy, Sublingual immunotherapy, SLIT, Patient reported outcome, Adherence, Real-world evidence

Background

Sublingual immunotherapy (SLIT) with Grazax® (ALK, Denmark) is well documented for the treatment of grass pollen allergy. The distinct effect comprises reduced symptom score in rhinoconjunctivitis, reduced medication score, an increased number of well days and a relevant improvement in quality of life [1–6]. Treatment with Grazax is also associated with a sustained and relevant increase of specific IgG4 [7]. Moreover, long-term follow-up has shown that the treatment effect is sustained after completion of the 3-year treatment course, hence the SLIT by means of this product has as the first one in the class demonstrated a disease-modifying effect on grass pollen-induced allergic rhinoconjunctivitis [7].

Irrespective of the severity of symptoms, patients suffering from transitory symptoms from seasonal hay fever during the grass pollen season, may find once daily treatment for 3 years somewhat challenging. Although subcutaneous immunotherapy is administered directly by physicians, the rate of adherence was found to be surprisingly low (< 70% [8]. The explanations for poor subcutaneous immunotherapy adherence in this study included inconvenience, lack of efficacy, costs and loss of working

*Correspondence: christer.janson@medsci.uu.se
[1] Department of Medical Sciences, Respiratory, Allergy and Sleep Research, Uppsala University Hospital, Uppsala University, Uppsala, Sweden
Full list of author information is available at the end of the article

hours [8]. The anticipation that orally administered once daily treatment may be easier to comply with for long-term treatment in chronic disease is confirmed to some extent as once daily oral dosing appears to be much easier than alternative dosing schedules and routes of administration [9]. Still, a WHO report has documented that treatment adherence in developed countries averages only 50%—and that low treatment adherence in chronic disease has a negative impact on patient outcome and health care costs [10].

For SLIT clinical trial data and post marketing surveys show favourable overall rates of adherence (>75%) [8], however, these rates may be inadequately reflected in a non-trial setting. Reasons for discontinuation of allergy immunotherapy comprised cost, inconvenience, feeling of inefficacy, and side effects. Reduction of costs and more efforts in education of patients and also specialists may improve the adherence to immunotherapy [8]. The real-world evidence on the long-term treatment persistence and patient reported outcome in patients allergic to grass pollen is scarce. The aim of this study was to study the patient reported outcome of SLIT against grass pollen allergy in a consecutive adult patient population at an allergy out-patient clinic at a Swedish University Hospital.

Methods
Patients
From 2006 to 2016 a total of 329 consecutive grass allergic patients started on Grazax (*Phleum pratense* 75.000 SQ-T/2800 BAU, ALK, Denmark) at the Allergy Department at Uppsala University Hospital at Uppsala University Hospital, Sweden. They were confirmed to be allergic to timothy grass by skin pricktest or measurement of specific IgE and subsequently they were prescribed sublingual immunotherapy (SLIT) (Grazax). In the autumn of 2016 all these patients were contacted by mail and invited to participate in the study.

Questionnaire
The patients received a questionnaire to be filled in online or in a hard copy. The questionnaire consisted of 22 questions and was based on questionnaires used in clinical follow-up of patients with allergen immunotherapy (http://www.alk.se). The questionnaire covered various aspects such as allergic symptoms during the most recent grass pollen season (summer of 2016), medication during this grass pollen season, month and year when starting and ending Grazax treatment and reason for discontinuation. Respondents were asked 'How were your allergic symptoms during the latest grass pollen season compared to the season before you started using Grazax?' with the opportunity to respond in five categories: much

improved, improved, similar, worse, much worse. The questionnaire also included information on whether patients who had asthma experienced that their asthma had improved or worsened during the treatment and questions about side effects. Two reminders were sent to participants not responding. The online data was collected through a web-based system (Webropol version 2.0, Helsinki, Finland).

Ethical approval was granted by the Regional Ethical Review Board in Uppsala, Sweden (Dnr 2016/266). The study was an observational study of the patient reported outcome of a standard treatment for grass pollen allergy; hence the study was not registered in public databases for clinical trial registration.

Statistics
All analyses were performed using STATA 14 (STAT Corp, College Station, Texas, USA). Descriptive statistics was used to analyse the data set, along with a Chi^2 test, unpaired t test. A p-value of < 0.05 was used as the level of statistical significance.

Results
The questionnaire was sent out to 329 patients whereof 207 (62.9%) responded. The responders had a higher mean age (39 ± 11 vs. 35 ± 10 years, $p = 0.001$) than the non-responders, whereas no significant difference was found in gender distribution. Of the responders 76 filled in the questionnaire by internet and 131 filled in a postal questionnaire. The female/male ratio was 105/102 with a mean age of 39 ± 11 years (range 19–70 years). One hundred and seven (52%) patients reported that they had completed the full 3-year treatment period, 55 (27%) were still on treatment, and 45 (22%) had discontinued treatment prematurely, before the end of the 3-year treatment period. The characteristics of the population are shown in Table 1

Subjects who fulfilled the treatment were older than those who discontinued the treatment before the full 3-year period ($p \leq .001$) had been completed, while no difference was found in gender distribution or in having asthma or other allergies than grass pollen allergy (Table 1).

Respondents who had completed the full treatment period reported that their allergy symptoms in the most recent grass pollen season had improved to a larger extent than subjects that were still on treatment or had discontinued the treatment prematurely (Fig. 1). There was also a significant difference when only comparing those that had fulfilled or discontinued the treatment ($p = 0.018$).

Table 1 Characteristics of participants (n (%) and mean ± SD

	Completed (n = 107)	On treatment (n = 55)	Discontinued (n = 45)
Female	53 (50%)	32 (58%)	20 (44%)
Age (years)	41 ± 11	37 ± 12	35 ± 9
Other allergies	77 (73%)	38 (72%)	30 (68%)
Asthma	47 (44%)	28 (53%)	20 (44%)
Year treatment started[a]			
2016	–	20 (39%)	9 (23%)
2015	–	18 (35%)	5 (13%)
2014	8 (8%)	13 (25%)	6 (15%)
2013	29 (30%)		4 (10%)
2012	14 (14%)		7 (18%)
2011	12 (12%)		3 (8%)
2010	7 (7%)		2 (5%)
2009	12 (12%)		1 (3%)
2008	8 (8%)		0
2007	–	–	–
2006	7 (7%)		2 (5%)

[a] Information missing for 20 patients

There was no significant difference between the groups in regard to the reported level of severity of allergic symptoms during the latest grass pollen season (Fig. 2).

The reported use of medication against allergy during the most recent grass pollen season is presented in Table 2.

For most medications, the lowest use was found in the group who completed the Grazax treatment with significant group difference for the use of montelukast and short acting beta-2-agonists. The difference in the use of montelukast remained significant when the analysis was restricted to those who completed and those who discontinued the treatment (p = 0.04).

Of the patients 145(71%) reported having another allergy besides grass pollen allergy. Almost half of these (n = 69) reported that this other allergy had improved compared with before the start of Grazax treatment, but there was no significant difference between the three groups (p = 0.62).

Of the 95 patients who reported that they had asthma before starting Grazax, 37% reported an improvement in their asthma and 16% a worsening. Having an improvement of asthma was twice as common among the patients who completed treatment compared to patients who discontinued (42 vs. 20%) and this difference was almost statistically significant (p = 0.08).

Oral and gastrointestinal side effects were reported by 31% of the patients. These side effects were significantly more common among those who discontinued the treatment compared to those who completed the whole

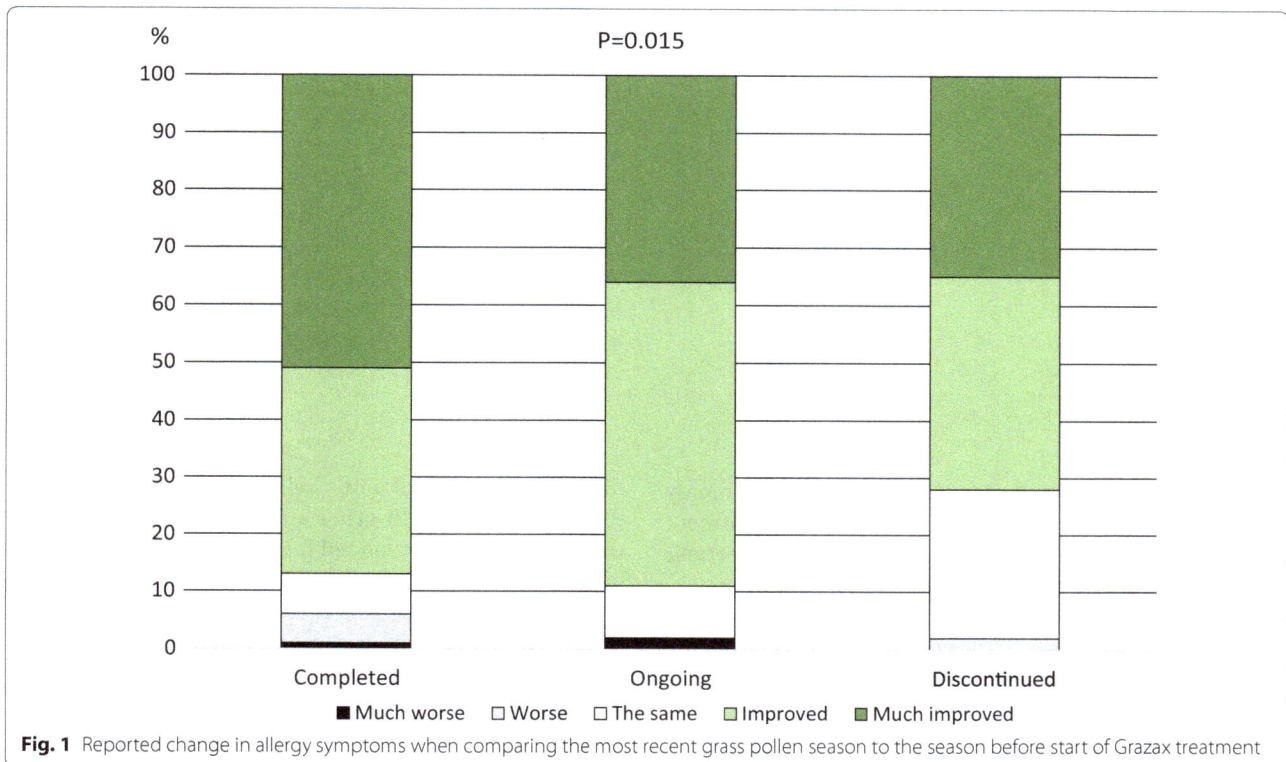

Fig. 1 Reported change in allergy symptoms when comparing the most recent grass pollen season to the season before start of Grazax treatment

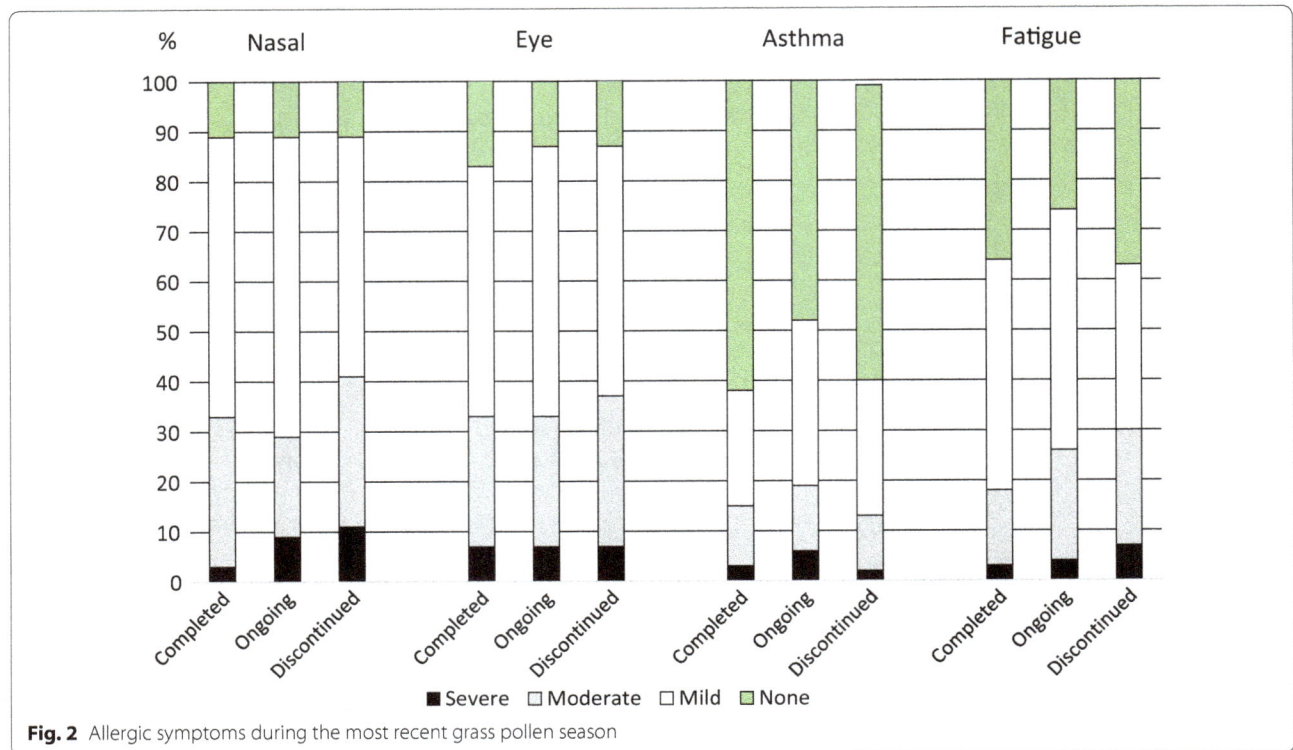

Fig. 2 Allergic symptoms during the most recent grass pollen season

Table 2 Use of medication against allergy during the most recent grass pollen season (n (%))

	Completed (n = 107)	On treatment (n = 55)	Discontinued (n = 45)	p-value
No medication	9 (8%)	3 (5%)	3 (7%)	0.78
Oral antihistamines	86 (80%)	50 (91%)	39 (87%)	0.19
Montelukast	9 (8%	14 (25%)	9 (20%)	0.01
Oral corticosteroids	6 (6%)	3 (5%)	3 (7%)	0.96
Nasal antihistamines	11 (10%)	13 (24%)	6 (13%)	0.07
Nasal corticosteroids	49 (46%)	33 (60%)	24 (53%)	0.22
Nasal cromoglycate	5 (5%)	1 (2%)	5 (11%)	0.11
Antihistamine eyedrops	31 (29%)	22 (40%)	17 (38%)	0.30
Cromone eyedrops	25 (23%)	16 (29%)	12 (27%)	0.72
Inhaled corticosteroids	35 (33%)	27 (49%)	15 (33%)	0.10
Short acting beta-2 agonists	16 (15%)	19 (35%)	11 (24%S)	0.02
Long acting beta-2 agonists	2 (2)	3 (5)	3 (7)	0.29

3-year period (49 vs. 24%, p = 0.02). The most commonly specific reason for discontinuing the Grazax treatment before the end of the 3-year period was that the patient forgot taking the treatment (Fig. 3).

Patients who completed the full treatment period were further analysed. Patients who reported having being much improved had a lower prevalence of asthma than those who did not (Table 3). There was also a trend that those with other allergies apart from allergy to grass pollen experienced less symptom improvement than those with only grass pollen allergy (p = 0.06). No significant difference was found in relation to sex, age, or to how long ago it was since the treatment was completed (Table 3).

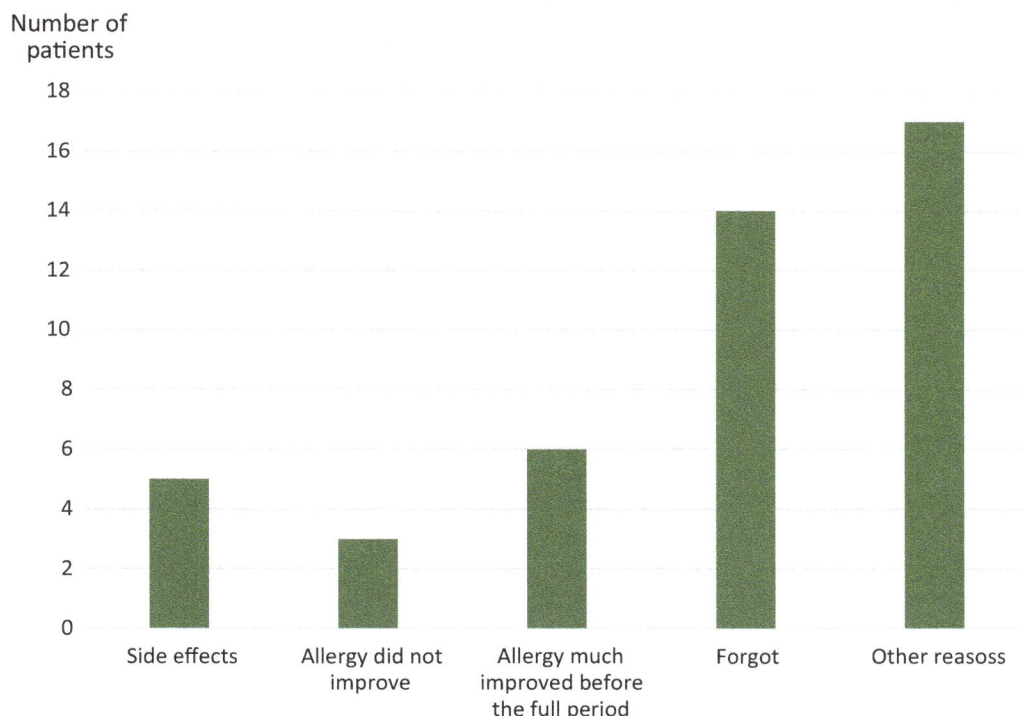

Fig. 3 Reported reason for discontinuation of Grazax treatment

Table 3 Comparison of patients that reported being much improved and those reporting less positive results after completing 3 years of Grazax treatment (n (%))

Allergic symptoms had much improved during the latest grass pollen season compared to the season before you started using

	Yes (n = 55)	No (n = 52)	p-value
Female	24 (45%)	29 (56%)	0.21
Age	42 ± 11	40 ± 11	0.39
Other allergies	35 (65%)	42 (81%)	0.06
Asthma	18 (33%)	29 (56%)	0.02
Year since treatment completion	3.5 ± 2.2	3.1 ± 2.3	0.36

Discussion

This real-world study of once daily treatment with SLIT against grass pollen allergy, based on the patient reported outcome among a Swedish consecutive population of adult grass pollen allergic patients at an outpatient allergy clinic. The majority of the patients completing a full 3-year period of SLIT against grass pollen allergy reported that their allergy was improved. This is in line with long-term clinical trial, where the effect rates compared to placebo (measured on symptom and medication score) where maintained at a steady level both during the 3-year treatment course and subsequently post treatment completion [7].

In this study 28% of a consecutive group of patients discontinued treatment. The adherence rate to SLIT is generally reported to be low with dropout rates ranging from 55–93% [11–13]. Allergen specific treatment with Grazax has in long-term follow-up of randomized clinical trial subjects demonstrated a distinct and sustained long-term effect over time—an effect that is withheld even after completion of the treatment course [7, 14]. In that, the treatment initiation holds promise to the grass pollen allergic patients of truly obtaining symptom relief or cure on a mid-term and long-term basis. Albeit this is the expectation among patients who start a treatment course of allergy immunotherapy, a proportion of patients never see the treatment course to the end as seen in this study and others [11–13, 15, 16]. One study reports that specific and timely measures taken in terms of an action plan, including patient education, frequent contacts, and strictly scheduled visits appeared to improve the rate of adherence, albeit not impressively [13]. Several studies stress the importance of close follow-up with patients and the need to implement patient education and utilizing technology-based tools, including online platforms, social media, e-mail, and a short message service by phone to improve the adherence and patient benefit along with the cost utility of SLIT to society [11, 13, 15, 16]. The data presented herein were retrospectively collected; hence there is no information on the follow-up with patients during the treatment course. However, it appears to be an interesting finding that the most frequent reason for discontinuation of treatment in this study was forgetfulness. Other authors report on side effects as the main reason [13, 16]. The randomized clinical trial setting may reflect a patient-doctor relationship that resembles concordance [15]. Daily clinical practice may seem far from ideal circumstances during a randomized clinical trial set-up. Still, it could it be argued that more consideration should be embraced in standard allergy practice towards partnering with the patient on a contract that aims at improving his or her health short-term and long-term—only with the efforts of the patient himself or herself [10, 11, 15, 16].

During clinical trials—as well as during this study—patients report an effect during the ongoing treatment period. However, the documented disease modifying effect, and an actual alteration of the immune system causing the symptoms, is expected to be associated with long-term treatment, requiring a high level of perseverance among patients. This data set demonstrates that treatment adherence is an issue that should be accounted for, and which is better reflected in real-world data than in randomized clinical trials. Real-world evidence may provide a more realistic view on treatment adherence than what is seen during a clinical trial set-up. Overall the respondents who completed the full treatment course matched the group of respondents who discontinued on female/male ratio, presence of other allergies, and concomitant asthma. Younger age and a higher prevalence of reported oral and/or gastrointestinal side effects characterised the group of subjects who terminated using SLIT. A lower adherence in younger patients is in accordance with a report using data from a Dutch pharmacy database [12]. In general, non-adherence of medications represents a major societal issue. Predictors of non-adherence and adherence include beliefs related to the benefits of medication for physical and mental disorders, complexities of systems of health care and treatment plans, and lifestyle and demographic characteristics of patients [17]. Acknowledging the problem appears to be relevant in any therapeutic area, including the management of allergic disorders in order to tailor the plan of care according to patient and system specific barriers.

Rhinoconjunctivitis very often coexists with asthma [18, 19]. In this study, approximately half of the patients had asthma along with seasonal rhinoconjunctivitis. The positive effect of Grazax on asthma symptoms and medicine scores has been demonstrated [20]. Moreover,

both sublingual and injection based immunotherapy have demonstrated a longstanding preventive effect in the development of asthma [21–23]. The data presented herein demonstrated that improvement of asthma was twice as common among the patients who completed treatment compared to patients who discontinued. The result reached only borderline statistically significance. Still, it points to an important point holding clinical relevance, in that it probably should be stressed heavily to patients that the effect of the long-term treatment with SLIT for seasonal symptoms is likely to improve existing asthma symptoms as well as rhinoconjunctivitis symptoms and may prevent the development of asthma.

Half of those who completed the treatment period reported that their allergic symptoms were much improved. This group was characterised by a lower prevalence of asthma and other allergies whereas the number of years that passed since the treatment ended was not related to this outcome. Other studies have shown that allergic patients tend to be polysensitized, and often polysensitization is associated with more severe disease [24]. This may be due to an inborn heterogeneity of the atopy in polysenzitised compared to the monosensitized patients [25, 26]. Rationally, it could be argued that monosensitized patients may demonstrate better effect than polysensitized patients in interventional investigations of specific allergen immunotherapy. This study tends to support this argument, albeit a series of studies argues against this and instead claiming equal effectiveness and safety of single-allergen sublingual SIT in mono- and polysensitized subjects [27–33]. Almost half of the patients that reported having another allergy besides grass pollen allergy reported that this other allergy had improved. Some of these patients may also have been on treatment with subcutaneous immunotherapy against birch allergens but unfortunately data on this matter is lacking.

Lack of efficacy has been reported as a reason for non-adherence in other studies [8]. In this study, a composite answer of 'other reasons' was most frequently reported as the reason for treatment discontinuation, followed by forgetfulness. Interestingly, pronounced effect appeared also to be a reason for treatment discontinuation, while lack of efficacy and adverse effect were more infrequent reasons for treatment discontinuation.

An advantage of a Real world investigation like this one is that controlled trials include more contact with healthcare professionals than the usual clinical care, which may lead to a selection of more compliant patient and alter patient behaviour compared with in a real world setting. Patient reported outcome appears particularly relevant in self-administered treatment of long duration. Additionally, treatment of seasonal symptoms in grass pollen allergic patients may present with specific issues related to perennial treatment and long-term treatment. This study represented a large proportion of consecutive patients, who were prescribed Grazax (62% responded), leaving the group of non-responders as a weakness to study. The questionnaire could be filled in online as well as on a hard copy that could be sent by mail. Furthermore, two reminders were sent to participants not responding, hence efforts were made to collect the information that would complete the data set. The non-responders were somewhat younger than the responders indicating that the proportion of patients not completing the full 3-year period was probably higher in the non-responders than the responders.

Conclusion

Treatment perseverance resulted in an improved patient reported outcome in comparison to patients who did not complete the treatment course as prescribed. Forgetfulness was more often the reason for discontinuation than e.g. adverse effects, leaving room for improvement on approaches that remind taking the medication, such as text messages, smart-phone applications, reminder features in the calendar etc.

Abbreviations
BAU: Bioequivalent Allergy Units; Ig: immunoglobin; SD: standard deviation; SLIT: sublingual immunotherapy; SQ-T: standardized quality-tablet; WHO: World Health Organization.

Authors' contributions
CJ drafted the analyses and manuscript. All authors provided feedback to the manuscript and approved the final version of the manuscript. All authors read and approved the final manuscript.

Author details
[1] Department of Medical Sciences, Respiratory, Allergy and Sleep Research, Uppsala University Hospital, Uppsala University, Uppsala, Sweden. [2] ALK Nordic, Kungsbacka, Sweden.

Acknowledgements
The authors were assisted in the preparation of the manuscript by Charlotte Strøm, MD, Ph.D., SharPen, Denmark. We are also grateful for the administrative work with the data set and the questionnaires done by Gun-Marie Bodman Lund, Maria Järvenson and Johan Järvenson, Sweden.

Funding
The study was financially supported by ALK Nordic.

References
1. Bachert C, Vestenbaek U, Christensen J, Griffiths UK, Poulsen PB. Cost-effectiveness of grass allergen tablet (GRAZAX) for the prevention of seasonal grass pollen induced rhinoconjunctivitis—a Northern European perspective. Clin Exp Allergy. 2007;37:772–9.
2. Dahl R, Kapp A, Colombo G, de Monchy JG, Rak S, Emminger W, et al. Sublingual grass allergen tablet immunotherapy provides sustained clinical benefit with progressive immunologic changes over 2 years. J Allergy Clin Immunol. 2008;121:512–8.
3. Durham SR, Riis B. Grass allergen tablet immunotherapy relieves individual seasonal eye and nasal symptoms, including nasal blockage. Allergy. 2007;62:954–7.
4. Durham SR. SQ-standardised grass tablet sublingual immunotherapy: persistent clinical benefit and progressive immunological changes during three years treatment. Arb Paul Ehrlich Inst Bundesinstitut Impfstoffe Biomed Arzneim Langen Hess. 2009;96:121–7.
5. Durham SR, Emminger W, Kapp A, Colombo G, de Monchy JG, Rak S, et al. Long-term clinical efficacy in grass pollen-induced rhinoconjunctivitis after treatment with SQ-standardized grass allergy immunotherapy tablet. J Allergy Clin Immunol. 2010;125:131–8.
6. Durham SR, Birk AO, Andersen JS. Days with severe symptoms: an additional efficacy endpoint in immunotherapy trials. Allergy. 2011;66:120–3.
7. Durham SR. Sustained effects of grass pollen AIT. Allergy. 2011;66(Suppl 95):50–2.
8. Senna G, Ridolo E, Calderon M, Lombardi C, Canonica GW, Passalacqua G. Evidence of adherence to allergen-specific immunotherapy. Curr Opin Allergy Clin Immunol. 2009;9:544–8.
9. Osterberg L, Blaschke T. Adherence to medication. N Engl J Med. 2005;353:487–97.
10. De GS, Sabate E. Adherence to long-term therapies: evidence for action. Eur J Cardiovasc Nurs. 2003;2:323.
11. Bender BG, Oppenheimer J. The special challenge of nonadherence with sublingual immunotherapy. J Allergy Clin Immunol Pract. 2014;2:152–5.
12. Kiel MA, Roder E, van Gerth WR, Al MJ, Hop WC, Rutten-van Molken MP. Real-life compliance and persistence among users of subcutaneous and sublingual allergen immunotherapy. J Allergy Clin Immunol. 2013;132:353–60.
13. Savi E, Peveri S, Senna G, Passalacqua G. Causes of SLIT discontinuation and strategies to improve the adherence: a pragmatic approach. Allergy. 2013;68:1193–5.
14. Durham SR, Emminger W, Kapp A, de Monchy JG, Rak S, Scadding GK, et al. SQ-standardized sublingual grass immunotherapy: confirmation of disease modification 2 years after 3 years of treatment in a randomized trial. J Allergy Clin Immunol. 2012;129:717–25.
15. Antico A. Long-term adherence to sublingual therapy: literature review and suggestions for management strategies based on patients' needs and preferences. Clin Exp Allergy. 2014;44:1314–26.
16. Incorvaia C, Mauro M, Leo G, Ridolo E. Adherence to sublingual immunotherapy. Curr Allergy Asthma Rep. 2016;16:12.
17. Wheeler KJ, Roberts ME, Neiheisel MB. Medication adherence part two: predictors of nonadherence and adherence. J Am Assoc Nurse Pract. 2014;26:225–32.
18. Linneberg A, Nielsen NH, Madsen F, Frolund L, Dirksen A, Jorgensen T. Secular trends of allergic asthma in Danish adults The Copenhagen Allergy Study. Respir Med. 2001;95:258–64.
19. Pite H, Pereira AM, Morais-Almeida M, Nunes C, Bousquet J, Fonseca JA. Prevalence of asthma and its association with rhinitis in the elderly. Respir Med. 2014;108:1117–26.
20. Dahl R, Stender A, Rak S. Specific immunotherapy with SQ standardized grass allergen tablets in asthmatics with rhinoconjunctivitis. Allergy. 2006;61:185–90.
21. Jacobsen L, Niggemann B, Dreborg S, Ferdousi HA, Halken S, Host A, et al. Specific immunotherapy has long-term preventive effect of seasonal and perennial asthma: 10-year follow-up on the PAT study. Allergy. 2007;62:943–8.

22. Niggemann B, Jacobsen L, Dreborg S, Ferdousi HA, Halken S, Host A, et al. Five-year follow-up on the PAT study: specific immunotherapy and long-term prevention of asthma in children. Allergy. 2006;61:855–9.

23. Valovirta E, Petersen TH, Piotrowska T, Laursen MK, Andersen JS, Sorensen HF, et al. Results from the 5-year SQ grass sublingual immunotherapy tablet asthma prevention (GAP) trial in children with grass pollen allergy. J Allergy Clin Immunol. 2018;141:529–38.

24. Kim KW, Kim EA, Kwon BC, Kim ES, Song TW, Sohn MH, et al. Comparison of allergic indices in monosensitized and polysensitized patients with childhood asthma. J Korean Med Sci. 2006;21:1012–6.

25. Kim CW, Kee JH, Jung HW, Choi SR, Cheong JW, Park JW, et al. Changing patterns of skin reactivity to inhalant allergens in asthmatic patients. J Asthma Allergy Clini Immunol. 2001;21:205–15.

26. Pene J, Rivier A, Lagier B, Becker WM, Michel FB, Bousquet J. Differences in IL-4 release by PBMC are related with heterogeneity of atopy. Immunology. 1994;81:58–64.

27. Amar SM, Harbeck RJ, Sills M, Silveira LJ, O'Brien H, Nelson HS. Response to sublingual immunotherapy with grass pollen extract: monotherapy versus combination in a multiallergen extract. J Allergy Clin Immunol. 2009;124:150–6.

28. Calderon MA, Cox L, Casale TB, Moingeon P, Demoly P. Multiple-allergen and single-allergen immunotherapy strategies in polysensitized patients: looking at the published evidence. J Allergy Clin Immunol. 2012;129:929–34.

29. Ciprandi G, Incorvaia C, Puccinelli P, Soffia S, Scurati S, Frati F. Polysensitization as a challenge for the allergist: the suggestions provided by the Polysensitization Impact on Allergen Immunotherapy studies. Expert Opin Biol Ther. 2011;11:715–22.

30. Didier A, Malling HJ, Worm M, Horak F, Jager S, Montagut A, et al. Optimal dose, efficacy, and safety of once-daily sublingual immunotherapy with a 5-grass pollen tablet for seasonal allergic rhinitis. J Allergy Clin Immunol. 2007;120:1338–45.

31. Lee JE, Choi YS, Kim MS, Han DH, Rhee CS, Lee CH, et al. Efficacy of sublingual immunotherapy with house dust mite extract in polyallergen sensitized patients with allergic rhinitis. Ann Allergy Asthma Immunol. 2011;107:79–84.

32. Malling HJ, Montagut A, Melac M, Patriarca G, Panzner P, Seberova E, et al. Efficacy and safety of 5-grass pollen sublingual immunotherapy tablets in patients with different clinical profiles of allergic rhinoconjunctivitis. Clin Exp Allergy. 2009;39:387–93.

33. Nelson H, Blaiss M, Nolte H, Wurtz SO, Andersen JS, Durham SR. Efficacy and safety of the SQ-standardized grass allergy immunotherapy tablet in mono- and polysensitized subjects. Allergy. 2013;68:252–5.

2

HIV-1 Nef promotes migration and chemokine synthesis of human basophils and mast cells through the interaction with CXCR4

Francesca Wanda Rossi[1]*, Nella Prevete[1], Felice Rivellese[1,2], Antonio Lobasso[1], Filomena Napolitano[1], Francescopaolo Granata[1], Carmine Selleri[3] and Amato de Paulis[1]

Abstract

Background: The Nef protein can be detected in plasma of HIV-1-infected patients and plays a role in the pathogenesis of HIV-1. Nef produced during the early stages of infection is fundamental in creating the ideal environment for viral replication, e.g. by reducing the ability of infected cells to induce an immune response.

Aim: Based on previous experience showing that both Tat and gp41 of HIV-1 are potent chemotactic factors for basophils and mast cells, and gp120 is a powerful stimulus for the release of histamine and cytokines (IL-4 and IL-13) from basophils, in this study we aimed to verify if the HIV Nef protein can exert some effects on basophils and mast cells purified from healthy volunteers through the interaction with the CXCL12 receptor, CXCR4.

Methods: Basophils purified from peripheral blood cells of 30 healthy volunteers and mast cells obtained from lung tissue of ten healthy volunteers were tested by flow cytometric analysis, chemotaxis and chemokine production by ELISA assays.

Results: Nef is a potent chemoattractant for basophils and lung mast cells obtained from healthy, HIV-1 and HIV-2 seronegative individuals. Incubation of basophils and mast cells with Nef induces the release of chemokines (CXCL8/IL-8 and CCL3/MIP-1α). The chemotactic activity of Nef on basophils and mast cells is mediated by the interaction with CXCR4 receptors, being blocked by preincubation of FcεRI+ cells with an anti-CXCR4 Ab. Stimulation with Nef or CXCL12/SDF-1α, a CXCR4 ligand, desensitizes basophils to a subsequent challenge with an autologous or heterologous stimulus.

Conclusions: These results indicate that Nef, a HIV-1-encoded α-chemokine homolog protein, plays a direct role in basophils and mast cell recruitment and activation at sites of HIV-1 replication, by promoting directional migration of human FcεRI+ cells and the release of chemokines from these cells. Together with our previous results, these data suggest that FcεRI+ cells contribute to the dysregulation of the immune system in HIV-1 infection.

Keywords: Mast Cells, Basophils, Nef, CXCR4, CXCL12/SDF-1α

*Correspondence: frawrossi@yahoo.it
[1] Department of Translational Medical Sciences and Center for Basic and Clinical Immunology Research (CISI), University of Naples Federico II, Via S. Pansini 5, 80131 Naples, Italy
Full list of author information is available at the end of the article

Background

The human immunodeficiency viruses HIV-1 and HIV-2 destroy CD4$^+$ lymphocytes, thus leading to AIDS [1]. Entry of HIV-1 into immune cells is mediated by the viral envelope glycoproteins (gp120 and gp41) [2] through their interaction with the CD4 glycoprotein, the primary receptor [3], the CC chemokine receptor 5 (CCR5) and the CXC chemokine receptor 4 (CXCR4), obligate coreceptors for virus entry [2].

Viral replication and host defence escape are regulated by HIV-1 proteins. The accessory protein Nef, is a crucial determinant of viral pathogenesis and disease progression to full-blown AIDS by optimizing the cellular environment for viral replication [4]. The key role of Nef is to control the expression levels of various cell surface molecules that play important roles in immunity and virus life cycle [5]. For example, Nef upregulates the surface expression of Tumor Necrosis Factor (TNF) and immature major histocompatibility complex class II (MHC-II). In contrast, Nef downregulates the surface expression of several other proteins including CD4, MHC-I, CD3, CD8, CD28, CXCR4, CCR5, CCR3, CD1, CD80/CD86, CTLA-4, mature (antigenic peptide-loaded) MHC-II [6]. Nef-mediated downregulation of MHC-I molecules, benefits the virus by interfering with the recognition and destruction of infected cells by cytotoxic T-cells [6]. Besides its well-studied effects on intracellular signaling, Nef also acts through its secretion in exosomes nanovesicles. Nef enhances exosome secretion and entry into uninfected CD4$^+$ T cells, thus leading to apoptotic death [7]. Nef is also responsible for the inhibition of T cell migration in vitro [8]. In addition, Nef affects the innate immune system by impairing phagocytosis, and augmenting the release of pro-inflammatory and chemotactic factors from macrophages [9]. Altogether, Nef activities support viral replication and survival while at the same time favor viral dissemination [10]. Many of these activities of extracellular Nef might be mediated indirectly or directly by the interaction with the chemokine receptor CXCR4 [2, 11, 12].

Basophils and mast cells are the only cells synthesizing histamine and expressing high affinity receptors for IgE (FcεRI) [13]. Immunologic activation of human basophils leads to the release of proinflammatory mediators and the synthesis of a restricted profile of cytokines (IL-4 and IL-13) and chemokines (CXCL8/IL-8 and CCL3/MIP-1α) [14, 15], while human mast cells express a wide spectrum of cytokines and chemokines [16, 17]. Besides being the effector cells of IgE-mediated responses, basophils and mast cells are implicated in many physiological and pathological processes, such as the response to infections [18, 19], inflammatory and autoimmune diseases [20, 21] and cancer [22, 23].

We have investigated the role of basophils and mast cells in the context of HIV infection, suggesting that FcεRI$^+$ cells may be a source of Th2 cytokines, thus contributing to the dysregulation of the immune system in HIV-1. Tat protein is a potent chemoattractant for human basophils and mast cells by interacting with the α-chemokine receptor CCR3 [24]. HIV-1 envelope gp41 peptide promotes migration of basophils and mast cells through interaction with formyl peptide receptors (FPRs) [25] and HIV-1 gp120 is a potent stimulus for IL-4 and IL-13 release from basophils [26, 27]. More recently, it has been reported that human mast cells can act as an inducible reservoir of persistent HIV infection [28] and that both mucosal mast cells and blood circulating basophils capture HIV-1 mediating viral trans-infection through the expression of multiple attachment factors (HAFs) [29, 30]. These findings indicate that human basophils and mast cells can contribute to the spread and persistence of HIV infection.

The results of our study further highlight the multiple interactions between HIV products and FcεRI$^+$ cells and confirm the relevance of these cells in the promotion of HIV-1 infection.

Methods

Purification of peripheral blood basophils

Basophils were purified from peripheral blood cells of 30 healthy, HIV-1 and HIV-2 seronegative, volunteers, aged 20–39 years (mean, 33.6 ± 4.9 years). Buffy coat cell packs from healthy volunteers, provided by the Hematology Unit of the University of Salerno, were reconstituted in PBS containing 0.5 g/L HSA and 3.42 g/L sodium citrate, and loaded onto a countercurrent elutriator (model J2-21; Beckman, Fullerton, CA). Several fractions were collected, and fractions containing large numbers of basophils (>20 × 10^6) and of good purity (>15%) were enriched by discontinuous Percoll gradients [16]. Basophils were further purified to near homogeneity (>98%) by depleting B cells, monocytes, NK cells, dendritic cells, erythrocytes, platelets, neutrophils, eosinophils, and T cells with a cocktail of hapten-conjugated CD3, CD7, CD14, CD15, CD16, CD36, CD45RA, and anti-HLA-DR Abs and MACS MicroBeads coupled to an anti-hapten mAb. The magnetically labeled cells were depleted by retaining them on a MACS column in the magnetic field of the Midi-MACS (Miltenyi Biotec, Bergisch Gladbach, Germany). Yields ranged from 3 to 10 × 10^6 basophils, with purity usually >98%, as assessed by basophil staining with Alcian Blue and counting in a Spiers-Levy eosinophil counter.

Isolation and purification of human lung mast cells (HLMC)

Lung tissue was obtained from ten patients undergoing thoracotomy and lung resection, after obtaining their informed consent according to the guidelines of the institutional review board. Macroscopically normal parenchyma was dissected free from pleura, bronchi, and blood vessels and minced into a single-cell suspension as previously described [31]. Yields ranged between 3×10^6 and 18×10^6 mast cells, with purity between 1 and 8%. Lung mast cells were purified by countercurrent elutriation (J2/21; Beckman) and then by discontinuous Percoll density gradient as previously described [31]. Mast cells were further purified to near homogeneity by positive selection and incubation with anti-FcεRI (IgG1) followed by the exposure to magnetic beads coated with MACS goat anti-mouse IgG. Labeled cells were enriched by positive selection columns (MACS system; Miltenyi Biotec). The final preparations contained >95% viable cells, as assessed by the trypan blue exclusion method, and purity was >98% mast cells.

Flow cytometric analysis of surface molecules

Flow cytometric analysis of cell surface molecules was performed as previously described [32]. Briefly, after saturation of non specific binding sites with total rabbit IgG, cells were incubated for 20 min at +4 °C with specific or isotype control antibodies. For indirect staining this step was followed by a second incubation for 20 min at +4 °C with an appropriate anti-isotype-conjugated antibody. Finally, cells were washed and analyzed with a FACSCalibur Cytofluorometer using Cell Quest software (Becton & Dickinson, San Fernando, CA). A total of 10^4 events for each sample were acquired in all cytofluorimetric analyses.

Chemotaxis assay

Basophil and mast cell chemotaxis was performed using a modified Boyden chamber technique as previously described [33]. Briefly, 25 µl of a Ca^{2+}-containing buffer or various concentrations of the chemoattractants in the same buffer were placed in triplicate in the lower compartment of a 48-well microchemotaxis chamber (Neuroprobe, Cabin John, MD). The lower compartments were covered with polycarbonate membranes with 5-µm pores (basophils) or with a two-filter sandwich constituted by 5-µm (lower) and 8-µm (upper) pore size polycarbonate membranes (mast cells) (Nucleopore, Pleasanton, CA). Fifty microliters of the cell suspensions (5×10^4/well) resuspended in a Ca^{2+}-containing buffer was pipetted into the upper compartments. The chemotactic chamber was then incubated for 1 h (basophils) or 3 h (mast cells) at 37 °C in a humidified incubator with 5% CO_2 (automatic CO_2 incubator, model 160 IR, ICN/Flow Laboratories). At the end of basophil incubation, the membrane was removed, washed with PBS on the upper side, fixed, and stained with May-Grunwald/Giemsa. When mast

cells were used, the upper polycarbonate filter was discarded, while the lower nitrate cellulose filter was fixed in methanol, stained with Alcian Blue, and then mounted on a microscope slide with Cytoseal (Stephen Scientific, Springfield, NJ). Basophil and mast cell chemotaxis was quantitated microscopically by counting the number of cells attached to the surface of the 5-µm cellulose nitrate filter. In each experiment 10 fields/triplicate filter were measured at ×40 magnification. The results were compared with buffer controls.

IL-4, IL-13, CXCL8/IL-8, CCL3/MIP-1α ELISA

IL-4, IL-13, CXCL8/IL-8, CCL3/MIP-1α release in the culture supernatants of basophils and HLMC cells were measured in duplicate determinations with a commercially available ELISA kit (R&D System, Minneapolis, MN) [32].

Statistical analysis

The results are expressed as the mean ± SEM. Statistical significance was analyzed by one-way ANOVA and, when the F value was significant, by Duncan's multiple range test [34]. Differences were considered significant at $p < 0.05$.

Results

CXCR4 expression on human basophils and mast cells

Extracellular Nef exerts several functions on immune cells via CXCR4 receptors [11, 12, 35]. We have therefore investigated at protein level, by flow cytometry, the expression of CXCR4 on human basophils and mast cells. Figure. 1 shows that the vast majority of basophils (~80%) (Fig. 1a) and HLMC (~65%) (Fig. 1b) expressed on their surface the chemokine receptor CXCR4. Figure 1c shows the mean fluorescence intensity of CXCR4 expression in basophils (grey column) and HLMC cells (black column) over basal.

Effect of HIV-1 r-Nef protein on human basophil *and mast cell* chemotaxis

Having found that FcεRI+ cells expressed the chemochine receptor CXCR4, we then assessed whether Nef was able to induce the chemotaxis of these cells. Figure 2a shows that r-Nef (3–300 ng/ml) (Abcam, Milton, Cambridge, UK) caused a concentration-dependent increase in chemotaxis of purified basophils. In a parallel series of experiments we compared the chemotactic activity of r-Nef with that of CXCL12/SDF-1α (R&D System (Minneapolis, MN) and of the formylated tripeptide N-formyl-methionyl-leucyl-phenylalanine (fMLF) (ICN Biomedicals) potent chemoattractants of human basophils through their interaction with the chemokine receptor CXCR4 and FPR1, respectively [19, 33]. Figure 2b

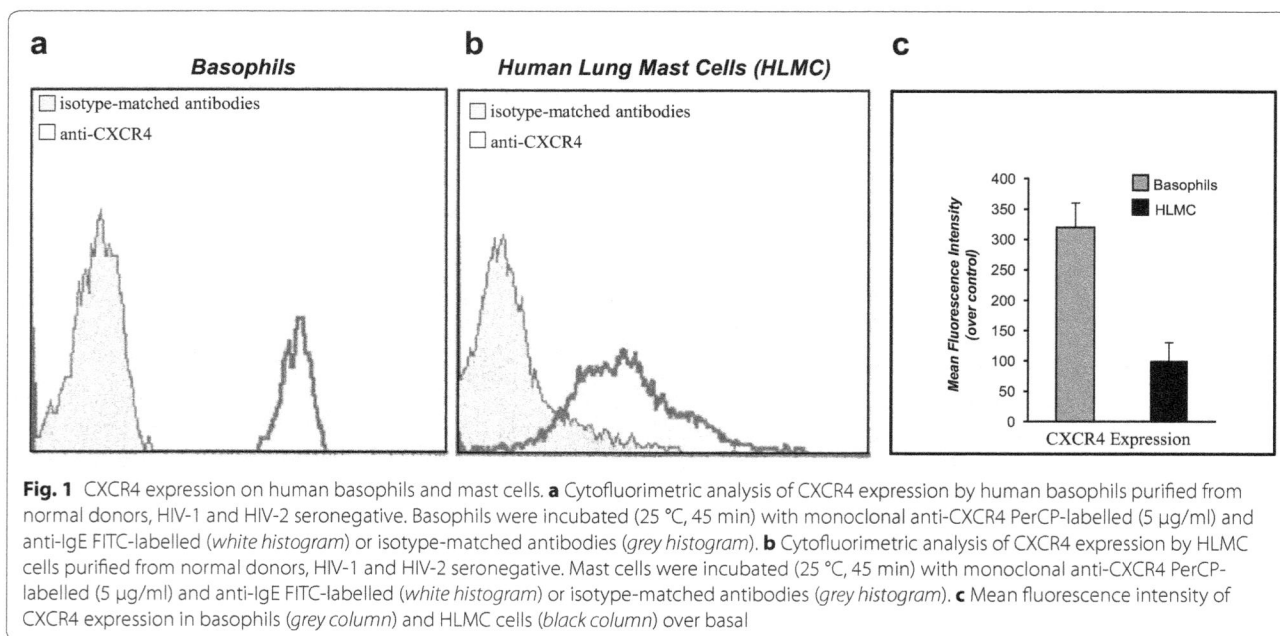

Fig. 1 CXCR4 expression on human basophils and mast cells. **a** Cytofluorimetric analysis of CXCR4 expression by human basophils purified from normal donors, HIV-1 and HIV-2 seronegative. Basophils were incubated (25 °C, 45 min) with monoclonal anti-CXCR4 PerCP-labelled (5 μg/ml) and anti-IgE FITC-labelled (*white histogram*) or isotype-matched antibodies (*grey histogram*). **b** Cytofluorimetric analysis of CXCR4 expression by HLMC cells purified from normal donors, HIV-1 and HIV-2 seronegative. Mast cells were incubated (25 °C, 45 min) with monoclonal anti-CXCR4 PerCP-labelled (5 μg/ml) and anti-IgE FITC-labelled (*white histogram*) or isotype-matched antibodies (*grey histogram*). **c** Mean fluorescence intensity of CXCR4 expression in basophils (*grey column*) and HLMC cells (*black column*) over basal

shows that CXCL12/SDF-1α (10 and 100 ng/ml) and fMLF (100 and 500 ng/ml) induced strong chemotaxis of human basophils. In the same experiments r-Nef (10 and 100 ng/ml) promoted comparable migratory effects on basophils.

Since a remarkable proportion of HLMC cells (65%) expressed CXCR4 receptor (Fig. 1b) and CXCR4 receptor on human mast cells was functionally active being involved in the chemotactic response to CXCL12/SDF-1α, we tested the chemotactic response to r-Nef of HLMC cells. Figure. 2c shows that r-Nef (3–300 ng/ml) induced a concentration-dependent increase in HLMC cells chemotaxis.

Checkerboard analysis was performed to discriminate between chemotaxis and nondirectional migration (chemokinesis) of basophils or mast cells. Cell migratory responses to specific stimuli were largely due to chemotaxis and not to chemokinesis (data not shown).

Nef-induced migration of basophils and mast cells through CXCR4

To establish whether the expression of CXCR4 on basophils was responsible for the chemoattractant effect of Nef, basophils were preincubated with an anti-CXCR4 antibody (5 μg/ml) and then assessed for their ability to migrate in response to Nef. Figure 3a shows that preincubation of basophils with an anti-CXCR4 antibody (R&D System, Minneapolis, MN) (5 μg/ml) inhibited the chemoattractant effect of Nef. Similarly, preincubation of basophils with an anti-CXCR4 antibody completely

suppressed the chemotactic activity of CXCL12/SDF-1α (100 ng/ml) on these cells. In contrast, the chemotactic effect of fMLF (500 ng/ml), which activates a specific seven-transmembrane receptor independent of the CXCR4 receptor [33, 36], was not affected by the anti-CXCR4 antibody.

We have previously demonstrated that Tat protein was an HIV-1-encoded α-chemokine homologous that promotes basophil migration through the interaction with the chemokine receptor CCR3 [24]. Figure 3b demonstrate that preincubation of basophils with anti-CCR3 antibody (R&D System, Minneapolis, MN) (5 μg/ml) inhibited the chemoattractant effect of Tat (60 ng/ml). In contrast, the chemotactic effects of both CXCL12/SDF-1α (100 ng/ml) and r-Nef (100 ng/ml) were not affected by anti-CCR3 antibody. In similar experiments, preincubation of mast cells with a monoclonal antibody against CXCR4 completely blocked the chemoattractant effect of Nef protein (data not shown).

Nef-induced heterologous desensitization of CXCR4

The relationship between CXCR4 receptors and Nef protein was further examined using CXCL12/SDF-1α to induce desensitization of CXCR4-mediated functions. In a first series of experiments, purified basophils (>98%) were incubated with buffer containing EDTA (4 mM), alone or in in the presence of CXCL12/SDF-1α (100 ng/ml) for 30 min at 37 °C. At the end of incubation, basophils were washed twice, resuspended in Ca^{2+}-containing buffer, and rechallenged with the chemotactic

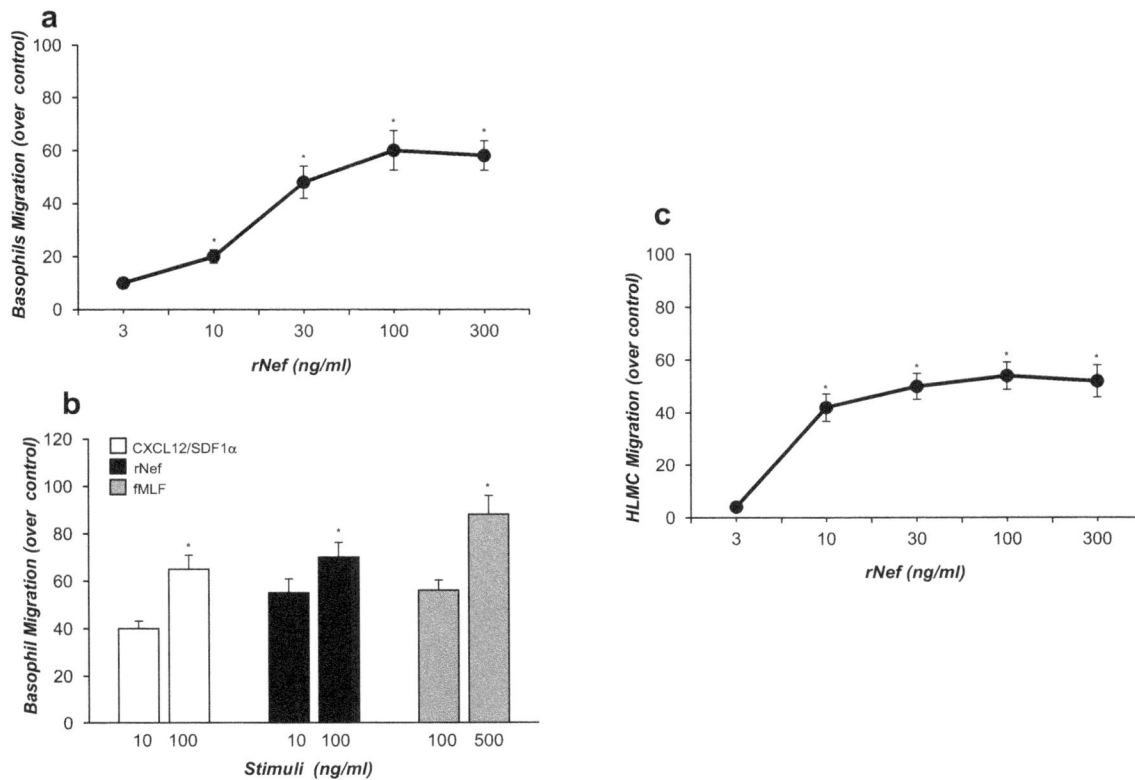

Fig. 2 Effect of r-Nef on chemotaxis of human basophils and mast cells. **a** Basophils were allowed to migrate toward r-Nef protein (3-300 ng/ml) for 1 h at 37 °C in the humidified incubator with 5% CO_2. Values are the mean $\pm$ SEM obtained from six independent experiments with different human basophil preparations. *$p < 0.05$ as compared to control. **b** Basophils were allowed to migrate toward the indicated concentrations of CXCL12/SDF-1α (*white histogram*), r-Nef (*black histogram*), and fMLF (*grey histogram*) for 1 h at 37 °C in a humidified incubator with 5% CO_2. Values are the mean $\pm$ SEM obtained from four experiments. *$p < 0.05$ as compared to control. **c** HLMC cells were allowed to migrate toward r-Nef protein (3-300 ng/ml) for 3 h at 37 °C in the humidified incubator with 5% CO_2. Values are the mean $\pm$ SEM obtained from six different experiments. *$p < 0.05$ as compared to control

stimuli (fMLF 500 ng/ml, CXCL12/SDF-α 100 ng/ml or r-Nef 100 ng/ml). Figure 4a shows that the response to CXCL12/SDF-1α or r-Nef was significantly reduced by the preincubation of cells with CXCL12/SDF-1α. By contrast, CXCL12/SDF-1α desensitization didn't affect fMLF-dependent chemotaxis.

In a second series of experiments, purified basophils (>98%) were incubated with a buffer containing EDTA (4 mM) in the presence or absence of CXCL12/SDF-1α (100 ng/ml) or r-Nef (100 ng/ml) for 30 min at 37 °C. At the end of the incubation, basophils were washed twice, resuspended in a Ca^{2+}-containing buffer, and rechallenged with the chemotactic stimuli (fMLF 500 ng/ml, CXCL12/SDF-1α 100 ng/ml or r-Nef 100 ng/ml). Figure 4b shows that the response to CXCL12/SDF-1α was significantly reduced by the preincubation with homologous or heterologous stimuli. Similarly, preincubation with r-Nef significantly reduced the chemotactic activity of both CXCL12/SDF-1α and r-Nef, indicating that

the two stimuli were using the same receptor. Again, the chemotactic response to fMLF was unaffected by the desensitization with CXCL12/SDF-1α or r-Nef.

Effect of Nef on chemokine release from human basophils and mast cells

r-Nef upregulates mRNA for MIP-1α/MIP-1α and several cytokines in human monocytes/macrophages [37]. We tested whether r-Nef could induce chemochine release by human basophils, which are known to release CXCL8/IL-8 and CCL3/MIP-1α upon immunological activation [38]. We therefore evaluated, at different timepoints, the release of CXCL8/IL-8 and CCL3/MIP-1α from basophils triggered with r-Nef. The results of three independent experiments showed a significant release of CXCL8/IL-8 after 4 h till 18 h of incubation (Fig. 5a), and CCL3/MIP-1α, after 4 h (Fig. 5b). Since the chemotaxis assay was performed after 1 h of incubation, it is likely that the chemotactic effect of Nef was not mediated by

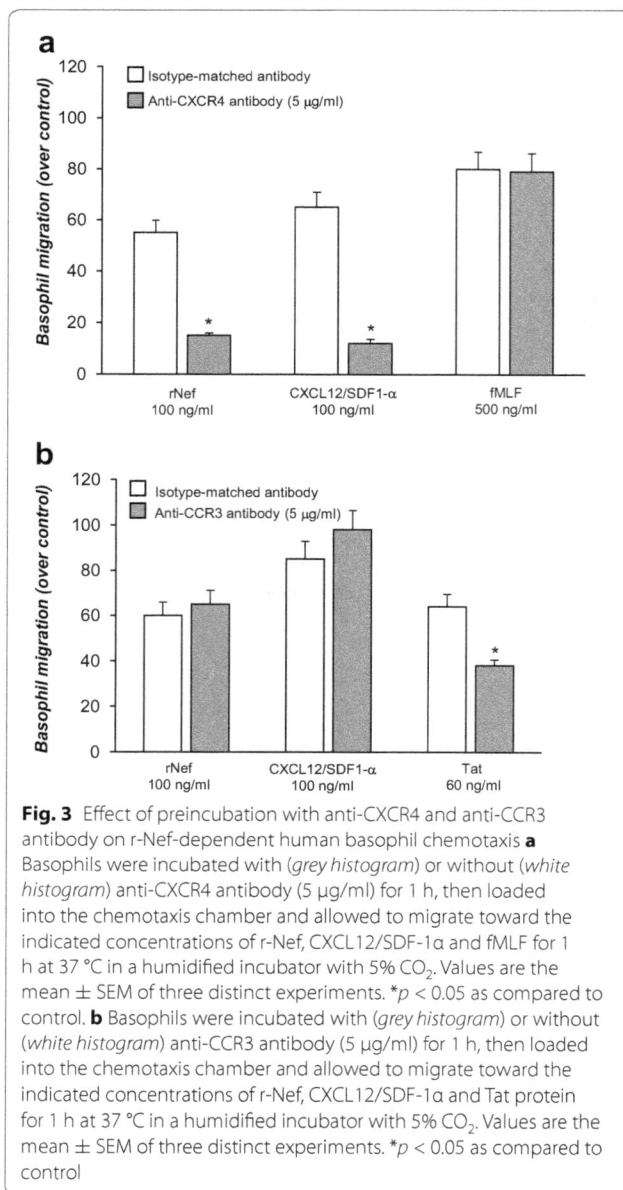

Fig. 3 Effect of preincubation with anti-CXCR4 and anti-CCR3 antibody on r-Nef-dependent human basophil chemotaxis **a** Basophils were incubated with (*grey histogram*) or without (*white histogram*) anti-CXCR4 antibody (5 µg/ml) for 1 h, then loaded into the chemotaxis chamber and allowed to migrate toward the indicated concentrations of r-Nef, CXCL12/SDF-1α and fMLF for 1 h at 37 °C in a humidified incubator with 5% CO_2. Values are the mean ± SEM of three distinct experiments. *$p < 0.05$ as compared to control. **b** Basophils were incubated with (*grey histogram*) or without (*white histogram*) anti-CCR3 antibody (5 µg/ml) for 1 h, then loaded into the chemotaxis chamber and allowed to migrate toward the indicated concentrations of r-Nef, CXCL12/SDF-1α and Tat protein for 1 h at 37 °C in a humidified incubator with 5% CO_2. Values are the mean ± SEM of three distinct experiments. *$p < 0.05$ as compared to control

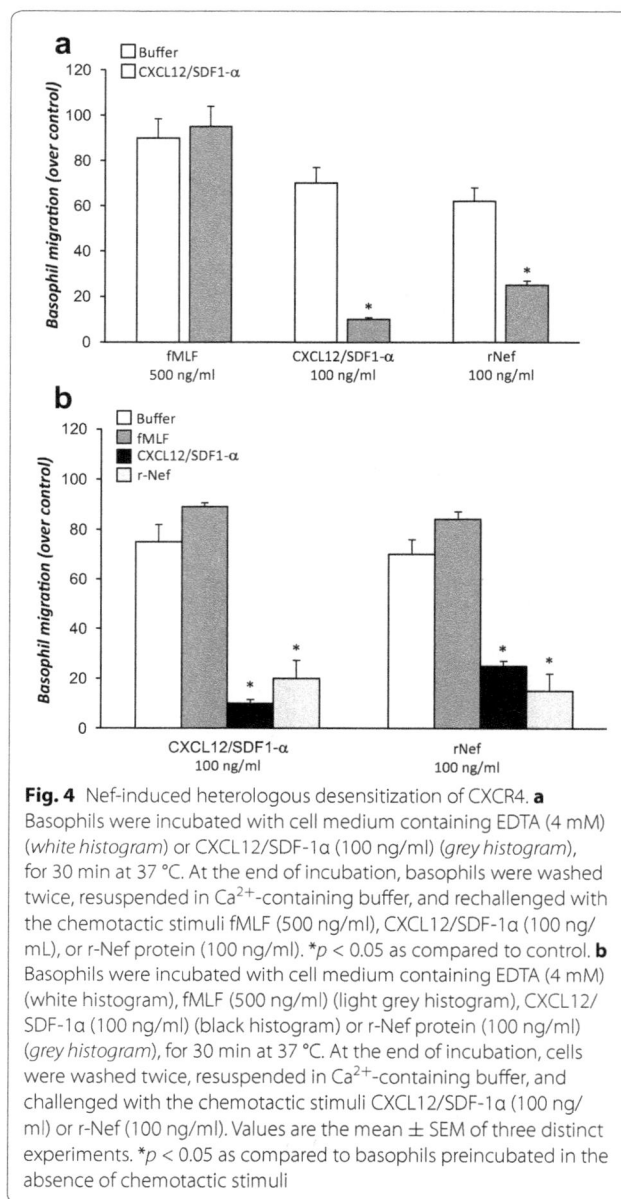

Fig. 4 Nef-induced heterologous desensitization of CXCR4. **a** Basophils were incubated with cell medium containing EDTA (4 mM) (*white histogram*) or CXCL12/SDF-1α (100 ng/ml) (*grey histogram*), for 30 min at 37 °C. At the end of incubation, basophils were washed twice, resuspended in Ca^{2+}-containing buffer, and rechallenged with the chemotactic stimuli fMLF (500 ng/ml), CXCL12/SDF-1α (100 ng/mL), or r-Nef protein (100 ng/ml). *$p < 0.05$ as compared to control. **b** Basophils were incubated with cell medium containing EDTA (4 mM) (white histogram), fMLF (500 ng/ml) (light grey histogram), CXCL12/SDF-1α (100 ng/ml) (black histogram) or r-Nef protein (100 ng/ml) (*grey histogram*), for 30 min at 37 °C. At the end of incubation, cells were washed twice, resuspended in Ca^{2+}-containing buffer, and challenged with the chemotactic stimuli CXCL12/SDF-1α (100 ng/ml) or r-Nef (100 ng/ml). Values are the mean ± SEM of three distinct experiments. *$p < 0.05$ as compared to basophils preincubated in the absence of chemotactic stimuli

the release of chemokines from basophils. In addition we also evaluated the effects of increasing concentrations of Nef and CXCL12/SDF-1α on cytokine (IL-4 and IL-13) release from basophils purified from healthy donors. In five experiments, both r-Nef (10 and 100 ng/ml) and CXCL12/SDF-1α (10 and 100 ng/ml) did not cause cytokine release from these cells (data not shown). We finally evaluated the kinetics of chemokine release induced by r-Nef from HLMC cells. Similarly to basophils, r-Nef induced a significant release of CXCL8/IL-8 at 12 and 24 h (Fig. 5c) and of CCL3/MIP-1α at 12 h (Fig. 5d).

Discussion

This study demonstrated that HIV-1 Nef protein is a chemoattractant for human basophils and mast cells (Fig. 2). The chemotactic activity of Nef protein was mediated by the interaction with the CXCR4 receptor present on a remarkable proportion of these cells (Figs. 1, 3). In addition, we found that Nef induced the production of chemokines (CXCL8/IL-8 and CCL3/MIP-1α) from basophils and mast cells (Fig. 5). This is the first demonstration that Nef protein is an HIV-1-encoded chemokine-homolog functionally active on human FcεRI[+] cells through the interaction with the CXCR4 receptor.

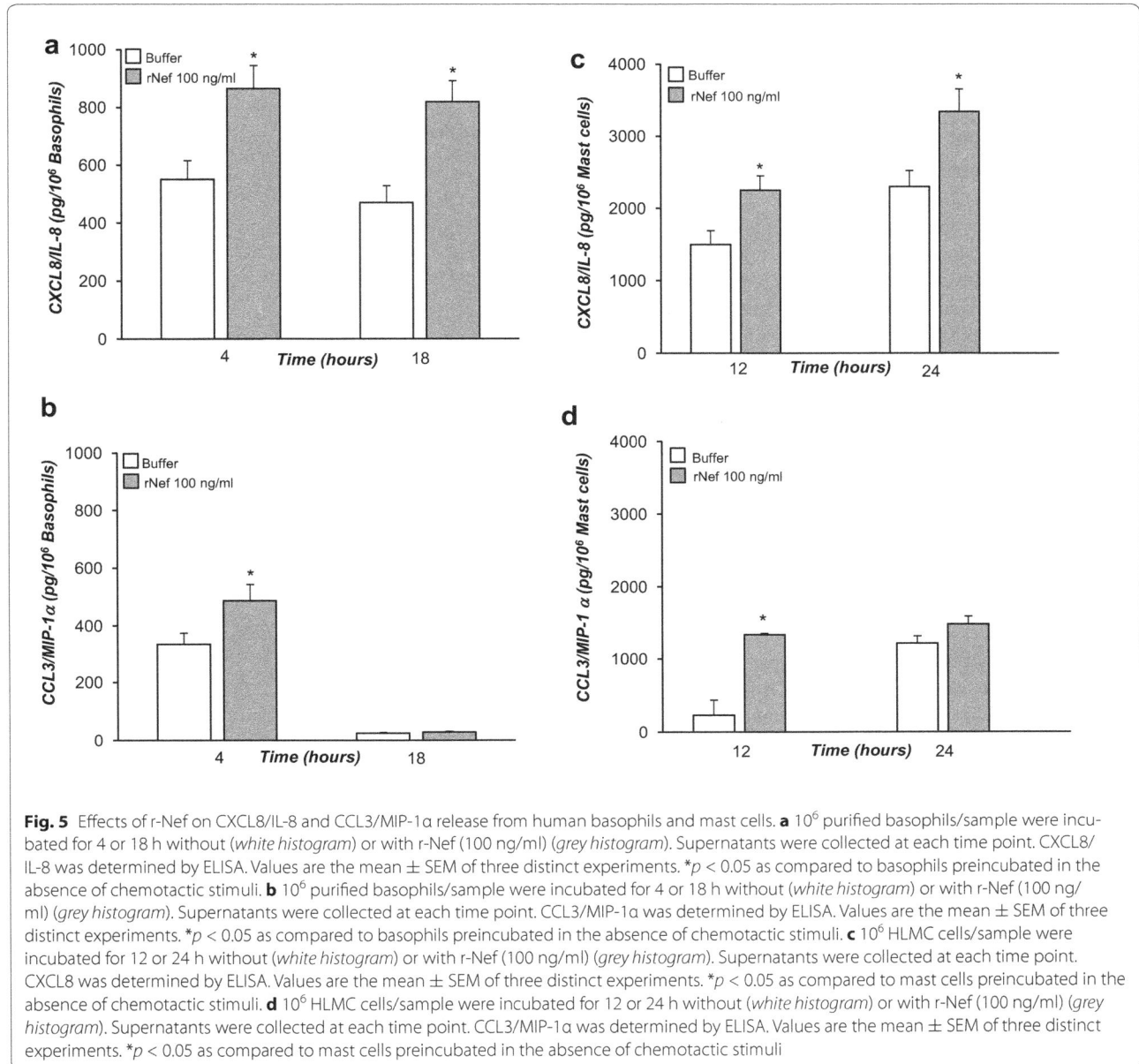

Fig. 5 Effects of r-Nef on CXCL8/IL-8 and CCL3/MIP-1α release from human basophils and mast cells. **a** 10^6 purified basophils/sample were incubated for 4 or 18 h without (*white histogram*) or with r-Nef (100 ng/ml) (*grey histogram*). Supernatants were collected at each time point. CXCL8/IL-8 was determined by ELISA. Values are the mean ± SEM of three distinct experiments. *$p < 0.05$ as compared to basophils preincubated in the absence of chemotactic stimuli. **b** 10^6 purified basophils/sample were incubated for 4 or 18 h without (*white histogram*) or with r-Nef (100 ng/ml) (*grey histogram*). Supernatants were collected at each time point. CCL3/MIP-1α was determined by ELISA. Values are the mean ± SEM of three distinct experiments. *$p < 0.05$ as compared to basophils preincubated in the absence of chemotactic stimuli. **c** 10^6 HLMC cells/sample were incubated for 12 or 24 h without (*white histogram*) or with r-Nef (100 ng/ml) (*grey histogram*). Supernatants were collected at each time point. CXCL8 was determined by ELISA. Values are the mean ± SEM of three distinct experiments. *$p < 0.05$ as compared to mast cells preincubated in the absence of chemotactic stimuli. **d** 10^6 HLMC cells/sample were incubated for 12 or 24 h without (*white histogram*) or with r-Nef (100 ng/ml) (*grey histogram*). Supernatants were collected at each time point. CCL3/MIP-1α was determined by ELISA. Values are the mean ± SEM of three distinct experiments. *$p < 0.05$ as compared to mast cells preincubated in the absence of chemotactic stimuli

It is well known that CXCR4 is a co-receptor for several strains of HIV-1 [39]. Here we demonstrated that soluble r-Nef specifically interacts with CXCR4 on human basophils and mast cells. Indeed, a monoclonal antibody anti-CXCR4 completely blocked the chemoattractant effect of Nef protein (Fig. 3). The specificity of this interaction was confirmed by the observation that preincubation of cells with anti-CCR3 antibody did not modify the chemotactic response of both r-Nef and CXCL12/SDF-1α (Fig. 3). Finally, the cross-desensitization of basophil chemotaxis with Nef provided the evidence that Nef interacts with the CXCR4 receptor on human FcεRI+ cells (Fig. 4).

These findings are relevant at different levels. Firstly, they suggest that during HIV-1 infection, Nef can influence the directional migration of human basophils and mast cells, thus contributing to the recruitment of these cells at sites of HIV-1 infection. Secondly, the chemotactic activity of Nef on human FcεRI+ cells might contribute to increase the local density of mast cells and basophils available for HIV-1 interaction through the virus-bound or shed gp120. In fact, we have previously demonstrated that gp120 from different clades interacts with the IgE V_H3^+ present on human FcεRI+ [26]. The superantigenic interaction between gp120 and IgE leads to the rapid synthesis and release of IL-4 and IL-13 from human FcεRI$^+$ cells [18]. This interaction might represent an initial source of cytokines, thereby favoring a shift from a Th0 toward a Th2 phenotype. The latter observation is relevant because HIV-1 is known to replicate preferentially in Th2 cells [40]. Finally, mast cells and basophils recruited at the site of HIV infection can directly contribute to the spread of the infection by acting as virus reservoir and mediating trans-infection of CD4$^+$ T cells, as recently demonstrated [28, 30].

The clinical relevance of our findings is confirmed by the observation that Nef was present in the serum of HIV-1-infected patients at concentrations as high as 10 ng/ml [41]. In tissues where viral replication occurs (e.g. the lymph nodes), local levels of Nef could exceed those found in serum. Because the early phases of infection are associated with high levels of viremia [1], and this, in turn, may be associated with high levels of Nef, chemokine-like activity of Nef on FcεRI$^+$ cells might be of clinical relevance in patients with HIV-1 infection.

Intriguingly, many viruses exploit the strategy of using homologs of cellular cytokines and chemokines to shield virus-infected cells from immune defenses and enhance virus survival in the host [42, 43]. The existence of these virus-encoded homologs of cellular proteins is indirect evidence of their relevant role in orchestrating the host immune response to invading pathogens [43]. Many large DNA viruses, including CMV and HHV-8, as well as the poxvirus *Molluscum contagiosum*, encode several α-chemokine homologs (virokines) acting on CCR3 or CCR8 receptors [44–46]. This novel observation may have several implications for a better understanding of the pathogenesis of HIV-1 infection.

In conclusion, we provided the first evidence that Nef protein is an HIV-1-encoded chemokine-homolog able to activate human FcεRI$^+$ cells, by interacting with the CXCR4 receptor on these cells. Because HIV-1 enters the body predominantly through mucosal surfaces and because early phases of infection are associated with high levels of viremia, both mast cells, in tissues, and basophils, in circulation, can be exposed to high local levels of Nef protein, which in turns induce their recruitement and activation in sites of infection. Overall, our results suggests a novel mechanism through which FcεRI$^+$ cells can contribute to the dysregulation of the immune system in HIV-1 infection.

Abbreviations

CXCR4: C-X-C motif chemokine receptor 4; CCR5: C-C motif chemokine receptor 5; CCR3: C-C motif chemokine receptor 3; CXCL12/SDF-1α: C-X-C motif chemokine 12/stromal cell-derived factor 1-alpha; TNF: tumor necrosis factor; CXCL8/IL-8: C-X-C motif chemokine ligand 8/interleukine 8; CCL3/MIP-1α: C-C motif chemokine ligand 3/macrophage inflammatory protein 1-alpha; HSA: human serum albumin; anti-FcεRI: mouse monoclonal IgG anti-α chain of high affinity receptor for IgE; anti-IgE: rabbit IgG anti-Fc fragment of human IgE; FcεRI: high affinity receptor for IgE; HLMC: human lung mast cells; P: 25 mM PIPES (pH 7.4), 110 mM NaCl, and 5 mM KCl; FPRs: formyl-peptide receptors; fMLF: formyl-methionyl-leucyl phenylalanine; r-Nef: recombinant-Nef.

Authors' contributions

FWR performed chemotaxis assays and was a major contributor in writing the manuscript, NP performed chemotaxis assays and FACS analysis, FR e AL purified peripheral basophils and isolated mast cells from tissue samples, FN performed ELISA assays, FPG interpreted the data, CS provided buffy coats from the Hematology Branch of the University of Salerno, ADP analyzed the data and was a contributor in writing the manuscript. All authors read and approved the final manuscript.

Author details

[1] Department of Translational Medical Sciences and Center for Basic and Clinical Immunology Research (CISI), University of Naples Federico II, Via S. Pansini 5, 80131 Naples, Italy. [2] Centre for Experimental Medicine and Rheumatology, William Harvey Research Institute, Barts and The London School of Medicine and Dentistry, Queen Mary University of London, London, UK. [3] Hematology Branch, Department of Medicine, University of Salerno, Salerno, Italy.

References

1. Moir S, Chun TW, Fauci AS. Pathogenic mechanisms of HIV disease. Annu Rev Pathol. 2011;6:223–48.
2. Barré-Sinoussi F, Ross AL, Delfraissy JF. Past, present and future: 30 years of HIV research. Nat Rev Microbiol. 2013;11:877–83.
3. Kwong PD, Wyatt R, Robinson J, Sweet RW, Sodroski J, Hendrickson WA. Structure of an HIV gp 120 envelope glycoprotein in complex with the CD4 receptor and a neutralizing human antibody. Nature. 1998;393:648–59.
4. Basmaciogullari S, Pizzato M. The activity of Nef on HIV-1 infectivity. Front Microbiol. 2014;5:232.
5. Fackler OT, Alcover A, Schwartz O. Modulation of the immunological synapse: a key to HIV-1 pathogenesis? Nat Rev Immunol. 2007;7:310–7.
6. Pereira EA, daSilva LL. HIV-1 Nef: taking control of protein trafficking. Traffic. 2016. doi:10.1111/tra.12412.
7. Aqil M, Mallik S, Bandyopadhyay S, Maulik U, Jameel S. Transcriptomic analysis of mrnas in human monocytic cells expressing the HIV-1 Nef protein and their exosomes. Biomed Res Int. 2015. doi:10.1155/2015/492395.
8. Vérollet C, Le Cabec V, Maridonneau-Parini I. HIV-1 Infection of T Lymphocytes and Macrophages Affects Their Migration via Nef. Front Immunol. 2015;6:514.
9. Olivetta E, Tirelli V, Chiozzini C, Scazzocchio B, Romano I, Arenaccio C. HIV-1 Nef impairs key functional activities in human macrophages through CD36 downregulation. PLoS ONE. 2014;9:e93699.
10. Ghiglione Y, Turk G. Nef performance in macrophages: the master orchestrator of viral persistence and spread. Curr HIV Res. 2011;9:505–13.
11. James CO, Huang MB, Khan M, Garcia-Barrio M, Powell MD, et al. Extracellular Nef protein targets CD4 + T cells for apoptosis by interacting with CXCR4 surface receptors. J Virol. 2004;78:3099–109.
12. Huang MB, Jin LL, James CO, Khan M, Powell MD, Bond VC. Characterization of Nef-CXCR4 interactions important for apoptosis induction. J Virol. 2004;78:11084–96.
13. Marone G, Lichtenstein LM, Galli SJ. Mast Cells and Basophils. San Diego: Academic Press; 2000.
14. Marone G, Borriello F, Varricchi G, Genovese A, Granata F. Basophils: historical reflections and perspectives. Chem Immunol Allergy. 2014;100:172–92.
15. Gessner A, Mohrs K, Mohrs M. Mast cells, basophils, and eosinophils acquire constitutive IL-4 and IL-13 transcripts during lineage differentiation that are sufficient for rapid cytokine production. J Immunol. 2005;174:1063–72.
16. Triggiani M, Giannattasio G, Balestrieri B, Granata F, Gelb MH, de Paulis A, et al. Differential modulation of mediator release from human basophils and mast cells by mizolastine. Clin Exp Allergy. 2004;34:241–9.

17. Marone G, Triggiani M, de Paulis A. Mast cells and basophils: friends as well as foes in bronchial asthma? Trends Immunol. 2005;26:25–31.

18. Marone G, Spadaro G, Liccardo B, Rossi FW, D'Orio C, Detoraki A. Superallergens: a new mechanism of immunologic activation of human basophils and mast cells. Inflamm Res. 2006;55(Suppl 1):S25–7.

19. Marone G, de Paulis A, Florio G, Petraroli A, Rossi FW, Triggiani M. Are mast cells MASTers in HIV-1 infection? Int Arch Allergy Immunol. 2001;125:89–95.

20. de Paulis A, Montuori N, Prevete N, Fiorentino I, Rossi FW, Visconte V, et al. Urokinase induces basophil chemotaxis through a urokinase receptor epitope that is an endogenous ligand for formyl peptide receptor-like 1 and -like 2. J Immunol. 2004;173:5739–48.

21. Prevete N, Rossi FW, Rivellese F, Lamacchia D, Pelosi C, Lobasso A, et al. Helicobacter pylori HP(2-20) induces eosinophil activation and accumulation in superficial gastric mucosa and stimulates VEGF-alpha and TGF-beta release by interacting with formyl-peptide receptors. Int J Immunopathol Pharmacol. 2013;26:647–62.

22. Melillo RM, Guarino V, Avilla E, Galdiero MR, Liotti F, Prevete N, et al. Mast cells have a protumorigenic role in human thyroid cancer. Oncogene. 2010;29:6203–15.

23. de Paulis A, Prevete N, Fiorentino I, Rossi FW, Staibano S, Montuori N, et al. Expression and functions of the vascular endothelial growth factors and their receptors in human basophils. J Immunol. 2006;177:7322–31.

24. de Paulis A, De Palma R, Di Gioia L, Carfora M, Prevete N, Tosi G, et al. Tat protein is an HIV-1-encoded beta-chemokine homolog that promotes migration and up-regulates CCR3 expression on human Fc epsilon RI+ cells. J Immunol. 2000;165:7171–9.

25. de Paulis A, Florio G, Prevete N, Triggiani M, Fiorentino I, Genovese A, et al. HIV-1 envelope gp41 peptides promote migration of human Fc epsilon RI+ cells and inhibit IL-13 synthesis through interaction with formyl peptide receptors. J Immunol. 2002;169:4559–67.

26. Patella V, Florio G, Petraroli A, Marone G. HIV-1 gp120 induces IL-4 and IL-13 release from human Fc epsilon RI + cells through interaction with the VH3 region of IgE. J Immunol. 2000;164:589–95.

27. Marone G, Florio G, Petraroli A, de Paulis A. Dysregulation of the IgE/Fc epsilon RI network in HIV-1 infection. J Allergy Clin Immunol. 2001;107:22–30.

28. Sundstrom JB, Ellis JE, Hair GA, Kirshenbaum AS, Metcalfe DD, Yi H, et al. Human tissue mast cells are an inducible reservoir of persistent HIV infection. Blood. 2007;109:5293–300.

29. Jiang AP, Jiang JF, Wei JF, Guo MG, Qin Y, Guo QQ, et al. Human Mucosal Mast Cells Capture HIV-1 and Mediate Viral trans-Infection of CD4+ T Cells. J Virol. 2015;90:2928–37.

30. Jiang AP, Jiang JF, Guo MG, Jin YM, Li YY, Wang JH. Human Blood-Circulating Basophils Capture HIV-1 and Mediate Viral trans-Infection of CD4 + T Cells. J Virol. 2015;89:8050–62.

31. de Paulis A, Minopoli G, Arbustini E, De Crescenzo G, Dal Piaz F, Pucci P, et al. Stem cell factor is localized in, released from, and cleaved by human mast cells. J Immunol. 1999;163:2799–808.

32. Prevete N, Salzano FA, Rossi FW, Rivellese F, Dellepiane M, Guastini L, et al. Role(s) of formyl-peptide receptors expressed in nasal epithelial cells. J Biol Regul Homeost Agents. 2011;25:553–64.

33. Rossi FW, Napolitano F, Pesapane A, Mascolo M, Staibano S, Matucci-Cerinic M, et al. Upregulation of the N-formyl Peptide receptors in scleroderma fibroblasts fosters the switch to myofibroblasts. J Immunol. 2015;194:5161–73.

34. Snedecor GW, Cochran WG. Statistical Methods Iowa State University Press, Ames; 1980.

35. Hrecka K, Swigut T, Schindler M, Kirchhoff F, Skowronski J. Nef proteins from diverse groups of primate lentiviruses downmodulate CXCR4 to inhibit migration to the chemokine stromal derived factor 1. J Virol. 2005;79:10650–9.

36. Rossi FW, Montuori N. FPRs: linking innate immune system and fibrosis. Oncotarget. 2015;6:18736–7.

37. Olivetta E, Percario Z, Fiorucci G, Mattia G, Schiavoni I, Dennis C, et al. HIV-1 Nef induces the release of inflammatory factors from human monocyte/macrophages: involvement of Nef endocytotic signals and NF-kappa B activation. J Immunol. 2003;170:1716–27.

38. Marone G, Galli SJ, Kitamura Y. Probing the roles of mast cells and basophils in natural and acquired immunity, physiology and disease. Trends Immunol. 2002;23:425–7.

39. Shen HS, Yin J, Leng F, Teng RF, Xu C, Xia XY, et al. HIV coreceptor tropism determination and mutational pattern identification. Sci Rep. 2016;6:21280.

40. Maggi E, Mazzetti M, Ravina A, Annunziato F, de Carli M, Piccinni MP, et al. Ability of HIV to promote a TH1 to TH0 shift and to replicate preferentially in TH2 and TH0 cells. Science. 1994;265:244–8.

41. Fujii Y, Otake K, Tashiro M, Adachi A. Soluble Nef antigen of HIV-1 is cytotoxic for human CD4 + T cells. FEBS Lett. 1996;393:93–6.

42. Kotenko SV, Saccani S, Izotova LS, Mirochnitchenko OV, Pestka S. Human cytomegalovirus arbors its own unique IL-10 homolog (cmvIL-10). Proc Natl Acad Sci USA. 2000;97:1695.

43. Lalani AS, Barrett JW, McFadden G. Modulating chemokines: more lessons from viruses. Immunol Today. 2000;21:100.

44. Vomaske J, Denton M, Kreklywich C, Andoh T, Osborn JM, Chen D, et al. Cytomegalovirus CC chemokine promotes immune cell migration. J Virol. 2012;86:11833–44.

45. Catusse J, Spinks J, Mattick C, Dyer A, Laing K, Fitzsimons C, et al. Immunomodulation by herpesvirus U51A chemokine receptor via CCL5 and FOG-2 down-regulation plus XCR1 and CCR7 mimicry in human leukocytes. Eur J Immunol. 2008;38:763–77.

46. Choi YB. Nicholas J Autocrine and paracrine promotion of cell survival and virus replication by human herpesvirus 8 chemokines. J Virol. 2008;82:6501–13.

3

Determinants of venom-specific IgE antibody concentration during long-term wasp venom immunotherapy

Valerio Pravettoni[1*], Marta Piantanida[1], Laura Primavesi[1], Stella Forti[2] and Elide A. Pastorello[3]

Abstract

Background: Venom immunotherapy (VIT) is an effective treatment for subjects with systemic allergic reactions (SR) to Hymenoptera stings, however there are few studies concerning the relevance of the venom specific IgE changes to decide about VIT cessation. We assessed IgE changes during a 5-year VIT, in patients stung and protected within the first 3 years (SP 0–3) or in the last 2 years (SP 3–5), and in patients not stung (NoS), to evaluate possible correlations between IgE changes and clinical protection.

Methods: Yellow jacket venom (YJV)-allergic patients who completed 5 years of VIT were retrospectively evaluated. Baseline IgE levels and after the 3rd and the 5th year of VIT were determined; all patients were asked about field stings and SRs.

Results: A total of 232 YJV-allergic patients were included and divided into the following groups: 84 NoS, 72 SP 0–3 and 76 SP 3–5. IgE levels decreased during VIT compared to baseline values ($\chi^2 = 346.029$, $p < 0.001$). Recent vespid stings accounted for significantly higher IgE levels despite clinical protection. IgE levels after 5 years of VIT correlated significantly with Mueller grade (F = 2.778, $p = 0.012$) and age (F = 6.672, $p = 0.002$). During follow-up from 1 to 10 years after VIT discontinuation, 35.2 % of the contacted patients reported at least one field sting without SR.

Conclusions: The yellow jacket-VIT temporal stopping criterion of 5 years duration did not result in undetectable IgE levels, despite a long-lasting protection. A mean IgE decrease from 58 to 70 % was observed, and it was less marked in elderly patients or in subjects with higher Mueller grade SR.

Keywords: Hymenoptera venom allergy, Hymenoptera venom immunotherapy, Specific IgE levels, VIT long-lasting protection, VIT discontinuation

Background

Venom immunotherapy (VIT) is an effective treatment for patients suffering from hymenoptera venom allergy (HVA) with severe systemic reaction (SR) and documented sensitization to the causative venom [1].

The optimal duration of VIT necessary to achieve long-term protection has been evaluated in several studies, aimed to identify useful parameters for a safe stopping [2–4]. The initially identified criterion was the development of negative skin tests and/or serum specific IgE

(sIgE) tests [5]. However, it was later noted that such outcome was rarely obtained, and that patients with positive sIgE were clinically protected from stings [2–6]. Thus, a VIT duration of at least 5 years was suggested, ideally accompanied by a decline in skin tests and sIgE levels [2–4, 7–11].

According to the latest guidelines, the decision to stop VIT must consider some risk factors for a future relapse, such as patient's age, type of venom, severity of pre-VIT reaction, occurrence of SR during VIT, and likelihood of future stings [12, 13]. Thus, the physician may be reluctant to stop VIT even when the temporal criterion is reached, because studies evaluating the relevance of the observed declines in sIgE to decide about VIT cessation

*Correspondence: v.pravettoni@policlinico.mi.it
[1] Clinical Allergy and Immunology Unit, Foundation IRCCS Ca' Granda, Ospedale Maggiore Policlinico, Milan, Italy
Full list of author information is available at the end of the article

are scarce, especially regarding patients not stung during VIT, in whom the actual clinical protection is unknown.

In this study, we retrospectively evaluated the decrease in sIgE over 5 years of VIT in 3 groups of yellow jacket venom (YJV)-allergic patients: subjects stung and protected within the first 3 years or within the last 2 years of VIT, and patients not stung during the VIT course. Furthermore, we followed these three groups of patients regarding further field stings after VIT cessation, to assess the long-lasting protection of VIT and the occurrence of reactions in patients who were not stung during VIT.

Methods

Patients

For this retrospective study, we used our hospital database and included YJV-allergic patients who completed 5 years of VIT without SR due to venom injections at any point of VIT. All patients met the VIT admission criteria and were treated in the Clinical Allergy and Immunology Unit, Foundation IRCCS Ca' Granda, Ospedale Maggiore Policlinico, Milan, Italy. Patients with elevated serum tryptase (>20 ng/mL) were excluded to avoid any mast cell disorder interference. Anamnesis were carefully documented, including the number of stings. SRs were classified according to Mueller grades [14].

All patients underwent VIT for at least 5 years with a maintenance dose of 100 µg of YJV (*Vespula spp.*) administered subcutaneously every 5 weeks, without changing the maintenance interval during the course of treatment. The VIT build-up phase was performed using a protocol that combines an initial rush session (first day $0.01 + 0.1 + 1 + 3$ µg, cumulative dose 4.11 µg) followed by weekly injections of 10, 20, 40, 70, 100 µg [15]. At the 3rd and the 5th year of VIT, the patients underwent subsequent diagnostic tests (skin tests and sIgE measurements). The occurrence of field stings and the patient's reaction were also documented.

The selected patients were divided into three groups: patients who were not stung (NoS) and patients who were stung and protected (SP) before the 3rd year (SP 0–3) or between the 3rd and the 5th year of VIT (SP 3–5); nobody among the SP patients experienced any SR after field stings.

Study design

The primary aims of the study were: (1) to evaluate the mean decrease in YJV-sIgE in all the patients and in patients stung in the first 3 years or in the last 2 years of VIT, and (2) to compare the mean YJV-sIgE decrease between patients stung and protected during VIT and patients not stung during VIT.

The secondary aims were: (1) to assess possible correlations between decrease in sIgE and patients' risk factors (age, reaction severity and number of stings), and (2) to assess the long-lasting protection in our patients by means of a phone follow-up.

Specific IgE level measurement

YJV-sIgE levels were measured in kUA/L by means of ImmunoCAP System (Phadia, Uppsala, Sweden) according to the manufacturer's instructions. Briefly, the allergen of interest is covalently coupled to ImmunoCAP and reacts with the sIgE in the patient sample; after washing, enzyme-labeled antibodies against IgE are added. After incubation and washing of the unbound enzyme-labeled anti-IgE, the bound complex is incubated with a developing agent, and finally the fluorescence of the eluate is measured. The higher the response value, the more sIgE is present in the serum sample. The responses are transformed into concentration by means of a calibration curve. The assay is highly automated and supplied of calibration curve and control curve, with a calibrator range 0–100 kUA/L. Clinical performance expressed as sensitivity (84–95 %) and specificity (85–94 %) and stability of the results have been reported from previous multicentric studies [16–18]. The tests were performed at baseline (CAP0) and after 3 (CAP3) and 5 (CAP5) years of VIT.

Statistical methods

We used: ANOVA analysis for repeated measures and the Wilcoxon post hoc test to evaluate the differences between the CAP values; ANOVA univariate analyses with the Bonferroni post hoc correction to evaluate the differences in each CAP value between the three groups; multivariate analysis for repeated measures (MANOVA) to evaluate the differences in the overall CAP values between the three groups as well as the effects of age, gender, Mueller grade and number of stings; Pearson's index to evaluate the correlations between continuous variables; the exact non-parametric Wilcoxon test to evaluate variables on small samples. A p value <0.05 was considered statistically significant. Data were analyzed using the SPSS® program release 17.0 (SPSS Inc., Chicago, IL).

Results

A total of 232 YJV-allergic patients (144 males, 88 females; mean age 45.05 ± 15.48 years) who completed 5 years of VIT were included in the study. Among them, 84 patients (53 males, 31 females) were never stung during VIT (group NoS), 72 patients (47 males, 25 females) were stung without SR by vespids within the first 3 years of VIT (group SP 0–3) and 76 patients (44 males, 32 females) were stung and protected during the last 2 years of VIT (group SP 3–5). No patient experienced SR during VIT as a result of field stings or as an adverse reaction to immunotherapy itself. The three groups had no statistically significant differences in mean age, number of stings before VIT or severity of sting reactions. The pre-VIT sting reactions were distributed as showed in Table 1. Considering other hypersensitivities, 22 patients had pollen allergies (11 NoS, 4 SP 0–3, 7 SP 3–5) and 17 had drug hypersensitivities (5 NoS, 9 SP 0–3, 3 SP 3–5).

Evolution of IgE values during 5 years of VIT

For the whole cohort (n = 232), YJV-sIgE levels decreased during VIT (Fig. 1) (χ^2 = 346.029, p < 0.001). This finding was confirmed by post hoc tests (CAP0–CAP3: Z = −12.173, p < 0.001; CAP3–CAP5: Z = −11.038, p < 0.001; CAP0–CAP5: Z = −12.850, p < 0.001).

CAP5 and CAP3 were significantly different among the three groups, whereas no significant differences were found between the three groups at baseline (Table 2).

The overall percentage reduction in CAP at the first (3rd year) and last (5th year) control were 44.2 and 34 %, respectively; the mean CAP percentage decrease between the baseline and the 5th year control reached 65.6 %, unlike the statistical analysis performed on skin test results that did not detect any significant differences (data not shown).

Considering CAP3 values, NoS patients had YJV-sIgE levels significantly lower than SP 0–3 patients; those who had experienced a more recent sting (SP 0–3) showed significantly higher CAP values than patients who were not stung (NoS). No significant difference was found between NoS and SP 3–5 patients, and between SP 0–3 and SP 3–5 (Table 2). The patients who were not stung during the first 3 years of VIT (NoS and SP 3–5) showed similar mean percentage reductions in CAP values, 48.2 and 53.7 %, respectively, while the reduction of the SP 0–3 patients was only 30.7 % (Table 3).

At the final VIT control (CAP5), the patients who were recently stung (SP 3–5) had significantly higher CAP values than those who were not stung or were stung during the first 3 years of VIT (Table 2). The sIgE final percentage reduction in the SP 3–5 group was less than 60 % when compared to baseline, while NoS and SP 0–3 patients presented a reduction of approximately 70 % (Table 3).

Influence of risk factors on the evolution of sIgE values

MANOVA analysis revealed that the CAP values were different during VIT (F = 28.872, p < 0.001) in the different groups (NoS, SP 0–3, SP 3–5). CAP values were also significantly related to Mueller grade (F = 2.778, p = 0.012) and age (F = 6.672, p = 0.002): a higher Mueller grade and a more advanced age were associated with higher CAP5 values. The Pearson's index confirmed a significant correlation between age and CAP 0–5 reduction (r = −0.609, p < 0.001). The other analyzed variables (gender and number of stings) were not statistically significant.

Follow-up after VIT discontinuation

All the patients were contacted by phone to determine if they had been stung after VIT cessation; results are reported in Table 4. We successfully contacted 159/232 (68.5 %) patients. Among the 84 NoS patients, we successfully contacted 70 (83 %) patients, 13 of which had been field-stung. 21 of the SP 0–3 patients and 22 of the SP 3–5 patients had been field-stung. A total of 56 (35.2 %) patients reported at least one field sting without any systemic reaction, from 1 to 10 years after VIT cessation. Some patients received multiple vespid stings from several months to several years after VIT cessation and did not experience any reactions.

Despite the clinicians recommendations to come back to our Centre for sIgE level determination in case of field sting after VIT discontinuation, only 13/56 (23.2 %) patients did. These patients (eight males, five females; mean age 43.54 ± 17.55) had a well tolerated field sting from few months to 4 years after VIT stopping. All of them had already been field stung during VIT, as seven patients belonged to SP 0–3 group and six to SP 3–5 group. As shown in Fig. 2, the mean IgE level determined about 2 months after the field sting resulted significantly different from the IgE level at baseline (Z = 2.342; p = 0.016) and at 5th year control (Z = −2.118; p = 0.034), while it did not differ from 3rd year control (Z = −0.235; p = 0.850).

Discussion

In this retrospective study, we selected 232 YJV-allergic patients. Serum sIgE levels determined before starting VIT, and at 3rd and 5th year controls, showed a significant decrease over time, which was an expected result. In fact, one of the immunological effects of VIT is the progressive reduction of sIgE levels [6, 19–21]. The reduction

Table 1 Patients' Mueller grade reaction

	Mueller I	Mueller II	Mueller III	Mueller IV
NoS	9	16	33	26
SP 0–3	8	18	25	21
SP 3–5	8	21	26	21
Total	25	55	84	68

Mueller grade reaction of our total study population, divided in patients never stung (NoS), stung in the first 3 years (SP 0–3), and stung in the last 2 years (SP 3–5) of venom immunotherapy

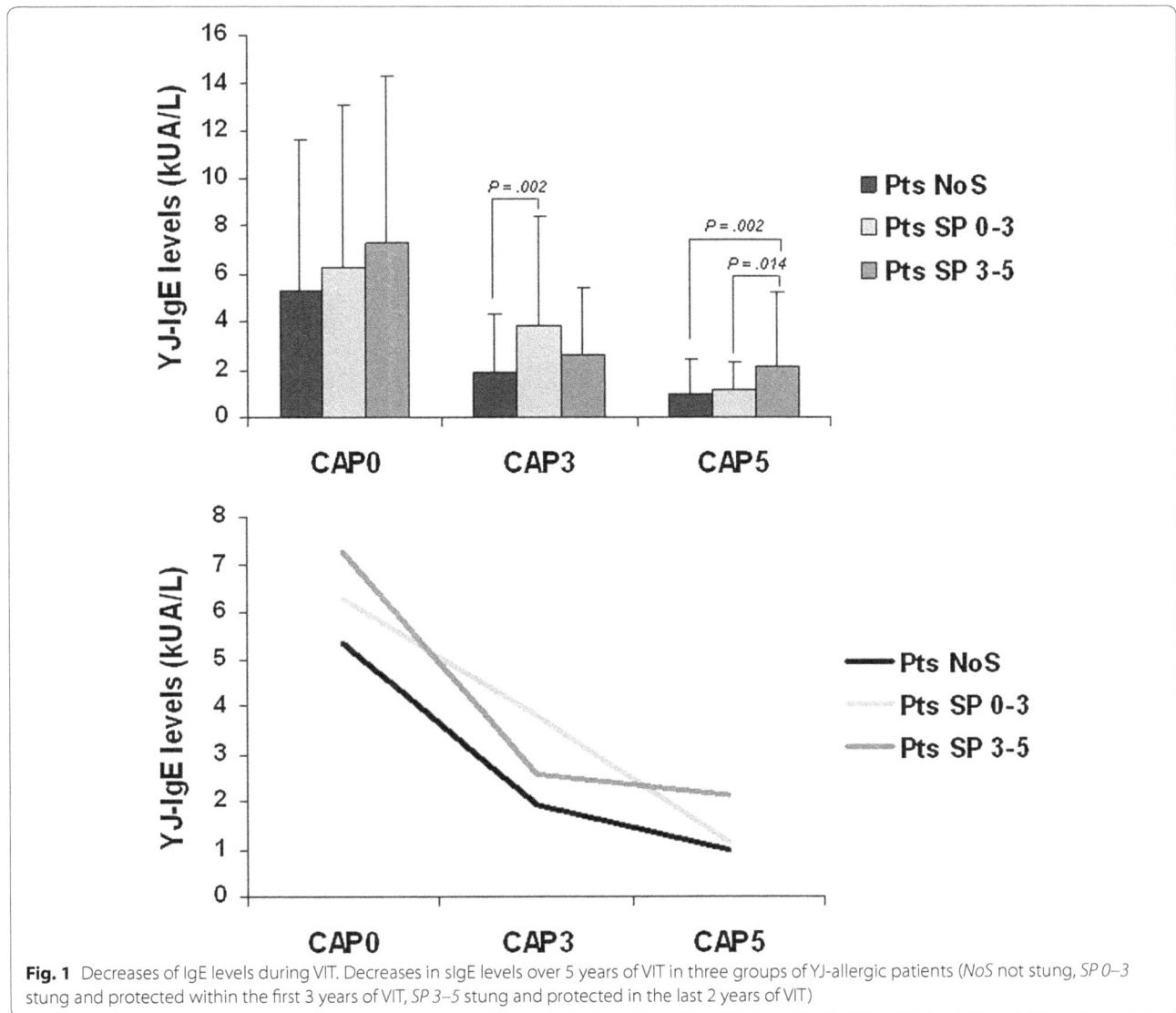

Fig. 1 Decreases of IgE levels during VIT. Decreases in sIgE levels over 5 years of VIT in three groups of YJ-allergic patients (*NoS* not stung, *SP 0–3* stung and protected within the first 3 years of VIT, *SP 3–5* stung and protected in the last 2 years of VIT)

Table 2 Statistical results of IgE variations during VIT

YJ-IgE levels (kUA/L)	Group			ANOVA		Post-Hoc test		
						NoS vs SP 0–3	NoS vs SP 3–5	SP 0–3 vs SP 3–5
	NoS	SP 0–3	SP 3–5	F	P	P (95 % CI)	P (95 % CI)	P (95 % CI)
CAP0	5.34 ± 6.26	6.27 ± 6.81	7.27 ± 7.05	1.663	0.192	1.00 (−3.53; 1.66)	0.209 (−4.49; 0.62)	1.00 (−3.65; 1.66)
CAP3	1.91 ± 2.42	3.81 ± 4.62	2.59 ± 2.80	6.261	*0.002*	*0.002* (−3.20; −0.59)	0.616 (−1.96; 0.61)	0.085 (−0.11; 2.55)
CAP5	0.97 ± 1.44	1.15 ± 1.17	2.13 ± 3.11	6.948	*0.001*	1.00 (−0.98; 0.63)	*0.002* (−1.95; −0.36)	*0.014* (−1.81; −0.16)

Statistically significant *P* values are in italics

Mean CAP values (±standard deviation) by group (*NoS* not stung, *SP 0–3*, stung and protected within the first 3 years of VIT, *SP 3–5* stung and protected in the last 2 years of VIT) and results of statistical analysis

Table 3 IgE percentage reduction during VIT related to field sting

YJ-IgE levels (kUA/L)	Group	Mean ± SD	Min	Max	Mean percentage reduction (%)
CAP0–CAP3	NoS	3.81 ± 5.13	0.01	27.59	48.2
	SP 0–3	2.61 ± 3.53	0.00	21.22	30.7
	SP 3–5	4.75 ± 5.32	0.00	25.07	53.7
CAP3–CAP5	NoS	0.97 ± 1.60	0.00	11.97	37.1
	SP 0–3	2.68 ± 4.13	0.00	20.97	50.3
	SP 3–5	0.82 ± 1.03	0.00	6.40	17.0
CAP0–CAP5	NoS	4.39 ± 5.48	0.00	27.54	68.6
	SP 0–3	5.15 ± 6.16	0.00	30.87	70.5
	SP 3–5	5.24 ± 5.55	0.12	25.30	57.7

Absolute (mean ± standard deviation SD, minimum and maximum) and percentage reductions of CAP values by group (*NoS* not stung, *SP 0–3* stung and protected within the first 3 years of VIT, *SP 3–5* stung and protected in the last 2 years of VIT)

Table 4 VIT discontinuation: restung patients' follow-up

Patients	NoS during VIT	SP during VIT
Total	84	148
Recalled	70	89
SP after VIT stopping	13/70	43/89
Within 1 year after	2	16[a]
After 2–3 years	–	11[a]
After 4–5 years	6	5[a]
After 7–8 years	3[a]	7 (4; 3[a])
After 9–10 years	2	4 (1; 3[a])

Follow-up after VIT discontinuation: number of patients stung and protected (SP) after stopping by group and period of time

[a] At least one patient received other field stings before or after

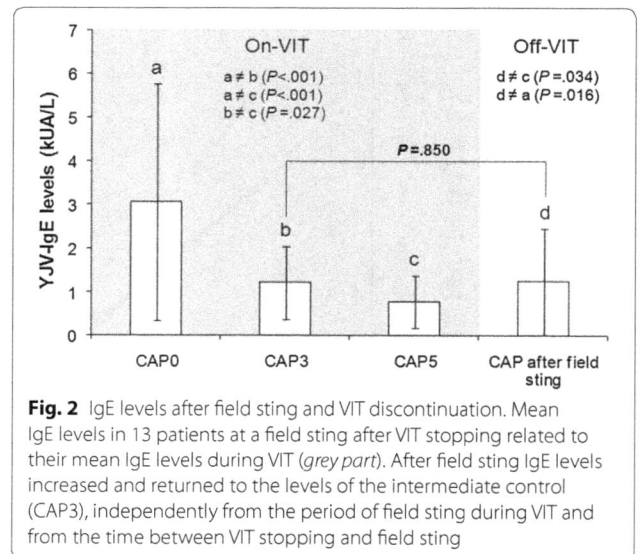

Fig. 2 IgE levels after field sting and VIT discontinuation. Mean IgE levels in 13 patients at a field sting after VIT stopping related to their mean IgE levels during VIT (*grey part*). After field sting IgE levels increased and returned to the levels of the intermediate control (CAP3), independently from the period of field sting during VIT and from the time between VIT stopping and field sting

of venom sIgE during VIT is a well known effect since 1983, when the loss of venom sensitivity due to VIT was described, with IgE levels showing an initial increase, and then followed by a reduction over the 3 years of VIT [6, 22]. The sIgE reduction over the course of VIT was confirmed by many studies, performed with both children and adults: after an initial increase at maintenance dose, venom sIgE fall after 3–5 years of venom immunotherapy [19–24]. Some Authors found a small decline in the mean venom sIgE levels also during the first year after VIT was stopped, suggesting both the duration of 5-year VIT and the passage of time can play a role in the decrease of sIgE [19]. The mechanism of specific IgE reduction during immunotherapy is likely due to the cytokine shift from a T-helper 2 to a T-helper 1 dominant pattern [25, 26]. Changes in cytokine production (decrease of IL-4, increase of IFN-gamma and IL-10) has been demonstrated for VIT, also during the early phase, with potential down regulation of mast cell and basophil reactivity, and rapid desensitization in rush VIT; in the longer term,

the immunological shift would result in an isotype switch from IgE to IgG [27–29].

Studies on natural history of insect sting allergy showed that, among patients with SRs and positive skin tests not treated with VIT, about 60 % had clinical re-sting reactions, with an higher rate of reactions in patients with more severe initial reactions [30]. Golden et al. [31] evaluated the changes in diagnostic tests and the risk of sting reactions in patients not admitted to VIT, demonstrating a 10–12 % per year loss in skin test positivity, with a negativization in 45 % of subjects after 4 years. Sensitization to venom may disappear in 30–50 % of cases after 5–10 years, but can also persist for many years even without sting exposure, with a 20 % chance of systemic reaction after 15 years in subject not treated with VIT. The risk of future systemic reactions depends on the severity of previous reactions: it is higher (60–70 %) in adults with severe anaphylaxis than in those with moderate (40 %) or mild (20 %) anaphylaxis [32]. In these studies, the reactivity of patients was assessed by spontaneous field stings or by deliberate sting challenges. Each method has its limitations: for field sting there is the uncertainty of the insect identification, for sting challenge (at least concerning vespids) there is the uncertainty of the amount of venom [33]. Indeed, there are studies demonstrating that a single negative sting challenge is not decisive to predict patient protection [33–35]. Up to now, in many European Countries, including Italy, the sting challenge is not recommended because is considered poorly reproducible and hazardous [12]. In one of the first surveys on VIT [6], 71 % of patients were clinically protected after a field sting, even though only a minority of them had negative sIgE after 3 years of VIT. Golden found a similar low percentage (approximately 30 %) of skin test negativization after 5 years of VIT, though all patients were sting challenge negative [36]. In the present study, at VIT cessation none of our patients exhibited a complete negativization of YJV-sIgE, even though the majority of them (63.8 %) had at least one well tolerated vespid field sting. Hence, a correlation between clinical protection and negativity of sIgE may not exist and should not be considered a reliable indicator of successful VIT.

To our knowledge, this is the first study investigating the associations of the risk factors for relapse after VIT with the evolution of sIgE levels during VIT. In our elderly patients and in patients with higher Mueller grade reactions, we observed a smaller decrease in sIgE during the VIT course; our results correlate well with the previously published data [7, 8, 11, 15]. A clinician evaluating the decision to stop VIT could take into consideration that patients with higher Mueller grade reactions and advanced age could present a smaller decrease of venom-sIgE, without necessarily invalidating the efficacy of VIT.

Analyzing the sIgE levels over time and the differences between the three groups (NoS, SP 0–3 and SP 3–5), we found a significant difference in CAP values at the 3rd year control between NoS and SP 0–3 patients, because of the sIgE increase associated to the recent vespid sting in the latter group. There was no significant difference between SP 0–3 and SP 3–5 patients, though the first group experienced a recent vespid sting, probably because of the higher CAP0 value presented by SP 3–5 patients. NoS and SP 3–5 patients exhibited a mean percentage reduction between CAP0 and CAP3 values of approximately 50 %, while SP 0–3 patients exhibited a less marked decrease (30 %).

At the 5th year control SP 0–3 patients had reduced CAP values, that were comparable with those of NoS patients. There was a significant difference between NoS,

SP 0–3 and SP 3–5 patients. Considering the mean percentage reduction between CAP3 and CAP5, SP 3–5 patients achieved only a 17 % reduction, while NoS and SP 0–3 patients experienced reductions of 37 and 50 %, respectively. Therefore, subjects who experienced a recent vespid sting, even if clinically protected, had significantly higher CAP values than patients who were not recently stung. Hence, higher than expected mean CAP values after 5 years of treatment in patients with recent field stings should not be considered as a criterion for VIT continuation. Despite sIgE levels has been evaluated after some years, we consider our CAP results to be reliable, as the stability, the reproducibility and the high degree of standardization of the ImmunoCAP assay have been previously demonstrated, retesting the same serum sample after storage at −20 °C over an 8-year period and confirming the reproducibility of the quantitative measurements of sIgE [18]. Furthermore, the coefficient of variation of the assay is very low (≤10 %) and independent of allergen specificity and IgE levels [37]. In our study the overall variability of sIgE detection at 3rd and 5th year of VIT is higher than 10 % of the coefficient of variation, so we can state that a real decrease in sIgE detection occurred.

After VIT stopping, 13 patients (seven belonging to SP 0–3 group and six to SP 3–5 group) underwent laboratory analyses after field stings. In this few patients sIgE levels increased after the field sting, resulting similar to the 3rd year control (Fig. 2).

We also performed phone interviews, asking patients if they had been stung after VIT stopping, to evaluate the protection rate. Among the 159 responders (70 NoS and 85 SP), 56 (35.2 %) reported one or more well-tolerated stings; almost all patients were clinically protected until 3 years after VIT cessation, and some were protected up to 10 years post-VIT. Only 19 % of NoS patients were stung after VIT termination; SP patients received more field stings than NoS patients after stopping VIT, most likely because they were less fearful to expose to risky outdoors situations. The follow-up survey after VIT cessation determined that all recalled patients, after 5 years VIT, were clinically protected for up to 10 years.

Considering the percentage reductions after 5 years of VIT, we observed that patients stung or not stung during the first 3 years showed a mean CAP reductions of roughly 70 % compared to their baseline values. For patients who were stung within the last 2 years of VIT, the mean CAP value decreased by roughly 58 % compared to baseline.

Conclusions

In conclusion, when a patient fulfills the temporal criterion for VIT duration (at least 5 years) but still has positive sIgE tests, a mean IgE decrease ranging from 58 to 70 % compared to baseline is likely to be expected. This decrease could be less striking in elderly patients or in subjects with a higher pre-treatment Mueller grade SR. Anyhow, the measurement of venom-specific IgE levels remains the best in vitro parameter to monitor VIT, as demonstrated by follow-up studies of patients with long-lasting protection.

Abbreviations
VIT: venom immunotherapy; SR: systemic reaction; YJV: yellow-jacket venom; YJ: yellow-jacket; sIgE: serum specific IgE; SP 0–3: patients stung and protected during the first 3 years of VIT; SP 3–5: patients stung and protected within the last 2 years of VIT; NoS: patients not stung during VIT; CAP: IgE levels detection by ImmunoCAP System; ANOVA: analysis of variance; MANOVA: multivariate analysis of variance.

Authors' contributions
VP, MP, LP and EAP participated in the design of the study, in interpretation of literature data, and contributed to drafting the manuscript and revising it critically. SF performed the statistical analysis. All authors read and approved the final manuscript.

Author details
[1] Clinical Allergy and Immunology Unit, Foundation IRCCS Ca'Granda, Ospedale Maggiore Policlinico, Milan, Italy. [2] Unit of Audiology, Foundation IRCCS Ca'Granda, Ospedale Maggiore Policlinico, Milan, Italy. [3] Unit of Allergology and Immunology, Niguarda Ca'Granda Hospital, Milan, Italy.

References
1. Hamilton RG. Diagnosis and treatment of allergy to hymenoptera venoms. Curr Opin Allergy Clin Immunol. 2010;10:323–9.
2. Golden DB, Kwiterovich KA, Kagey-Sobotka A, Lichtenstein LM. Discontinuing venom immunotherapy: extended observations. J Allergy Clin Immunol. 1998;101:298–305.
3. Golden DB. Discontinuing venom immunotherapy. Curr Opin Allergy Clin Immunol. 2001;1:353–6.
4. Graft DF. Venom immunotherapy: when to start, when to stop. Allergy Asthma Proc. 2000;21:113–6.
5. Bousquet J, Müller UR, Dreborg S, Jarisch R, Malling HJ, Mosbech H, Urbanek R, Youlten L. Immunotherapy with hymenoptera venoms. Position paper of the Working Group on immunotherapy of the European Academy of Allergy and Clinical Immunology. Allergy. 1987;42:401–13.
6. Thurnheer U, Müller U, Stoller R, Lanner A, Hoigne R. Venom immunotherapy in hymenoptera sting allergy. Comparison of rush and conventional hyposensitization and observations during long-term treatment. Allergy. 1983;38:465–75.
7. Urbanek R, Forster J, Kuhn W, Ziupa J. Discontinuation of bee venom immunotherapy in children and adolescents. J Pediatr. 1985;107:367–71.
8. Reisman RE. Duration of venom immunotherapy: relationship to the severity of symptoms of initial insect sting anaphylaxis. J Allergy Clin Immunol. 1993;92:831–6.
9. Müller U, Helbling A, Berchtold E. Immunotherapy with honeybee venom and yellow jacket venom is different regarding efficacy and safety. J Allergy Clin Immunol. 1992;89:529–35.
10. Lerch E, Müller UR. Long-term protection after stopping venom immunotherapy: results of re-stings in 200 patients. J Allergy Clin Immunol. 1998;101:606–12.
11. Golden DB, Johnson K, Addison BI, Valentine MD, Kagey-Sobotka A, Lichtenstein LM. Clinical and immunologic observations in patients who stop venom immunotherapy. J Allergy Clin Immunol. 1986;77:435–42.
12. Bonifazi F, Jutel M, Bilò BM, Birnbaum J, Müller U, EAACI Interest Group on Insect Venom Hypersensitivity. Prevention and treatment of hymenoptera venom allergy: guidelines for clinical practice. Allergy. 2005;60:1459–70.
13. Moffitt JE, Golden DB, Reisman RE, Lee R, Nicklas R, Freeman T, deshazo R, Tracy J, Bernstein IL, Blessing-Moore J, Khan DA, Lang DM, Portnoy JM, DE Schuller, Spector SL, Tilles SA. Stinging insect hypersensitivity: a practice parameter update. J Allergy Clin Immunol. 2004;114:869–86.
14. Mueller HL. Diagnosis and treatment of insect sensitivity. J Asthma Res. 1966;3:331–3.
15. Pucci S, Arsieni A, Biale C, Ciccarelli A, Incorvaia C, Parzanese I, Passalacqua G, Pravettoni V, Severino M, Venuti A. Diagnosis and treatment of Hymenoptera sting hypersensitivity. Guidelines of Italian Society of Allergy and Clinical Immunology. Ital J Allergy Clin Immunol. 2005;15:139–61.
16. Johansson SGO, editor. Clinical Workshop. IgE antibodies and the Pharmacia CAP System in allergy diagnosis. Lidköping: Landströms; 1988.
17. Pastorello EA, Incorvaia C, Pravettoni V, Bonini S, Canonica GW, Ortolani C, Romagnani S, Tursi A, Zanussi C. A multicentric study on sensitivity and specificity of a new in vitro test for measurement of IgE antibodies. Ann Allergy. 1991;67:365–70.
18. Paganelli R, Ansotegui IJ, Sastre J, Lange CE, Roovers MH, Groot H, Lindholm NB, Ewan PW. Specific IgE antibodies in the diagnosis of atopic disease. Clinical evaluation of a new in vitro test system, UniCAP, in six European allergy clinics. Allergy. 1998;53:763–8.
19. Keating MU, Kagey-Sobotka A, Hamilton RG, Yunginger JW. Clinical and immunologic follow-up of patients who stop venom immunotherapy. J Allergy Clin Immunol. 1991;88:339–48.
20. Reisman RE, Lantner R. Further observations of stopping venom immunotherapy: comparison of patients stopped because of a fall in serum venom-specific IgE to insignificant levels with patients stopped prematurely by self-choice. J Allergy Clin Immunol. 1989;83:1049–54.
21. Randolph CC, Reisman RE. Evaluation of decline in serum venom-specific IgE as a criterion for stopping venom immunotherapy. J Allergy Clin Immunol. 1986;77:823–7.
22. Clayton WF, Reisman RE, Georgitis JW, Wypych JI, Arbesman CE. Effect of prolonged venom immunotherapy on serum venom-specific IgE and IgG. Clin Allergy. 1983;13:301–7.
23. Graft DF, Schuberth KC, Kagey-Sobotka A, Kwiterovich KA, Niv Y, Lichtenstein LM, Valentine MD. The development of negative skin tests in children treated with venom immunotherapy. J Allergy Clin Immunol. 1984;73:61–8.
24. Graft DF, Schuberth KC, Kagey-Sobotka A, Kwiterovich KA, Niv Y, Lichtenstein LM, Valentine MD. Assessment of prolonged venom immunotherapy in children. J Allergy Clin Immunol. 1987;80:162–99.
25. Akdis M, Akdis CA. Mechanisms of allergen-specific immunotherapy. J Allergy Clin Immunol. 2007;119:780–91.
26. Bellinghausen I, Klostermann B, Bottcher I, Knop J, Saloga J. Importance of the inducible costimulator molecule for the induction of allergic immune responses and its decreased expression on T helper cells after venom immunotherapy. Immunology. 2004;112:80–6.
27. McHugh SM, Deighton J, Stewart AG, Lachmann PJ, Ewan PW. Bee venom immunotherapy induces a shift in cytokine responses from a TH-2 to a TH-1 dominant pattern: comparison of rush and conventional immunotherapy. Clin Exp Allergy. 1995;25:828–38.
28. Bellinghausen I, Metz G, Enk AH, Christmann S, Knop J, Saloga J. Insect venom immunotherapy induces interleukin-10 production and a Th2-to-Th1 shift, and changes surface marker expression in venom-allergic subjects. Eur J Immunol. 1997;27:1131–9.
29. Mamessier E, Birnbaum J, Dupuy P, Vervloet D, Magnan A. Ultra-rush venom immunotherapy induces differential T cell activation and regulatory patterns according to the severity of allergy. Clin Exp Allergy. 2006;36:704–13.
30. Reisman RE. Natural history of insect sting allergy: relationship of severity of symptoms of initial sting anaphylaxis to re-sting reactions. J Allergy Clin Immunol. 1992;90:335–9.
31. Golden DB, Marsh DG, Freidhoff LR, Kwiterovich RN, Addison B, Kagey-Sobotka A, Lichtenstein LM. Natural history of Hymenoptera venom sensitivity in adults. J Allergy Clin Immunol. 1997;100:760–6.

32. Golden DB. Insect sting allergy and venom immunotherapy: a model and mystery. J Allergy Clin Immunol. 2005;115:439–47.

33. Franken HH, Dubois AE, Minkema HJ, van der Heide S, de Monchy JG. Lack of reproducibility of a single negative sting challenge response in the assessment of anaphylactic risk in patients with suspected yellow jacket hypersensitivity. J Allergy Clin Immunol. 1994;93:431–6.

34. Hauk P, Friedl K, Kaufmehl K, Urbanek R, Forster J. Subsequent insect stings in children with hypersensitivity to Hymenoptera. J Pediatr. 1995;126:185–90.

35. Ruëff F, Przybilla B, Müller U, Mosbech H. The sting challenge test in Hymenoptera venom allergy. Position paper of the Subcommittee on Insect Venom Allergy of the European Academy of Allergology and Clinical Immunology. Allergy. 1996;51:216–25.

36. Golden DB, Addison BI, Gadde J, Kagey-Sobotka A, Valentine MD, Lichtenstein LM. Prospective observations on stopping prolonged venom immunotherapy. J Allergy Clin Immunol. 1989;84:162–7.

37. Lambert C, Sarrat A, Bienvenu F, Brabant S, Nicaise-Roland P, Alyanakian MA, Apoil PA, Capron C, Couderc R, Evrard B, Jaby D, Hémont C, Lainé C, Lelong M, Mariotte D, Martinet J, Rénier G, Sainte-Laudy J, Tabary T, Treiner E, Uring-Lambert B, Vigneron C, Vivinus M, Witthuhn F, Vitte J, AllergoBioNet sIgE Accreditation Interest Group. The importance of EN ISO 15189 accreditation of allergen-specific IgE determination for reliable in vitro allergy diagnosis. Allergy. 2015;70:180–6.

4

Comparing the ability of molecular diagnosis and CAP-inhibition in identifying the really causative venom in patients with positive tests to Vespula and Polistes species

Eleonora Savi[1], Silvia Peveri[1], Elena Makri[2], Valerio Pravettoni[3] and Cristoforo Incorvaia[2*]

Abstract

Background: Cross-reactivity among Hymenoptera venoms is an important issue when prescribing venom immunotherapy (VIT). Using all venoms eliciting a positive response results in treatment excess and unjustified cost increase. The first in vitro method that helped to identify the really causative venom was RAST-inhibition, but in latest years also molecular allergy (MA) diagnostics, that detects specific sIgE to single venom allergens, was introduced. We compared the two methods in patients with double sensitization to *Vespula* spp. and *Polistes* spp.

Methods: Fifty-four patients with anaphylactic reactions to Hymenoptera stings and positive results to skin tests and sIgE measurement with whole venom from *Vespula* spp. and *Polistes dominula* were included in the study. Sera from all patients were analyzed by CAP-inhibition (Thermo Fisher Scientific, Uppsala, Sweden) and MA diagnostics with recombinant Ves v 1, Ves v 5 and Pol d 5.

Results: By the data obtained from MA technique, VIT would have been prescribed to 7 patients for *Polistes*, to 6 for *Vespula*, and to 41 for both venoms. With the data from CAP inhibition, it would have been a prescription to 15 patients for *Polistes*, to 28 for *Vespula*, and to 11 for both venoms. A good concordance between the results of MA and CAP-inhibition was found only when the value in kU/l of Ves v 5 were about twice those of Pol d 5, and vice versa.

Conclusions: These findings suggest that in the choice of the venom to be used for VIT CAP-inhibition remains a pivotal tool, because the significance of in vitro inhibition is definite and provides a diagnostic importance higher than MA in patients with positive tests to both *Vespula* and *Polistes* spp.

Keywords: Hymenoptera venom allergy, Vespids, Diagnosis, CAP inhibition, Molecular allergy

Background

Stings by Hymenoptera, including honeybees (*Apis mellifera*), yellow jackets (*Vespula species*), paper wasps (*Polistes species*), and hornets (*Dolicho vespula, Vespa crabro*) cause systemic allergic reactions in 1–5 % of the population in Europe and North America [1]. The mechanism of these reactions is an IgE-mediated sensitization to proteins of the venoms injected with the stings, particularly enzymes like phospholipase A and hyaluronidase, and for vespids antigen 5 [2]. A common issue in diagnosis of Hymenoptera venom allergy (HVA) is the occurrence of multiple positive results to the different venoms, mainly due to cross-reactivity between phospholipase A1 for vespids, and hyaluronidase, that may concern all venoms; another important cross-reactivity source is common cross-reactive carbohydrate determinants (CCD) [3]. This has led to perform very often venom immunotherapy (VIT) with all venoms eliciting a positive response to tests. However, in the 1990s Hamilton et al. demonstrated by the technique of RAST-inhibition that one third of 305 patients with HVA with

---

*Correspondence: cristoforo.incorvaia@gmail.com
[2] Allergy/Pulmonary Rehabilitation, ICP Hospital, Via Bignami 1, 20100 Milan, Italy
Full list of author information is available at the end of the article

positive *Vespula*- and *Polistes*-reactive IgE in the skin and/or serum were identified as candidates for exclusion of *Polistes* from immunotherapy because their IgE anti-*Polistes* was more than 95 % cross-inhibitable with *Vespula* venom [4]. After the demonstration that CAP system had better performances than RAST [5], CAP-inhibition was used instead to assess cross-reactivity. Concerning Hymenoptera venom, CAP-inhibition studies allowed to detect the importance of CCD as a cause for the double positivity to *A. mellifera* and *Vespula* venom [6], and the extent of cross-reactivity between *Vespa crabro* and *Vespula* venom [7]. Two studies focused the role of CAP-inhibition in suggesting the correct choice of the venom to be used for VIT in patients with apparent poly-sensitization [8, 9].

In the latest decade, the technique of molecular allergy (MA), that makes possible to measure specific IgE (sIgE) to single venom allergens was introduced as a further in vitro method to identify with precision the causative venom [10]. In fact, in patients with positive tests to *A. mellifera* and *Vespula* venom the detection of sIgE to Api m 1, Ves v 1 and Ves v 5 allowed recognition of double sensitization from cross-reactions [11]. Indeed, double positivity to tests with *Vespula* and *Polistes species* is very frequent. In 2012, a MA-based study on patients with such kind of sensitization found that *Polistes* and *Vespula* were the culprit insect in 49 and 20 %, respectively [12], but this was in contrast with the general knowledge on the importance of these species in HVA [13].

The aim of this study was to compare the capacity of MA technique and CAP-inhibition to identify the culprit vespid in patients positive to both *Vespula* and *Polistes* whole venoms.

Methods

Fifty-four outpatients with anaphylactic reactions to Hymenoptera stings of at least Mueller grade II [14] in the last 6 months and double positive response to tests with *Vespula* and *Polistes* spp. were included in the study. All patients did not recognize the culprit insect and thus were unable to provide data to identify the really causative species. Skin tests were performed with *Vespula* spp. and *Polistes dominula* venom (ALK-Abellò Horsholm, Denmark) for *Vespula species* and *P. dominula*, with an initial prick test at 100 mcg/ml, followed, if negative, by intradermal testing at 0.1 and 1 mcg/ml [15]. Venom-specific serum IgE measurement was done by CAP system (Thermo Fisher Scientific, Uppsala, Sweden) to whole venom of *Vespula* spp. and *P. dominula*, as well to recombinant Ves v 1, Ves v 5 and Pol d 5.

All patients sample sera were analyzed by CAP-inhibition to identify the actual sensitization by the laboratory method previously described by Caruso et al. [9].

Briefly, two 100 mcL aliquots of patient's serum were incubated separately for 12 h at 4 °C with 200 ml of *P. dominula* or *Vespula* venoms at increasing dilutions (0; 25 mcg; 50 mcg; 100 mcg/ml). Subsequently, sIgE against each of the venoms were determined in the samples prepared as above. The extent of homologous (blockage of venom-sIgE by the same venom) and heterologous (blockage of the venom-sIgE by the other venom) inhibition was computed with the following formula: % inhibition = 100 − [IgE inhibited sample (kU/l) × 100/ IgE anti-venom (kU/l) at zero concentration of venom]. According to Straumann et al. [8] a percentage of homologous inhibition >70 % was required to perform heterologous inhibition. The same percentage was considered suggestive of cross-reactivity among *Vespula* and *Polistes* venom. The venom preparations tested were the same used for skin tests. For statistical analysis was used the Cohen (k) concordance index, that establishes the grade of concordance based on the following k values: <0, no concordance, 0–0.4 poor concordance, 0.4–0.6, fair concordance, 0.6–0.8, good concordance, and 0.8–1, excellent concordance.

All patients gave their consent to the use of the data obtained from the diagnostic procedures for scientific research.

Results

The patients had similar reactivity by skin testing to *Vespula* and *Polistes* spp. venom. An homologous inhibition higher than 70 % was detected in all sera. Table 1 shows the data obtained from measurement of sIgE to whole venom by CAP and to single allergens by MA technique. By such data, based on MA results VIT would have been prescribed to 7 patients with *Polistes*, to 6 patients with *Vespula*, and to 41 patients with both venoms. Based on CAP inhibition data VIT would have prescribed to 15 patients with *Polistes*, to 28 patients with *Vespula*, and to 11 patients with both venoms. The concordance between the results of MA with Ves v 1, Ves v 5, Pol d 5 and the results of CAP-inhibition was very poor, showing a value of k = 0.01. A good concordance was found only when the value in kU/l of Ves v 5 were about twice those of Pol d 5, and vice versa.

Discussion

A number of studies demonstrated that VIT prevents any kind of reaction to insect stings in most patients and is completely effective in preventing fatal reactions [16]. To expect the same outcome in the daily practice, the allergist must choice the appropriate venom for VIT, but this is often complicated by the issue of cross-reactivity, which concerns all venoms but is particularly common for vespids [13]. The first in vitro technique that helped

Table 1 Results obtained with MA technique and CAP-inhibition and choice of VIT for each method. The same choices for MA and CAP-inhibition are highlighted in italics

No	Age/sex	Whole venom extracts		Recombinant allergens (kUA/L)			Venom used for VIT		CAP inhibition (% of inhibition)				Venom used for VIT	
		Vespula spp.	*Polistes dominula*	Ves v 5	Ves v 1	Pol d 5	*Vespula*	*Polistes*	*Vespula* spp. sIgE *Vespula* spp. venom	P. dominula sIgE *Vespula* spp. venom	*Vespula* spp. sIgE by P. dominula venom	P. dominula sIgE by P. dominula venom	*Vespula*	*Polistes*
1	45/m	5.54	4.65	1.15	3	0.57	X		88	72	80	87	X	
2	56/f	5.14	9.3	47.2	3	81.4	X	X	80	50	35	78	X	X
3	68/f	1.73	1.94	9.66	0	14.6	X	X	100	35	80	92		X
4	57/m	0.63	1.41	1.7	1	2.59	X	X	100	50	50	80	X	X
5	74/m	>100	>100	5.21	0.09	4.28	X	X	88	80	65	90	X	X
6	76/m	55.3	80.3	17.3	41.3	17.6	X	X	75	35	70	95		X
7	35/m	2.51	1.17	17.5	0.04	21.4	X	X	80	50	50	77	X	X
8	61/m	1.28	2.62	2.93	0	5.57	X	X	95	50	95	92		X
9	48/m	9.49	1.99	1.88	7.31	1.17	X	X	95	75	55	82	X	
10	71/m	6.04	1.73	12.1	1.68	8.73	X	X	100	73	40	78	X	
11	52/m	10.4	7.36	10.5	10.7	11.1	X	X	75	73	82	93		X
12	62/m	0.53	1.08	2.47	0	4.44	X	X	95	60	97	99		X
13	23/m	13.3	9.76	14.9	6	8.34	X	X	90	40	40	90	X	X
14	45/m	1.89	1.93	1.48	1.8	1.93	X	X	90	60	65	86	X	X
15	44/f	3.65	1.34	20.1	0.06	18.1	X	X	93	35	27	90	X	X
16	64/f	2.59	1.73	32.3	0.01	38.7	X	X	99	86	78	93	X	
17	66/m	2.2	10.1	3.8	0.42	7.28	X	X	93	60	35	92	X	X
18	42/m	29.2	46.3	5.31	24.9	22.2	X	X	95	60	87	94	X	X
19	58/m	3.2	3.82	5.72	1.6	4.26	X	X	80	58	50	85	X	X
20	34/m	6.23	5.79	4.36	4.31	3.76	X	X	75	69	55	90	X	
21	55/f	4.54	9.71	5.86	0.74	10.2	X	X	74	33	50	80	X	X
22	55/m	13.8	7.48	12.8	4.33	5.19	X		90	75	33	82	X	
23	43/m	7.71	6.45	2.78	22.2	0.94	X		88	80	65	88	X	
24	51/f	6.37	7.16	6.5	0.02	7.4	X	X	94	80	73	93	X	
25	67/m	1.82	1.79	0.4	0.78	0.39	X	X	94	70	60	92	X	
26	72/m	5.52	12.7	4.49	0.92	9.93		X	86	50	87	75		X
27	75/m	4.88	5.39	3.97	0.05	4.77	X	X	75	63	79	94		X
28	55/m	75.6	1.3	76.8	1.11	66.1	X	X	98	96	70	75	X	
29	57/f	5.35	2.33	4.2	0	1.3	X	X	96	94	30	78	X	

Table 1 continued

No	Age/sex	Whole venom extracts		Recombinant allergens (kUA/L)			Venom used for VIT		CAP inhibition (% of inhibition)				Venom used for VIT	
		Vespula spp.	Polistes dominula	Ves v 5	Ves v 1	Pol d 5	Vespula	Polistes	Vespula spp. sIgE Vespula spp. venom	P. dominula sIgE Vespula spp. venom	Vespula spp. sIgE by P. dominula venom	P. dominula sIgE by P. dominula venom	Vespula	Polistes
30	66/m	3.14	02:34	2.89	0.04	0.04	X		99	92	54	80	X	
31	47/m	40	32	99	0.17	98	X	X	83	93	36	78	X	
32	65/f	8.16	5.15	7.1	2.3	4.6	X	X	98	99	56	75	X	
33	59/m	3.51	3	1.73	0.7	2	X	X	84	78	52	79	X	
34	60/m	1.43	1.2	46	0.1	4.23	X	X	97	70	67	76	X	
35	21/m	1.6	2.3	1.9	0.46	2	X	X	95	66	61	93	X	X
36	55/m	6.04	5.93	5.18	0.82	5.17	X	X	97	70	57	75	X	
37	46/f	1.35	3.11	5.89	0.02	10.8	X	X	92	83	59	83	X	
38	32/f	1.05	1.83	0.88	0.8	2.25		X	76	45	82	76		X
39	50/f	4.01	2.33	94.8	9.22	81.4	X	X	99	96	64	87	X	
40	47/m	1.2	1.8	3.14	0	5.48	X	X	85	40	80	75		X
41	56/m	2.14	2.98	27.6	0.39	45.2	X	X	92	86	75	76	X	
42	41/m	>100	>100	99	0.16	98.5	X	X	99	95	60	92	X	
43	51/f	1.74	1.7	0.6	0.08	0.59	X	X	90	81	52	76	X	
44	74/m	19.2	17.5	16.8	0.19	19.2	X	X	95	85	47	85	X	
45	45/m	1.06	2.27	1.3	0.09	5.8		X	94	44	91	91		X
46	67/m	22.8	83.6	21	18	63		X	95	42	96	98		X
47	25/m	3.9	5.59	1.5	2.3	5.6		X	75	30	65	70		X
48	22/m	5.02	12	5.49	0.92	19.93		X	86	50	87	75		X
49	68/m	4.15	3.38	5.6	1.3	1.6	X		90	65	45	78	X	
50	59/f	3.83	5.02	3.53	0.1	4.98	X	X	96	52	83	90		X
51	61/m	17.3	15.8	15.8	0.3	14.3	X	X	98	76	59	86	X	
52	63/m	6.15	8.9	7.03	8.14	9.45	X	X	96	54	61	90	X	X
53	16/m	5.46	3.76	6.08	3.92	6.18	X	X	81	83	29	82	X	
54	52/f	1.33	1.34	0.56	0.05	0.75	X	X	94	86	37	75	X	

to identify the really causative venom was RAST-inhibition, followed by CAP-inhibition, whose reagents allow more accurate measurements [5–8]. In recent years the technique of MA diagnostics was introduced and detects the IgE antibodies to single molecules contained in allergen sources [17]. Assessing sIgE to recombinant and natural venom components from each vespid species in 45 patients with allergic reactions to stings and positive ImmunoCAP and/or intradermal tests to vespid venoms, Monsalve et al. found that 9 of these patients had clearly higher IgE values to nVes v 1 or nVes v 5 or both, thus indicating that *Vespula* was most probably the sensitizing species for these patients, while the probable sensitization could be clearly assigned to *P. dominula* in 22/45 cases, because of the higher values of Pol d 1 and/or Pol d 5. In 14/45, the quantitative response did not allow to identify the possible sensitizing species [12]. For such cases, the authors suggested that, "unless complex inhibition studies or sting challenges are performed", double sensitization should be considered to prescribe a correct immunotherapy. More recently, Hemmer stated that "The identification of the primary venom in patients testing positive for *Vespula* and *Polistes* (paper wasps) is particularly important in Mediterranean areas. MA technique with the marker allergens Ves v 5 and Pol d 5 may directly identify the causative venom in the majority of patients" [18].

Actually, our findings show that MA would have indicated 7 treatments with *Polistes* and 6 with *Vespula*, while information obtained by CAP-inhibition would have indicated 15 treatments with *Polistes* and 28 with *Vespula*, thus reducing the number of double treatments from 41 to 11, and confirming the observation from Hamilton et al. on the capacity of this in vitro method to avoid unnecessary VIT treatments [4]. This suggests that in the choice of the venom to be used in immunotherapy CAP-inhibition remains a pivotal tool, because the significance of in vitro inhibition is definite and provides a diagnostic importance higher than MA in patients with positive tests to both *Vespula* and *Polistes* spp. who failed to recognize the culprit vespid. The availability of additional molecules, such as Pol d 1, will probably improve the ability of MA in vespid allergy, but this warrants to be demonstrated by further studies. Both MA and CAP-inhibition studies thus far available were not tested against a gold standard for diagnosis of HVA. Indeed, differently from other fields of allergy, for example with the double-blind placebo-controlled food challenge for the diagnosis of food allergy [19], no gold standard is definitely accepted for HVA. In particular, the sting challenge test is not recommended for vespid allergy due to the variable amounts of venom injected with the sting [20]. The actual demonstration of the tolerance to venom induced

by VIT is based on the outcome of field stings, but follow-up studies investigating the proof of the results of MA or CAP-inhibition by field stings are not available.

Indeed, in times of spending review also the cost-effectiveness of VIT is questioned [21]. Nobody can argue its life-saving role when the culprit venom is used, but avoiding additional treatments with unnecessary venoms, as obtained by CAP-inhibition, that in our study spared 30 additional treatments in 54 patients, may allow to significantly reduce the costs.

Authors' contributions

ES conceived the study, ES and SP performed the in vitro testing, EM and CI contributed to literature search and to the writing of the manuscript. CI provided the final revision of the manuscript, VP revised the language and remade the Table 1. All authors read and approved the final manuscript.

Author details

[1] Allergy Unit, G. Da Saliceto Hospital, AUSL Piacenza, Piacenza, Italy. [2] Allergy/Pulmonary Rehabilitation, ICP Hospital, Via Bignami 1, 20100 Milan, Italy. [3] Department of Internal Medicine, Clinical Allergy and Immunology, IRCCS Foundation Ca' Granda Ospedale Maggiore Policlinico, Milan, Italy.

Competing interests

ES has received fees by Thermofisher, Stallergenes and ALK for lectures in medical congresses; SP has received fee by Thermofisher for a lecture in a medical congress; VP has received fee by Alk-Abellò for consultancy; CI is a scientific consultant for Stallergenes.

References

1. Bilò BM, Bonifazi F. Epidemiology of insect venom anaphylaxis. Curr Opin Allergy Clin Immunol. 2008;8:330–7.
2. Muller UR. Hymenoptera venom proteins and peptides for diagnosis and treatment of venom allergic patients. Inflamm Allergy Drug Targets. 2011;10:420–8.
3. Spillner E, Blank S, Jakob T. Hymenoptera allergens: from venom to "venome". Front Immunol. 2014;5:77.
4. Hamilton RG, Wisenauer JA, Golden DB, Valentine MD, Adkinson NF Jr. Selection of Hymenoptera venoms for immunotherapy on the basis of patient's IgE antibody cross-reactivity. J Allergy Clin Immunol. 1993;92:651–9.
5. Pastorello EA, Incorvaia C, Pravettoni V, Marelli A, Farioli L, Ghezzi M. Clinical evaluation of CAP System and RAST in the measurement of specific IgE. Allergy. 1992;47:463–6.
6. Hemmer W, Focke M, Kolarich D, Wilson IB, Altmann F, Wöhrl S, et al. Antibody binding to carbodydrate is a frequent cause for double positivity to honeybee and yellow jacket venom in patients with stinging-insect allergy. J Allergy Clin Immunol. 2001;108:1045–52.
7. Severino MG, Caruso B, Bonadonna P, Labardi D, Macchia D, Campi P, et al. Cross reactivity between European hornet and yellow racket venoms. Eur Ann Allergy Clin Immunol. 2010;42:141–5.
8. Straumann F, Bucher C, Wüthrich G. Double sensitization to honeybee and wasp venom: immunotherapy with one or with both venoms? value of FEIA inhibition for the identification of the cross-reacting IgE antibodies in double-sensitized patients to honeybee and wasp venom. Int Arch Allergy Immunol. 2000;123:268–74.
9. Caruso B, Bonadonna P, Severino MG, Manfredi M, Dama A, Schiappoli M, et al. Evaluation of the IgE cross-reactions among vespid venoms. A possible approach for the choice of immunotherapy. Allergy. 2007;62:561–4.
10. Incorvaia C, Mauro M, Pravettoni V, Pucci S. Hypersensitivity to Hymenoptera venom: advances in diagnosis and implications for treatment. Recent Pat Inflamm Allergy Drug Discov. 2011;5:128–35.

11. Muller U, Schmid-Grandelmeier P, Hausmann O, Helbling A. IgE to recombinant allergens Api m 1, Ves v 1 and Ves v 5 distinguish double sensitization from crossreaction in venom allergy. Allergy. 2012;67:1069–73.

12. Monsalve RI, Vega A, Marques L, Miranda A, Fernandez J, Soriano V, et al. Component resolved diagnosis of vespid venom-allergic individuals: phospholipases and antigen 5s are necessary to identify *Vespula* or *Polistes* sensitization. Allergy. 2012;67:528–36.

13. Incorvaia C, Mauro M. Can component resolved diagnosis overturn the current knowledge on vespid allergy? Allergy. 2012;67:966.

14. Mueller HL. Diagnosis and treatment of insect sensitivity. J Asthma Res. 1966;3:331–3.

15. Pucci S, Arsieni A, Biale C, Ciccarelli A, Incorvaia C, Parzanese I, et al. Diagnosis and treatment of Hymenoptera sting hypersensitivity. guidelines of the Italian Society of Allergy and Alinical Immunology. It J Allergy Clin Immunol. 2005;15:139–61.

16. Boyle RJ, Elremeli M, Hockenhull J, Cherry MG, Bulsara MK, Daniels M, et al. Venom immunotherapy for preventing allergic reaction to insect stings. Cochrane Database Syst Rev. 2012;10:CD008838.

17. Treudler R, Simon JC. Overview of component resolved diagnostics. Curr Allergy Asthma Rep. 2013;13:110–7.

18. Hemmer W. Cross-reactions between Hymenoptera venoms from different families, genera and species. Hautarzt. 2014;65:775–9.

19. Macchia D, Melioli G, Pravettoni V, Nucera E, Piantanida M, Caminati M, et al. Food Allergy Study Group (ATI) of the Italian Society of allergy, asthma and clinical immunology (SIAAIC). Guidelines for the use and interpretation of diagnostic methods in adult food allergy. Clin Mol Allergy. 2015;13:27.

20. Ruëff F, Przybilla B, Müller U, Mosbech H. The sting challenge test in Hymenoptera venom allergy. Position paper of the subcommittee on insect venom allergy of the European Academy of Allergology and Clinical Immunology. Allergy. 1996;51:216–25.

21. Boyle RJ, Dickson R, Hockenhull J, Cherry MG, Elremeli M. Immunotherapy for Hymenoptera venom allergy: too expensive for European health care? Allergy. 2013;68:1341–2.

5

Drug induced exfoliative dermatitis: state of the art

Mona-Rita Yacoub[1,2]*, Alvise Berti[2], Corrado Campochiaro[2], Enrico Tombetti[2], Giuseppe Alvise Ramirez[2], Andrea Nico[3], Elisabetta Di Leo[3], Paola Fantini[3], Maria Grazia Sabbadini[1,2], Eustachio Nettis[3] and Giselda Colombo[1,2]

Abstract

Drug induced exfoliative dermatitis (ED) are a group of rare and severe drug hypersensitivity reactions (DHR) involving skin and usually occurring from days to several weeks after drug exposure. Erythema multiforme (EM), Stevens–Johnson syndrome (SJS) and toxic epidermal necrolysis (TEN) are the main clinical presentations of drug induced ED. Overall, T cells are the central player of these immune-mediated drug reactions. Here we provide a systematic review on frequency, risk factors, pathogenesis, clinical features and management of patients with drug induced ED.

Keywords: Exfoliative dermatitis, Drug hypersensitivity, Stevens–Johnson syndrome, Lyell's syndrome, Toxic epidermal necrolysis, Erythema multiforme, Delayed type hypersensitivity, Pathogenesis, Clinical features, Therapy

Background

Cutaneous drug eruptions are one of the most common types of adverse reaction to medications, with an overall incidence of 2–3 % in hospitalized patients [1]. In particular, drug induced exfoliative dermatitis (ED) are a group of rare and more severe drug hypersensitivity reactions (DHR) involving skin and mucous membranes and usually occurring from days to several weeks after drug exposure [2]. Erythema multiforme (EM), Stevens–Johnson syndrome (SJS) and toxic epidermal necrolysis (TEN) are the main clinical presentations of drug induced ED. Important data on ED have been obtained by RegiSCAR (European Registry of Severe Cutaneous Adverse Reactions to Drugs: www.regiscar.org), an ongoing pharmaco-epidemiologic study conducted in patients with SJS and TEN. Overall, T cells are the central player of these immune-mediated drug reactions. Immune-histopathological features allow to distinguish generalized bullous drug eruption from SJS/TEN [3–6]. Still, treatment indication, choice and dosage remain unclear, and efficacy yet unproven. Here we provide a systematic review of frequency, risk factors, molecular and cellular mechanisms of reactions, clinical features, diagnostic work-up and therapy approaches to drug induced ED.

Epidemiology

Epidemiological studies on EM, SJS and TEN syndromes report different results, probably related to several biases, such as ethnical differences, diagnostic criteria and drug consumption patterns in different socio-economic systems. Albeit the lack of epidemiologic data regarding EM, its reported prevalence is less than 1 % [7–10]. Several authors report the incidence of hospitalization for EM ranging from 0.4–6 cases per million people per year of northern Europe [11] to almost 40 cases per million people per year of United States [12]. EM usually occurs in young adults of 20–40 years of age [13], with women affected more frequently than men (1.5:1.0) [14]. Recurrence occurs in around one-third of cases [15] and there is a genetic predisposition for certain Asian groups [16]. Mucosal involvement could achieve almost 65 % of patients [17]. EM's mortality rate is not well reported.

Overall, incidence of SJS/TEN ranges from 2 to 7 cases per million person per year [9, 18–20], with SJS the commonest [21]. In HIV patients, the risk of SJS and TEN have been reported to be thousand-fold higher, roughly 1 per 1000 per year [19]. Prevalence is low, with mortality

*Correspondence: yacoub.monarita@hsr.it
[1] Department of Allergy and Clinical Immunology, IRCCS San Raffaele Hospital, Via Olgettina 60, 20132 Milan, Italy
Full list of author information is available at the end of the article

of roughly 5–12.5 % for SJS and 50 % for TEN [1, 2]. In general, they occur more frequently in women, with a male to female ratio of 0.6 [22]. The overall mortality rate is roughly 30 %, ranging from 10 % for SJS to more than 30 % for TEN, with the survival rate worsening until 1 year after disease onset [9, 18–21].

Pharmacogenetics studies have found an association between susceptibility to recurrent EM in response to several stimuli and human leukocyte antigen (HLA) haplotypes of class II, in particular HLA DQB1*0301 [23].

On the other hand, it has been demonstrated that genetic predisposition may increase the risk for sulphonamide-induced [24] and carbamazepine-induced TEN and SJS [25]. Scientific evidences suggest a role for HLAs and drug-induced SJS/TEN, although some racial differences have been found that can be due to variation of frequencies of these alleles and to the presence of other susceptibility genes [26]. These studies have confirmed an association between carbamazepine-induced SJS/TEN with HLA-B*1502 allele among Han Chinese [27], carbamazepine and HLA-A*3101 and HLA-B*1511 [16], phenytoin and HLA-B*1502 [28], allopurinol and HLA-B*5801 [29]. For carbamazpine, several studies have found a common link between specific HLAs and different kinds of cutaneous adverse reactions, as for HLA-A*3101 in Japanese [30] and Europeans [31]. Because a certain degree of cross-reactivity between the various aromatic anti-epileptic drugs exists, some HLAs have been found to be related to SJS/TEN with two drugs, as the case of HLA-B*1502 with both phenytoin and oxcarbazepine [32].

Pathogenesis

Apoptosis-inducing factors and lymphocyte-mediated cytotoxicity have been deeply investigated in ED. Four main pathways have been found to play important roles in the pathogenesis of keratinocyte death: (1) Fas-FasL interaction, (2) Perforin/granzyme B pathway, (3) Granulysin and (4) Tumor necrosis factor α (TNF-α) [26].

1. *Fas-FasL interaction*: Fas is a membrane-bound protein that after interaction with Fas-ligand (FasL) induces a programmed cell death, through the activation of intracellular caspases. T and NK lymphocytes can produce FasL that eventually binds to target cells. In ED increased levels of FasL have been detected in patients' sera [33]. The exact source of FasL production has not been yet identified as different groups have postulated that the production might be sought in keratinocytes themselves [33] or in peripheral blood mononuclear cells [34]. In any case all authors concluded that the blockage of FasL prevents keratinocyte apoptosis [35]. The exact role of FasL

in the pathogenesis of toxic epidermal necrolysis is still questionable especially because a correlation between serum FasL levels and disease severity has not been established and because its levels have been found to be increased also in drug-induced hypersensitivity syndrome and maculopapular eruption [36].

2. *Perforin/granzyme* B pathway: Nassif and colleagues have proposed a role for perforin/grazyme B in keratinocyte death [37]. They found that the inhibition of these molecules could attenuate the cytotoxic effect of lymphocytes toward keratinocytes. A correlation between increased levels of perforin/granzyme B and the severity of TEN was also described [38].

3. *Granulysin*: Granulysin is a pro-apoptotic protein that binds to the cell membrane by means of charge interaction without the need of a specific receptor, producing a cell membrane disruption, and leading to possible cell death. Chung and colleagues found an high expression of this molecule in TEN blister fluid [39] and confirmed both in vitro and in vivo its dose-dependent cytotoxicity [39]. Moreover, after granulysin depletion, they observed an increase in cell viability. The serum levels of granulysin were also found to be increased in the early stage of SJS/TEN, but not in other cutaneous DHR [40].

4. *Tumor necrosis factor* α: TNF-α seems also to play an important role in TEN [41]. The fluid of blisters from TEN patients was found to be rich in TNF-α, produced by monocytes/macrophages present in the epidermis [42], especially the subpopulation expressing CD16, known to produce higher levels of inflammatory cytokines [43]. TNF-α has a dual role: interacts with TNF-R1 activating Fas pathway and activates NF-κB leading to cell survival. Although the final result of this dual interaction is still under investigation, it seems that the combination of TNF-α, IFN-γ (also present in TEN patients) and the activation of other death receptors such as TWEAK can lead to apoptosis of keratinocytes [44].

A central role in the pathogenesis of ED is played by CD8+ lymphocytes and NK cells. Even though there is not a significant increase in the number of T cells infiltrating the skin of TEN patients, it was found that their role is crucial, even more than HLAs types. In fact, it was demonstrated that the specificity of the TCR is a required condition for the self-reaction to occur. In particular, a specific T cell clonotype was present in the majority of patients with carbamazepine-induced SJS/TEN and that this clonotype was absent in all patients tolerant to the drug who shared the same HLA with the SJS/TEN patients [45]. The enhanced activation of CD8 T cells seems also to be influenced by the impaired function of

CD4 + CD25 + FoxP3 + Treg cells found in the peripheral blood of TEN patients in the acute phase [46].

In addition to all these mechanisms, alarmins, endogenous molecules released after cell damage, were found to be transiently increased in SJS/TEN patients, perhaps amplifying the immune response, including α-defensin, S100A and HMGB1 [47]. These molecules may play a role in amplifying the immune response and in increasing the release of other toxic metabolites from inflammatory cells [48].

Histologic features

Given the different histopathological features of the EM, SJS and TEN, we decided to discuss them separately.

EM

In EM a lymphocytic infiltrate (CD8+ and macrophages), associated with vacuolar changes and dyskeratosis of basal keratinocytes, is found along the dermo-epidermal junction, while there is a moderate lymphocytic infiltrate around the superficial vascular plexus [20]. Partial to full thickness epidermal necrosis, intraepidermal vesiculation or subepidermal blisters, due to spongiosis and to the cellular damage of the basal layer of the epidermis, can be present in the advanced disease [49] Occasionally, severe papillary edema is also present [20]. The dermis shows an inflammatory infiltrate characterized by a high-density lichenoid infiltrate rich in T cells (CD4+ more than CD8+) with macrophages, few neutrophils and occasional eosinophils; the latter especially seen in cases of DHR [5, 50].

SJS

The SJS histology is characterized by a poor dermal inflammatory cell infiltrate and full thickness necrosis of epidermis [20, 49]. The epidermal-dermal junction shows changes, ranging from vacuolar alteration to subepidermal blisters [20]. The dermo-epidermal junction and epidermis are infiltrated mostly by CD8+ T lymphocytes whereas dermal infiltrate, mainly made from CD4+ T lymphocytes, is superficial and mostly perivascular [20, 51].

TEN

TEN is characterized by full-thickness epidermal necrosis with an evident epidermal detachment and sloughing caused by necrosis of keratinocytes following apoptosis [49, 52]. It's also characterized by a cell-poor infiltrate, where macrophages and dendrocytes with a strong TNF-α immunoreactivity predominate [6, 50].

Clinical manifestations and culprit agents

EM is a self-limited skin condition mainly associated with infections and drugs [53, 54]. It has a wide spectrum of severity, and it is divided in minor and major (EMM). The former is usually a recurring, localized eruption of the skin characterized by pathognomonic target or iris lesions, with minimal or no mucosal involvement (Fig. 1). EMM is a clinically severe, potentially life-threatening, extensive sloughing of epidermis, generally involving mucosal tissue. In EMM lesions typically begin on the extremities and sometimes spread to the trunk. Infectious agents are the major cause of EM, in around 90 % of cases, especially for EM minor and in children. Herpes simplex virus (HSV) 1 and 2 are the main triggers in young adults (>80 % of cases), followed by Epstein-Barr virus (EBV), and Mycoplasma pneumonia [55–58]. Among drug related cases, the main triggering factors are sulfonamides, nonsteroidal anti-inflammatories (NSAIDs), penicillins, and anticonvulsants (Table 1) [59]. Neoplastic conditions (renal and gastric carcinoma), autoimmune disease (inflammatory bowel disease), HIV infection, radiation, and food additives/chemicals have been reported to be predisposing factor [59].

SJS and TEN are two overlapping syndromes resembling severe burn lesions and characterized by skin detachment. When less than 10 % of the body surface area (BSA) is involved, it is defined SJS, when between 10 and 30 % of BSA it is defined overlapping SJS/TEN, when more than 30 % of BSA, TEN [2] (Additional file 1: Figure S1, Additional file 2: Figure S2). SJS/TEN syndrome is associated with severe blistering, mucocutaneous peeling, and multi-organ damage and could be life threatening. TEN is also known as "Lyell syndrome", since it was first described by Alan Lyell in 1956 [2, 60].

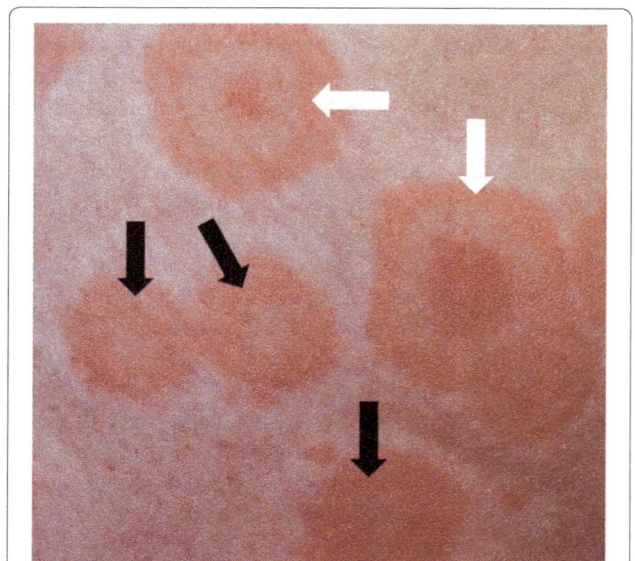

Fig. 1 Erythema multiforme (photo reproduced with permission of Gary White, MD): typical target lesions (*white arrows*) together with atypical two-zoned lesions (*black arrows*)

Table 1 Most common culprit drugs in SJS/TEN and EM

Drugs associated with Stevens–Johnson syndrome and toxic epidermal necrolisis

	Risk a priori	Prevalence in SJS/TEN registries	Extension of employment	Probable/very probable causality in multicenter trials
Allopurinol	Very high	Very high	Widespread	Frequent
Anticonvulsants Carbamazepine Lamotrigine Phenobarbital Phenytoin Valproic Acid	Very high	Very high	Widespread	Frequent
NSAIDs	Variable	High	Widespread	Variable
Oxicam NSAIDs	Very high	Low	Limited	Frequent
Sulfonamides Cotrimoxazole Sulfadiazine Sulfasalazine Others	High	High	Widespread	Frequent
Non-sulfa antibiotics				
Aminopenicillins	Low	Medium	Widespread	Non frequent
Cephalosporins	Medium	Medium	Widespread	Non frequent
Quinolones	Medium	Medium	Widespread	Moderately frequent
Macrolides	Medium	Medium	Widespread	No
Tetraciclines	Medium	Low	Medium	Frequent
Nevirapine	High	High	Limited	Frequent
Pantoprazole	Unknown	Low	Widespread	ND
Paracetamol	Low	High	Widespread	Non freqeuent
Furosemide	Low	Variable	Widespread	ND
Sertraline	High	Low	Medium	Frequent
Drugs associated with erythema multiforme				
Sulfonamides				
NSAIDs				
Anticonvulsants				
Antibiotics (mainly penicillins)				

Unlike EMM, SJS and TEN are mainly related to medication use. The strength of association with the development of SJS/TEN may vary among countries and historical periods, reflecting differences in ethnicities and prescription habits among the studied populations [61–64]. Exposure to anticonvulsivants (phenytoin, phenobarbital, lamotrigine), non-nucleoside reverse transcriptase inhibitors (nevirapine), cotrimoxazole and other sulfa drugs (sulfasalazine), allopurinol and oxicam NSAIDs [2] confers a higher risk of developing SJS/TEN. Several authors reported also an increased incidence for aminopenicillins, cephalosporins, and quinolones [61, 62]. Drugs such as paracetamol, other non-oxicam NSAIDs

and furosemide, bringing a relatively low risk of SJS/TEN a priori, are also highly prevalent as putative culprit agents in large SJS/TEN registries, due to their widespread use in the general population [63, 64] (Table 1). Rarely, *Mycoplasma pneumoniae*, dengue virus, cytomegalovirus, and contrast media may be the causative agent of SJS and TEN [22, 65–67].

It is not completely clear whether EM and SJS are separate clinical entities or if they represent two different expressions of a single disease process. However, according to a consensus definition [54], EMM syndrome has been separated from SJS/TEN spectrum.

Diagnosis E prognosis
Prodromal and acute phase
During the acute reaction, diagnosis of ED is mainly based on clinical parameters. Initial symptoms could be aspecific, as fever, stinging eyes and discomfort upon swallowing, occurring few days before the onset of mucocutaneous involvement. Early sites of skin involvement include trunk, face, palms and soles and rapidly spread to cover a variable extension of the body. EMM is characterizes by target lesions, circular lesions of 1-2 cm of diameter, that are defined as typical or atypical that tends to blister. Typical target lesions consist of three components: a dusky central area or blister, a dark red inflammatory zone surrounded by a pale ring of edema, and an erythematous halo on the periphery. Atypical target lesions manifest as raised, edematous, palpable lesions with only two zones of color change and/or an extensive exanthema with a poorly defined border darker in the center (Fig. 1). In SJS and TEN mucosal erosions on the lips, oral cavity, upper airways, conjunctiva, genital tract or ocular level are frequent [60, 68–70].

Allergy workout
In acute phase it is crucial to assess the culprit agent, in particular when the patient was assuming several drugs at time of DHR. First of all, Sassolas and coauthors proposed an algorithm of drug causality (ALDEN) in order to improve the individual assessment of drug causality in TEN and SJS [71]. ALDEN has shown a good accuracy to assess drug causality compared to data obtained by pharmacovigilance method and case–control results of the EuroSCAR case–control analysis for drugs associated with TEN.

In vivo tests
Diagnosis in a routine setting is based on patch test (PT) while skin test (prick and intradermal tests) with a delayed reading are contraindicated in these patients [72]. PTs have to be performed at least 6 months after the recovery

of the reaction, and show a variable sensitivity considering the implied drug, being higher for beta-lactam, glycopeptide antibiotics, carbamazepine, lamotrigine, proton pump inhibitors, tetrazepam, trimethoprim—sulfametoxazole, pseudoephedrine and ramipril [73–76].

In vitro tests

Lymphocyte transformation test (LTT) performed as described by Pichler and Tilch [77] shows a lower sensitivity in severe DHR compared to less severe DHR [78] but, if available, should be performed within 1 week after the onset of skin rash in SJS and TEN [79]. A promising and complementary in vitro tool has been used by Polak ME et al. [80], which consists of the determination of IFNγ and IL4 by ELISpot (Enzyme-linked immunospot assay), allowing to increase the sensitivity of LTT during acute DHR (82 versus 50 % if compared to LPA).

Prognosis

A severity-of-Illness score for toxic epidermal necrolysis (SCORTEN) has been proposed and validated to predict the risk of death at admission [81]. The SCORTEN scale is based on a minimal set of parameters as described in the following table. For the calculation, available values on vital and laboratory parameters within the first 3 days after admission to the first hospital are considered when the reaction started outside the hospital (community patients) or at the date of hospitalization for in-hospital patients. Considered variables in SCORTEN are shown in Table 2. Mortality rate of patients with TEN has shown to be directly correlated to SCORTEN, as shown in Fig. 2.

Differential diagnosis

As described in Table 3, major differential diagnosis of EM and SJS/TEN are (1) staphylococcal scalded skin syndrome (SSSS), (2) autoimmune blistering diseases and disseminated fixed bullous drug eruption, (3) others severe delayed DHR [6, 70, 82] (4) Graft versus host disease

1) *SSSS* is characterized by periorificial face scabs, deepithelialization of friction zones and conspicuous desquamation after initial erythroderma. Trigger is

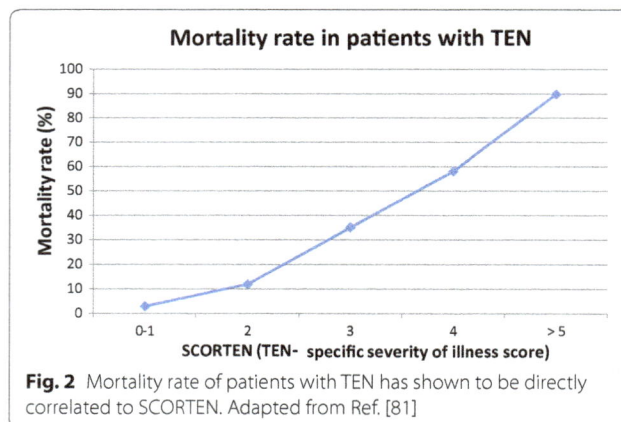

Fig. 2 Mortality rate of patients with TEN has shown to be directly correlated to SCORTEN. Adapted from Ref. [81]

an exotoxin released by *Staphylococcus aureus* [83]. A useful sign for differential diagnosis is the absence of mucosal involvement, except for conjunctiva. Main discriminating factors between EMM, SJS, SJS-TEN, TEN and SSSS is summarized in Table 3 [84].

2) *Pemphigus vulgaris, paraneoplastic pemphigus, bullous pemphigoid and linear IgA dermatosis* have to be considered. In order to rule out autoimmune blistering diseases, direct immune fluorescence staining should be additionally performed to exclude the presence of immunoglobulin and/or complement deposition in the epidermis and/or the epidermal-dermal zone, absent in ED. The Nikolsky's sign is not specific for SJS/TEN, in fact it is present also in auto-immune blistering diseases like pemphigus vulgaris. *Bullous pemphigoid* is characterized by large, tense bullae, but may begin as an urticarial eruption. Linear IgA dermatosis most commonly presents in patients older than 30 years. The lesions consist of pruritic, annular papules, vesicles, and bullae that are found in groups, clinically it is similar to dermatitis herpetiformis, without a gluten-sensitive enteropathy [85]. Bullous dermatoses can be debilitating and possibly fatal. Pemphigus vulgaris usually starts in the oral mucosa followed by blistering of the skin, which is often painful. Paraneoplastic pemphigus is associated with neoplasms, most commonly of lymphoid tissue, but also Waldenström's macroglobulinemia, sarcomas, thymomas and Castleman's disease.

3) *Other delayed DHR*

a. Acute generalized exanthematous pustulosis (AGEP) is characterized by acute erythematous skin lesions, generally arising in the face and intertriginous areas, subsequently sterile pinhead-sized nonfollicular pustules arise and if they coalesce, may sometimes mimic a positive Nikolsky's sign and in this case the condition may be misinterpreted as TEN [86].

Table 2 The SCORTEN variables

SCORTEN variables	
Age ≥40 years	1
Involved BSA at day 1 ≥10 %	1
Presence of cancer or malignancy	1
Heart rate ≥120 beats per minute	1
Serum urea level ≥10 mmol/L	1
Serum bicarbonate level <20 mmol/L	1
Serum glucose ≥14 mmol/L	1

Table 3 Differential diagnosis in a patient with suspected exfoliative dermatitis

Pathological condition	Pattern of skin lesions	Body surface area with epidermal detachment (%)	Trigger	Distribution of lesions
Erythema multiforme major (EMM)	Typical and atypical target papules and plaques, minimum involvement of mucous membranes (especially oral mucosae)	<10	Infection (*Mycoplasma pneumoniae, Herpes simplex*), drugs	Predominantly acrally distributed, i.e., begin on hands and feet
Stevens–Johnson syndrome (SJS)	No target lesions typical/atypical target lesions flattened, cotton wool spots purple confluent in the skin of the face and trunk, serious eruptions mucous membranes at the level of one or more sites	<10	Drugs	Diffuse. The eruption begins on the trunk
Overlap syndrome between Stevens–Johnson and Toxic Epidermal Necrolysis (SJS/TEN)	No target lesions/typical target lesions/atypical target lesions flattened	Between 10 and 30	Drugs	Diffuse. The eruption begins on the trunk
Toxic epidermal necrolysis (TEN)	No target lesions/typical target lesions/atypical target lesions flattened; begins with severe mucosal erosions and progresses to a detachment spread and generalized epidermis.	>30	Drugs	Diffuse. The eruption begins on the trunk
Staphylococcical scalded skin syndrome (SSSS)	Variable detachment between the stratum granulosum and the stratum corneum	Variable	Bacterial infection (*Staphylococci*)	Diffuse. No mucosal involvement except for conjunctiva

b. Drug reaction with Eosinophilia and systemic symptoms (DRESS) syndrome can mimic SJS and TEN in the early phases, since ED can occur together with the typical maculo-papular rash. In contrast with DRESS, eosinophilia and atypical lymphocytes are not described in patients with SJS or TEN. Both DRESS and SJS may have increased liver enzymes and hepatitis, but they occur in only 10 % of cases of SJS compared to 80 % of DRESS. Interstitial nephritis is common in DRESS syndrome, occurring roughly in 40 % of cases, whereas pre-renal azotemia may occur in SJS and TEN.

4) *Graft versus host disease (GVHD)* Acute GVHD usually happens within the first 6 months after a transplant. Common acute symptoms include abdominal pain or cramps, nausea, vomiting, and diarrhea, jaundice, skin rash and eyes dryness and therefore could mimic the prodromal and early phase of ED. The diagnosis of GVDH requires histological confirmation [87].

Management and therapy

The therapeutic approach of EMM, SJS, TEN depends on extension of skin, mucosal involvement and systemic patient's conditions. A multidisciplinary team is fundamental in the therapeutic management of patients affected by exfoliative DHR. The team should include not only physicians but also dedicated nurses,

physiotherapists and psychologists and should be instituted during the first 24 h after patient admission. Patients present an acute high-grade of skin and mucosal insufficiency that obviously leads to great impairment in the defenses against bacteria that normally live on the skin, increasing the high risk of systemic infections. Moreover, transpiration and thermoregulation are greatly impaired with an elevated loss of fluids, proteins and electrolytes through the damaged skin and mucosae. For these reasons, patients should be admitted to intensive burn care units or in semi-intensive care units where they may have access to sterile rooms and to dedicated medical personnel [49, 88].

Patients can be extremely suffering because of the pain induced by skin and mucosal detachment. They usually have fever, are dyspneic and cannot physiologically feed. The most important actions to do are listed in Fig. 2, and described below.

a) Immediate individuation and interruption of the culprit agent

As written before, Sassolas B. et al. [71] realized an algorhitm named ALDEN (algorithm of drug causality for epidermal necrolysis) which helps to establish a cause/effect relationship as "probable" or "very probable" in 70 % of cases. All non-indispensable drugs have to be stopped because they could alter the metabolism of the culprit agent.

b) Evaluation of the skin and mucosal involvement

Dermatologist and/or allergist should confirm the diagnosis, individuate the culprit agent, give indications about skin management and necessity to obtain the consultation of the ENT specialist, the gynecologist/urologist, the ophthalmologist and/or the pulmonologist in the case of mucosal involvement.

c) First-line interventions

Patient must be placed in an antidecubitus fluidized bed and room temperature must be kept at 30–32 °C in order to slow catabolism and reduce the loss of calories through the skin [89]. All the linen must be sterile. It is necessary to obtain as soon as possible a central venous access and to start a continuous monitoring of vital signs. In case of an oral mucositis that impairs nutrition, it is indicated to position a nasogastric tube. Also a vesical catheter should be placed to avoid urethral synechiae and to have a precise fluid balance. In case of a respiratory failure, oxygen should be administrated and a NIMV may be required. Temporary tracheostomy may be necessary in case of extended mucosal damage. In serious cases invasive ventilation can be necessary for ARDS. It is also extremely important to obtain within the first 24 h cultural samples from skin together with blood, urine, nasal, pharyngeal and bronchus cultures. Ophthalmologic consultations must be repeated at fixed intervals to avoid the appearance of conjunctival irreversible complications such as chronic conjunctivitis with squamous metaplasia, trichiasis, symblepharon, punctate keratitis and sicca syndrome. Gynecologist consultation is required for avoiding the appearance of vaginal phimosis or sinechias.

d) Prophylactic, supportive and complications therapy

1. *Hydration and hemodynamic balance.* Fluid balance is a main focus. Once established the percentage of the involved skin, lactate Ringer infusion of 1–2 mL/Kg/ % of involved skin must be started during the first 24 h [91]. The velocity of infusion should be regulated according to patients arterial pressure with the aim of 30 mL/h urinary output (1 mL/kg/h in case of a child). Blood gas analysis, glucose and creatinine levels together with electrolytes should be evaluated and therapy should be modified accordingly. Vasoactive amines may be necessary in case of shock. Albumin is recommended only is albumin serum level is <2.5 mg/dL. Furosemide or ethacrynic acid may be required to maintain an adequate urinary output [90].

2. *Nutritional support.* An increased metabolism is typical of patients with extended disepithelized areas. This hypermetabolic state is also furtherly increased by the inflammation present in affected areas. Early enteral nutrition has also a protective effect on the intestinal mucosa and decreases bacterial colonization. Usually the amount of calories is 1500–2000 kcal/day and the velocity of infusion is gradually increased based on patients tolerability [92].

3. *Gastric protection.* To avoid the appearance of gastric stress ulcer it is recommended to start a therapy with intravenous proton pump inhibitors.

4. *Anticoagulation therapy.* For the prevention of deep venous thrombosis; usually low molecular weight heparin at prophylactic dose are used.

5. *Antipyretic therapy.* It is recommended to use 1.5 mg/kg hydrocortisone. If necessary, it can be repeated every 6–8 h. NSAIDs should be avoided as they can induce ED as well.

6. *Painkiller therapy.* Intravenous administration is recommended. In more severe cases continuous iv therapy can be necessary. Most common used drugs are: morphine, fentanyl, propofol and midazolam.

7. *Antibiotic therapy.* It is not recommended to use prophylactic antibiotic therapy. It should be used only in case of a documented positivity of cultural samples. If there is a high suspicion of infection without a documented source of infection, broad range empiric therapy should be started.

8. *Antiviral therapy.* Ganciclovir and cidofovir should be used when polymerase-chain reactions (PCR) on peripheral blood or other biological sample identifies a viral reactivation (HHV6, HHV7, EBV and CMV). In more severe cases antiviral therapies should be given together with intravenous immunoglobulins [93].

9. *Growth-factors (G-CSF).* It recommended to used G-CSF in patients with febrile neutropenia [94, 95].

10. *Plasmapheresis.* It should be considered only once the patient is stable and if the skin damage is still ongoing and doesn't respond to other conventional therapies (corticosteroids or IVIG). Plasmapheresis may have a role in the treatment of ED because it removes Fas-L [96], other cytokines known to be implied in the pathogenesis (IL-6, IL-8, TNF-α) [97, 98]. Moreover Mawson A and colleagues hypothesized that the efficacy of plasmapheresis is able to reduce serum level of vitamin A. In patients with SJS/TEN increased serum levels of retinoid acid have been found. These levels could reflect the interaction between culprit drugs and aldehyde dehydrogenase that is the enzyme which metabolizes retinoid acid. Increased level of retinoid acid could be responsible for keratinocytes apoptosis [99].

11. *Topical treatment.* Patients must be cleaned in the affected areas until epithelization starts. In spared areas it is necessary to avoid skin detachment. It is also recommended to void larger vesicles with a

syringe. It is important to protect the damaged skin with sterile fat dressing especially in the genital area. 5 % silver nitrate compresses have antiseptic properties. Synthetic bilaminar membranes with silver nitrate have also a role in skin repairing and avoid protein loss through the damaged skin [100, 101]. It is advised against the use of silver sulfadiazine because sulphonamide can be culprit agents. Autologous transplantation of mesenchymal umbilical cord cells seems also to be highly efficacious [102]. Accurate eye cleaning with saline solution is fundamental for the prevention of synechiae and for reducing corneal damage. In more severe cases corneal protective lens can be used. It could also be useful to use artificial tears and lubricating antiseptic gels. The applications of topical cyclosporine and autologous serum have also been showed to be useful in refractory cases [103]. Oral hygiene with antiseptic and painkiller mouthwash (chlorhexidine + lidocaine + aluminum hydroxide) together with aerosol therapy with saline and bronchodilators can reduce upper airways symptoms.

e) Anti-inflammatory and systemic immunosuppressive therapy

It is important to take into consideration the mechanism of action of the different drugs in the pathogenesis of ED [104].

Systemic corticosteroids: These are the most common used drugs because of their known anti-inflammatory and immunosuppressive effect through the inhibition of activated cytotoxic T-cells and the production of cytokines. Corticosteroids could also reduce the amount of keratinocytes apoptosis and the activation of caspases [105]. In EMM their efficacy is demonstrated in controlling the evolution of the disease [106]. In SJS, SJS/TEN and TEN the efficacy of corticosteroids is far from being demonstrated. Recently, a meta-analysis based on 6 retrospective studies evaluating the role of corticosteroids alone or together with IVIG has been published [107]. In this study, 965 patients were reviewed. The authors concluded that they couldn't demonstrate corticosteroids efficacy in monotherapy, but the use of steroid alone is not linked to an increased risk of mortality due to infective complications [108, 109].

The most commonly used steroids were methylprednisolone, prednisolone and dexamethasone. The induction dosage in EMM is usually 1 mg/kg/day that should be maintained until a complete control of the skin is obtained. The taper of steroid therapy should be gradual [93]. In most severe cases the suggested dosage is iv 1–1.5 mg/kg/day. Iv bolus of steroid (dexamethasone

100–300 mg/day or methylprednisolone 250–1000 mg/day) for 3 consecutive days with a gradual taper steroid therapy is sometimes advised. A switch to oral therapy can be performed once the mucosal conditions improve.

If after 4 days there is not an improvement it is advised to consider the association of steroid or its replacement with one of the following drugs [49, 93]:

Intravenous immunoglobulins (IVIG): play their role through the inhibition of Fas–Fas ligand interaction that it is supposed to be the first step in keratinocytes apoptosis [33]. A recently published meta-analysis by Huang [110] and coworkers on IVIG in SJS/SJS-TEN/TEN reviewed 17 studies with 221 patients and compared the results obtained with high-dosage IVIG (>2 g/kg) compared to lower-dosage IVIG (<2 g/kg). 12 out of 17 studies concluded for a positive role of IVIG in ED. In the 5 studies that concluded negatively for IVIG, the dosage was below 0.4 g/kg/day and treatment was maintained for less than 5 days. Schwartz RA et al. [49] confirmed these results and even suggested that higher dosage regimen with 2.7–4 g/kg seem to be more effective in survival outcome. A recent review [111] on 33 pediatric cases of TEN and 6 cases of SJS/TEN overlap showed that therapy with IVIG with a dosage of 0.25–1.5 g/kg for 5 days resulted in 0 % mortality rate and faster epithelization. In conclusion, therapy wth IVIG should be started within the first 5 days and an high-dosage regimen should be preferred (2.5–4 g/kg for adults and 0.25–1.5 g/kg in children divided in 3–5 days).

Cyclosporine A (Cys A): Cys A works through the inhibition of calcineurin, that is fundamental for cytotoxic T lymphocytes activation. In an open trial on cyclosporine in 29 patients with TEN, the use of Cys A for at least 10 days led to a rapid improvement without infective complications [112]. Kirchhof MG et al. [113] retrospectively compared mortality in 64 patients with ED treated either with iv or oral Cys A (3–5 mg/kg) or IVIG (2–5 g/Kg). The authors concluded for a potential beneficial effect of Cys A and a possible improvement in survival compared to IVIG. In conclusion we suggest that therapy with cyclosporine is valuable option with a dosage of 3–5 mg/kg oral or iv for 7 days.

Anti-TNF-alpha drugs:

–   Infliximab: chimeric IgG monoclonal anti-TNF-α antibody. It was used with success in different case reports [114–116]. The administration of a single dose of 5 mg/kg was able to stop disease progression in 24 h and to induce a complete remission in 6–14 days. Infliximab was used in cases refractory to high-dosage steroid therapy and/or IVIG.

– Etanercept: monoclonal antibody against the TNF-α receptor. Paradisi et al. [117] described a cohort of ten patients affected by TEN treated with a single dose of etanercept 50 mg sc with a rapid and complete resolution and without adverse events.

Even though there is a strong need for randomized trials, anti-TNF-α drugs, in particular a single dose of infliximab 5 mg/kg ev or 50 mg etanercept sc should be considered in the treatment of SJS and TEN, especially the most severe cases when IVIG and intravenous corticosteroids don't achieve a rapid improvement.

Conclusions

EDs are serious and potentially fatal conditions. Their occurrence can be prevented by avoiding drug over-prescription and drug associations that interfere with the metabolism of the most frequent triggers [118]. This is particularly true for patients with many comorbidities and poli-drug therapy, where it is advisable to monitor liver and kidney toxicity and to avoid Vitamin A excess [99]. Genotyping is recommended in specific high-risk ethnic groups (e.g. asiatic) before starting therapies with possible triggers (e.g. HLA-B1502, HLA-B5701, HLA-B5801 and carbamazepine, abacavir, and allopurinol, respectively).

Once ED has occurred, it has to be managed in the adequate setting with a multidisciplinary approach, and every effort has to be made to identify and avoid the trigger and to prevent infectious and non-infectious complications. Supportive and specific care includes both local and systemic measures, as represented in Fig. 3. For SJS/TEN, corticosteroids are the cornerstone of treatment albeit efficacy remains unclear. Despite improved knowledge of the immunopathogenesis of these conditions, immune-modulatory therapies currently used have not been definitively proved to be efficacious [49, 107], and new strategies are urgently needed.

Abbreviations

AGEP: acute generalized exanthematous pustulosis; ALDEN: algorithm of drug causality for epidermal necrolysis; BSA: body surface area; CMV: cytomegalovirus; Cys A: cyclosporine A; DHR: drug hypersensitivity reactions; EBV: Epstein–Barr virus; ED: exfoliative dermatitis; EM(M): erythema multiforme (major); ENT: ear-nose-throat; G-CSF: granulocyte-colony stimulating factor; GVHD: graft versus host disease; HHV: human herpes virus; HIV: human immunodeficiency virus; HMGB1: high mobility group box 1; HSV: herpes simplex virus; IVIG: intravenous immunoglobulins; LPA: lymphocyte proliferation assay; LTT: lymphocyte transformation test; NSAIDs: non steroidal anti-inflammatory drugs; PCR: polimerase chain reaction; PPI: proton pump inhibitors; PT: patch test; RegiSCAR: European registry of severe cutaneous adverse reactions to drugs; SSSS: staphylococcal scalded skin syndrome; SJS: Steven–Johnson syndrome; TEN: toxic epidermal necrolysis; TNF-α: tumor necrosis factor α.

Authors' contributions

MRY, MGS, EN and GC designed the study, selected scientifically relevant information, wrote and revised the manuscript. AB, CC, ET, GAR, AN, EDL, PF performed a critical revision on the current literature about the described topic, wrote and revised the manuscript. All authors read and approved the final manuscript.

Author details

[1] Department of Allergy and Clinical Immunology, IRCCS San Raffaele Hospital, Via Olgettina 60, 20132 Milan, Italy. [2] Vita-Salute San Raffaele University, Milan, Italy. [3] Section of Allergy and Clinical Immunology, Dept. of Internal Medicine, University of Bari, Bari, Italy.

Acknowledgements

The authors wish to thank Dr. Gary White for the picture of EM showed in Fig. 1.

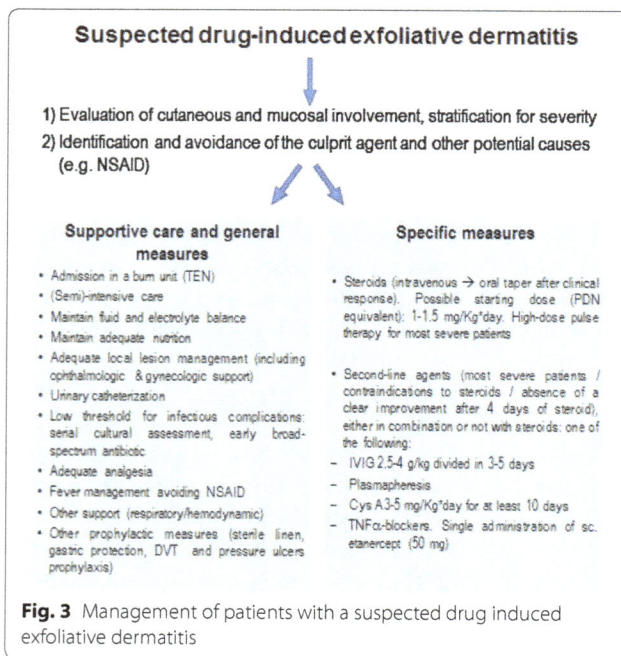

Suspected drug-induced exfoliative dermatitis

1) Evaluation of cutaneous and mucosal involvement, stratification for severity
2) Identification and avoidance of the culprit agent and other potential causes (e.g. NSAID)

Supportive care and general measures

- Admission in a burn unit (TEN)
- (Semi-)intensive care
- Maintain fluid and electrolyte balance
- Maintain adequate nutrition
- Adequate local lesion management (including ophthalmologic & gynecologic support)
- Urinary catheterization
- Low threshold for infectious complications: serial cultural assessment, early broad-spectrum antibiotic
- Adequate analgesia
- Fever management avoiding NSAID
- Other support (respiratory/hemodynamic)
- Other prophylactic measures (sterile linen, gastric protection, DVT and pressure ulcers prophylaxis)

Specific measures

- Steroids (intravenous → oral taper after clinical response). Possible starting dose (PDN equivalent): 1-1.5 mg/Kg*day. High-dose pulse therapy for most severe patients

- Second-line agents (most severe patients / contraindications to steroids / absence of a clear improvement after 4 days of steroid), either in combination or not with steroids: one of the following:
  - IVIG 2.5-4 g/kg divided in 3-5 days
  - Plasmapheresis
  - Cys A 3-5 mg/Kg*day for at least 10 days
  - TNFα-blockers. Single administration of sc. etanercept (50 mg)

Fig. 3 Management of patients with a suspected drug induced exfoliative dermatitis

References

1. Nayak S, Acharjya B. Adverse cutaneous drug reaction. Indian J Dermatol. 2008;53(1):2–8.
2. Schwartz RA, McDonough PH, Lee BW. Toxic epidermal necrolysis: Part I Introduction, history, classification, clinical features, systemic manifestations, etiology, and immunopathogenesis. J Am Acad Dermatol. 2013;69(2):173–4.
3. Fritsch PO. Erythema multiforme Stevens–Johnson syndrome and toxic epidermal necrolysis. In: Eisen AZ, Wolff K, editors. Fitzpatrick's dermatology in general medicine. New York: McGraw-Hill; 2003. p. 543–57.
4. Fritsch PO. Erythema multiforme and toxic epidermal necrolysis. In: Eisen AZ, Wolff K, editors. Fitzpatrick's dermatology in general medicine. New York: McGraw-Hill; 2003. p. 585–600.
5. Wetter DA, Camilleri MJ. Clinical, etiologic, and histopathologic features of Stevens–Johnson syndrome during an 8-year period at Mayo Clinic. Mayo Clin Proc. 2010;85(2):131–8.
6. Cho YT, et al. Generalized bullous fixed drug eruption is distinct from Stevens–Johnson syndrome/toxic epidermal necrolysis by immunohistopathological features. J Am Acad Dermatol. 2014;70(3):539–48.
7. Chan HL, et al. The incidence of erythema multiforme, Stevens–Johnson syndrome, and toxic epidermal necrolysis. A population-based study with particular reference to reactions caused by drugs among outpatients. Arch Dermatol. 1990;126(1):43–7.
8. Kamaliah MD, et al. Erythema multiforme, Stevens–Johnson syndrome and toxic epidermal necrolysis in northeastern Malaysia. Int J Dermatol. 1998;37(7):520–3.
9. Schopf E, et al. Toxic epidermal necrolysis and Stevens–Johnson syndrome. An epidemiologic study from West Germany. Arch Dermatol. 1991;127(6):839–42.
10. Huff JC, Weston WL, Tonnesen MG. Erythema multiforme: a critical review of characteristics, diagnostic criteria, and causes. J Am Acad Dermatol. 1983;8(6):763–75.
11. Roujeau JC, Stern RS. Severe adverse cutaneous reactions to drugs. N Engl J Med. 1994;331(19):1272–85.
12. Strom BL, et al. A population-based study of Stevens–Johnson syndrome. Incidence and antecedent drug exposures. Arch Dermatol. 1991;127(6):831–8.
13. Carrozzo M, Togliatto M, Gandolfo S. Erythema multiforme. A heterogeneous pathologic phenotype. Minerva Stomatol. 1999;48(5):217–26.
14. Manganaro AM. Erythema multiforme. Gen Dent. 1996;44(2):164–6.
15. Oliveira L, Zucoloto S. Erythema multiforme minor: a revision. Am J Infect Dis. 2008;4(4):224–31.
16. Lonjou C, et al. A marker for Stevens–Johnson syndrome…: ethnicity matters. Pharmacogenomics J. 2006;6(4):265–8.
17. Wetter DA, Davis MD. Recurrent erythema multiforme: clinical characteristics, etiologic associations, and treatment in a series of 48 patients at Mayo Clinic, 2000 to 2007. J Am Acad Dermatol. 2010;62(1):45–53.
18. Roujeau JC, et al. Toxic epidermal necrolysis (Lyell syndrome). Incidence and drug etiology in France, 1981-1985. Arch Dermatol. 1990;126(1):37–42.
19. Mittmann N, et al. Incidence of toxic epidermal necrolysis and Stevens–Johnson Syndrome in an HIV cohort: an observational, retrospective case series study. Am J Clin Dermatol. 2012;13(1):49–54.
20. Rzany B, et al. Histopathological and epidemiological characteristics of patients with erythema exudativum multiforme major, Stevens–Johnson syndrome and toxic epidermal necrolysis. Br J Dermatol. 1996;135(1):6–11.
21. Sekula P, et al. Comprehensive survival analysis of a cohort of patients with Stevens–Johnson syndrome and toxic epidermal necrolysis. J Invest Dermatol. 2013;133(5):1197–204.
22. Fournier S, et al. Toxic epidermal necrolysis associated with *Mycoplasma pneumoniae* infection. Eur J Clin Microbiol Infect Dis. 1995;14(6):558–9.
23. Khalil I, et al. HLA DQB1* 0301 allele is involved in the susceptibility to erythema multiforme. J Invest Dermatol. 1991;97(4):697–700.
24. Wolkenstein P, et al. A slow acetylator genotype is a risk factor for sulphonamide-induced toxic epidermal necrolysis and Stevens–Johnson syndrome. Pharmacogenet Genom. 1995;5(4):255–8.
25. Chang CC, et al. Association of HLA-B*1502 allele with carbamazepine-induced toxic epidermal necrolysis and Stevens–Johnson syndrome in the multi-ethnic Malaysian population. Int J Dermatol. 2011;50(2):221–4.
26. Chung WH, Hung SI. Recent advances in the genetics and immunology of Stevens–Johnson syndrome and toxic epidermal necrosis. J Dermatol Sci. 2012;66(3):190–6.
27. Chung WH, et al. Medical genetics: a marker for Stevens–Johnson syndrome. Nature. 2004;428(6982):486.
28. Locharernkul C, et al. Carbamazepine and phenytoin induced Stevens–Johnson syndrome is associated with HLA-B* 1502 allele in Thai population. Epilepsia. 2008;49(12):2087–91.
29. Hung S-I, et al. HLA-B* 5801 allele as a genetic marker for severe cutaneous adverse reactions caused by allopurinol. Proc Natl Acad Sci USA. 2005;102(11):4134–9.
30. Ozeki T, et al. Genome-wide association study identifies HLA-A* 3101 allele as a genetic risk factor for carbamazepine-induced cutaneous adverse drug reactions in Japanese population. Hum Mol Genet. 2011;20(5):1034–41.
31. McCormack M, et al. HLA-A* 3101 and carbamazepine-induced hypersensitivity reactions in Europeans. N Engl J Med. 2011;364(12):1134–43.
32. Man CB, et al. Association between HLA-B* 1502 allele and antiepileptic drug-induced cutaneous reactions in Han Chinese. Epilepsia. 2007;48(5):1015–8.
33. Viard I, et al. Inhibition of toxic epidermal necrolysis by blockade of CD95 with human intravenous immunoglobulin. Science. 1998;282(5388):490–3.
34. Abe R. Toxic epidermal necrolysis and Stevens–Johnson syndrome: soluble Fas ligand involvement in the pathomechanisms of these diseases. J Dermatol Sci. 2008;52(3):151–9.
35. Downey A, et al. Toxic epidermal necrolysis: review of pathogenesis and management. J Am Acad Dermatol. 2012;66(6):995–1003.
36. Tohyama M, et al. A marked increase in serum soluble Fas ligand in drug-induced hypersensitivity syndrome. Br J Dermatol. 2008;159(4):981–4.
37. Nassif A, et al. Drug specific cytotoxic T-cells in the skin lesions of a patient with toxic epidermal necrolysis. J Invest Dermatol. 2002;118(4):728–33.
38. Posadas SJ, et al. Delayed reactions to drugs show levels of perforin, granzyme B, and Fas-L to be related to disease severity. J Allergy Clin Immunol. 2002;109(1):155–61.
39. Chung W-H, et al. Granulysin is a key mediator for disseminated keratinocyte death in Stevens–Johnson syndrome and toxic epidermal necrolysis. Nat Med. 2008;14(12):1343–50.
40. Abe R, et al. Granulysin as a marker for early diagnosis of the Stevens–Johnson syndrome. Ann Intern Med. 2009;151(7):514–5.
41. Tohyama M, Hashimoto K. Immunological mechanisms of epidermal damage in toxic epidermal necrolysis. Curr Opin Allergy Clin Immunol. 2012;12(4):376–82.
42. Paquet P, et al. Immunoregulatory effector cells in drug-induced toxic epidermal necrolysis. Am J Dermatopathol. 2000;22(5):413–7.
43. Tohyama M, et al. Possible involvement of CD14 + CD16 + monocyte lineage cells in the epidermal damage of Stevens–Johnson syndrome and toxic epidermal necrolysis. Br J Dermatol. 2012;166(2):322–30.
44. De Araujo E, et al. Death ligand TRAIL, secreted by CD1a + and CD14 + cells in blister fluids, is involved in killing keratinocytes in toxic epidermal necrolysis. Exp Dermatol. 2011;20(2):107–12.
45. Ko TM, et al. Shared and restricted T-cell receptor use is crucial for carbamazepine-induced Stevens-Johnson syndrome. J Allergy Clin Immunol. 2011;128(6):1266–76.
46. Takahashi R, et al. Defective regulatory T cells in patients with severe drug eruptions: timing of the dysfunction is associated with the pathological phenotype and outcome. J Immunol. 2009;182(12):8071–9.
47. Morel E, et al. Expression of alpha-defensin 1-3 in T cells from severe cutaneous drug-induced hypersensitivity reactions. Allergy. 2011;66(3):360–7.
48. Morel E, et al. CD94/NKG2C is a killer effector molecule in patients with Stevens-Johnson syndrome and toxic epidermal necrolysis. J Allergy Clin Immunol. 2010;125(3):703–10.
49. Schwartz RA, McDonough PH, Lee BW. Toxic epidermal necrolysis: Part II Prognosis, sequelae, diagnosis, differential diagnosis, prevention, and treatment. J Am Acad Dermatol. 2013;69(2):187.
50. Paquet P, Pierard GE. Erythema multiforme and toxic epidermal necrolysis: a comparative study. Am J Dermatopathol. 1997;19(2):127–32.

51. Nassif A, et al. Toxic epidermal necrolysis: effector cells are drug-specific cytotoxic T cells. J Allergy Clin Immunol. 2004;114(5):1209–15.

52. Paul C, et al. Apoptosis as a mechanism of keratinocyte death in toxic epidermal necrolysis. Br J Dermatol. 1996;134(4):710–4.

53. Sokumbi O, Wetter DA. Clinical features, diagnosis, and treatment of erythema multiforme: a review for the practicing dermatologist. Int J Dermatol. 2012;51(8):889–902.

54. Bastuji-Garin S, et al. Clinical classification of cases of toxic epidermal necrolysis, Stevens–Johnson syndrome, and erythema multiforme. Arch Dermatol. 1993;129(1):92–6.

55. Huff JC. Erythema multiforme and latent herpes simplex infection. Semin Dermatol. 1992;11(3):207–10.

56. Orton PW, et al. Detection of a herpes simplex viral antigen in skin lesions of erythema multiforme. Ann Intern Med. 1984;101(1):48–50.

57. Gonzalez-Delgado P, et al. Erythema multiforme to amoxicillin with concurrent infection by Epstein-Barr virus. Allergol Immunopathol (Madr). 2006;34(2):76–8.

58. Grosber M, et al. Recurrent erythema multiforme in association with recurrent Mycoplasma pneumoniae infections. J Am Acad Dermatol. 2007;56(5 Suppl):S118–9.

59. Samim F, et al. Erythema multiforme: a review of epidemiology, pathogenesis, clinical features, and treatment. Dent Clin North Am. 2013;57(4):583–96.

60. Stern RS. Clinical practice. Exanthematous drug eruptions. N Engl J Med. 2012;366(26):2492–501.

61. Roujeau JC, et al. Medication use and the risk of Stevens–Johnson syndrome or toxic epidermal necrolysis. N Engl J Med. 1995;333(24):1600–7.

62. Mockenhaupt M, et al. Stevens–Johnson syndrome and toxic epidermal necrolysis: assessment of medication risks with emphasis on recently marketed drugs. The EuroSCAR-study. J Invest Dermatol. 2008;128(1):35–44.

63. Abe J, et al. Stevens–Johnson syndrome and toxic epidermal necrolysis: the Food and Drug Administration adverse event reporting system, 2004-2013. Allergol Int. 2015;64(3):277–9.

64. Abe J, et al. Analysis of Stevens–Johnson syndrome and toxic epidermal necrolysis using the Japanese Adverse Drug Event Report database. J Pharm Health Care Sci. 2016;2:14.

65. Grieb G, et al. A rare case of toxic epidermal necrolysis with unexpected Fever resulting from dengue virus. Case Rep Dermatol. 2010;2(3):189–94.

66. Garza A, Waldman AJ, Mamel J. A case of toxic epidermal necrolysis with involvement of the GI tract after systemic contrast agent application at cardiac catheterization. Gastrointest Endosc. 2005;62(4):638–42.

67. Khalaf D, et al. Toxic epidermal necrolysis associated with severe cytomegalovirus infection in a patient on regular hemodialysis. Mediterr J Hematol Infect Dis. 2011;3(1):e2011004.

68. Ardern-Jones MR, Friedmann PS. Skin manifestations of drug allergy. Br J Clin Pharmacol. 2011;71(5):672–83.

69. Verma R, Vasudevan B, Pragasam V. Severe cutaneous adverse drug reactions. Med J Armed Forces India. 2013;69(4):375–83.

70. Harr T, French LE. Toxic epidermal necrolysis and Stevens–Johnson syndrome. Orphanet J Rare Dis. 2010;5:39.

71. Sassolas B, et al. ALDEN, an algorithm for assessment of drug causality in Stevens–Johnson Syndrome and toxic epidermal necrolysis: comparison with case-control analysis. Clin Pharmacol Ther. 2010;88(1):60–8.

72. Barbaud A. Skin testing and patch testing in non-IgE-mediated drug allergy. Curr Allergy Asthma Rep. 2014;14(6):442.

73. Barbaud A. Skin testing in delayed reactions to drugs. Immunol Allergy Clin North Am. 2009;29(3):517–35.

74. Barbaud A, et al. A multicentre study to determine the value and safety of drug patch tests for the three main classes of severe cutaneous adverse drug reactions. Br J Dermatol. 2013;168(3):555–62.

75. Wolkenstein P, et al. Patch testing in severe cutaneous adverse drug reactions, including Stevens–Johnson syndrome and toxic epidermal necrolysis. Contact Dermatitis. 1996;35(4):234–6.

76. Lin YT, et al. A patch testing and cross-sensitivity study of carbamazepine-induced severe cutaneous adverse drug reactions. J Eur Acad Dermatol Venereol. 2013;27(3):356–64.

77. Pichler WJ, Tilch J. The lymphocyte transformation test in the diagnosis of drug hypersensitivity. Allergy. 2004;59(8):809–20.

78. Tang YH, et al. Poor relevance of a lymphocyte proliferation assay in lamotrigine-induced Stevens–Johnson syndrome or toxic epidermal necrolysis. Clin Exp Allergy. 2012;42(2):248–54.

79. Kano Y, et al. Utility of the lymphocyte transformation test in the diagnosis of drug sensitivity: dependence on its timing and the type of drug eruption. Allergy. 2007;62(12):1439–44.

80. Polak ME, et al. In vitro diagnostic assays are effective during the acute phase of delayed-type drug hypersensitivity reactions. Br J Dermatol. 2013;168(3):539–49.

81. Bastuji-Garin S, et al. SCORTEN: a severity-of-illness score for toxic epidermal necrolysis. J Invest Dermatol. 2000;115(2):149–53.

82. Harr T, French LE. Stevens–Johnson syndrome and toxic epidermal necrolysis. Chem Immunol Allergy. 2012;97:149–66.

83. Napoli B, et al. Staphylococcal Scalded Skin Syndrome: criteria for Differential Diagnosis from Lyell's Syndrome. Two Cases in Adult Patients. Ann Burns Fire. Disasters. 2006;19(4):188–91.

84. Ayangco L, Rogers RS 3rd. Oral manifestations of erythema multiforme. Dermatol Clin. 2003;21(1):195–205.

85. Bickle K, Roark TR, Hsu S. Autoimmune bullous dermatoses: a review. Am Fam Physician. 2002;65(9):1861–70.

86. Paulmann M, Mockenhaupt M. Severe drug-induced skin reactions: clinical features, diagnosis, etiology, and therapy. J Dtsch Dermatol Ges. 2015;13(7):625–45.

87. Wu PA, Cowen EW. Cutaneous graft-versus-host disease–clinical considerations and management. Curr Probl Dermatol. 2012;43:101–15.

88. Kaffenberger BH, Rosenbach M. Toxic epidermal necrolysis and early transfer to a regional burn unit: is it time to reevaluate what we teach? J Am Acad Dermatol. 2014;71(1):195–6.

89. Letko E, Papaliodis DN, Papaliodis GN, Daoud YJ, Ahmed AR, Foster CS. Stevens–Johnson syndrome and toxic epidermal necrolysis: a review of the literature. Ann Allergy Asthma Immunol. 2005;94(4):419–23.

90. Fernando SL. The management of toxic epidermal necrolysis. Australas J Dermatol. 2012;53(3):165–71.

91. Shiga S, Cartotto R. What are the fluid requirements in toxic epidermal necrolysis? J Burn Care Res. 2010;31(1):100–4.

92. Mayes T, et al. Energy requirements of pediatric patients with Stevens–Johnson syndrome and toxic epidermal necrolysis. Nutr Clin Pract. 2008;23(5):547–50.

93. Descamps V, Ranger-Rogez S. DRESS syndrome. Joint Bone Spine. 2014;81(1):15–21.

94. Goulden V, Goodfield MJ. Recombinant granulocyte colony-stimulating factor in the management of toxic epidermal necrolysis. Br J Dermatol. 1996;135(2):305–6.

95. Jarrett P, et al. Toxic epidermal necrolysis treated with cyclosporin and granulocyte colony stimulating factor. Clin Exp Dermatol. 1997;22(3):146–7.

96. Yamada H, Takamori K. Status of plasmapheresis for the treatment of toxic epidermal necrolysis in Japan. Ther Apher Dial. 2008;12(5):355–9.

97. Kostal M, et al. Beneficial effect of plasma exchange in the treatment of toxic epidermal necrolysis: a series of four cases. J Clin Apher. 2012;27(4):215–20.

98. Narita YM, et al. Efficacy of plasmapheresis for the treatment of severe toxic epidermal necrolysis: is cytokine expression analysis useful in predicting its therapeutic efficacy? J Dermatol. 2011;38(3):236–45.

99. Mawson AR, Eriator I, Karre S. Stevens–Johnson syndrome and toxic epidermal necrolysis (SJS/TEN): could retinoids play a causative role? Med Sci Monit. 2015;21:133–43.

100. Huang SH, et al. AQUACEL Ag in the treatment of toxic epidermal necrolysis (TEN). Burns. 2008;34(1):63–6.

101. Smith SD, et al. Role of nanocrystalline silver dressings in the management of toxic epidermal necrolysis (TEN) and TEN/Stevens–Johnson syndrome overlap. Australas J Dermatol. 2015;56(4):298–302.

102. Li X, et al. Umbilical cord mesenchymal stem cell transplantation in drug-induced Stevens–Johnson syndrome. J Eur Acad Dermatol Venereol. 2013;27(5):659–61.

103. Gueudry J, et al. Risk factors for the development of ocular complications of Stevens–Johnson syndrome and toxic epidermal necrolysis. Arch Dermatol. 2009;145(2):157–62.

104. Paquet P, Pierard GE, Quatresooz P. Novel treatments for drug-induced toxic epidermal necrolysis (Lyell's syndrome). Int Arch Allergy Immunol. 2005;136(3):205–16.

105. Trautmann A, et al. Targeting keratinocyte apoptosis in the treatment of atopic dermatitis and allergic contact dermatitis. J Allergy Clin Immunol. 2001;108(5):839–46.

106. Bourgeois GP, et al. A review of DRESS-associated myocarditis. J Am Acad Dermatol. 2012;66(6):e229–36.

107. Law EH, Leung M. Corticosteroids in Stevens–Johnson Syndrome/toxic epidermal necrolysis: current evidence and implications for future research. Ann Pharmacother. 2015;49(3):335–42.

108. Schneck J, et al. Effects of treatments on the mortality of Stevens–Johnson syndrome and toxic epidermal necrolysis: a retrospective study on patients included in the prospective EuroSCAR Study. J Am Acad Dermatol. 2008;58(1):33–40.

109. Pehr K. The EuroSCAR study: cannot agree with the conclusions. J Am Acad Dermatol. 2008;59(5):898–9.

110. Huang YC, Li YC, Chen TJ. The efficacy of intravenous immunoglobulin for the treatment of toxic epidermal necrolysis: a systematic review and meta-analysis. Br J Dermatol. 2012;167(2):424–32.

111. Del Pozzo-Magana BR, et al. A systematic review of treatment of drug-induced Stevens–Johnson syndrome and toxic epidermal necrolysis in children. J Popul Ther Clin Pharmacol. 2011;18:e121–33.

112. Valeyrie-Allanore L, et al. Open trial of ciclosporin treatment for Stevens–Johnson syndrome and toxic epidermal necrolysis. Br J Dermatol. 2010;163(4):847–53.

113. Kirchhof MG, et al. Retrospective review of Stevens–Johnson syndrome/toxic epidermal necrolysis treatment comparing intravenous immunoglobulin with cyclosporine. J Am Acad Dermatol. 2014;71(5):941–7.

114. Fischer M, et al. Antitumour necrosis factor-alpha antibodies (infliximab) in the treatment of a patient with toxic epidermal necrolysis. Br J Dermatol. 2002;146(4):707–9.

115. Kreft B, et al. Etoricoxib-induced toxic epidermal necrolysis: successful treatment with infliximab. J Dermatol. 2010;37(10):904–6.

116. Patmanidis K, et al. Combination of infliximab and high-dose intravenous immunoglobulin for toxic epidermal necrolysis: successful treatment of an elderly patient. Case Rep Dermatol Med. 2012;2012:915314.

117. Paradisi A, et al. Etanercept therapy for toxic epidermal necrolysis. J Am Acad Dermatol. 2014;71(2):278–83.

118. Stamp LK, Chapman PT. Gout and its comorbidities: implications for therapy. Rheumatology (Oxford). 2013;52(1):34–44.

6

Biomarkers and severe asthma: a critical appraisal

Alessandra Chiappori[1†], Laura De Ferrari[1†], Chiara Folli[1], Pierluigi Mauri[2], Anna Maria Riccio[1] and Giorgio Walter Canonica[1*]

Abstract

Severe asthma (SA) is a clinically and etiologically heterogeneous respiratory disease which affects among 5–10 % of asthmatic patients. Despite high-dose therapy, a large patients percentage is not fully controlled and has a poor quality of life. In this review, we describe the biomarkers actually known in scientific literature and used in clinical practice for SA assessment and management: neutrophils, eosinophils, periostin, fractional exhaled nitric oxide, exhaled breath condensate and galectins. Moreover, we give an overview on clinical and biological features characterizing severe asthma, paying special attention to the potential use of these ones as reliable markers. We finally underline the need to define different biomarkers panels to select patients affected by severe asthma for specific and personalized therapeutic approach.

Keywords: Severe asthma, Biomarkers, Exhaled nitric oxide, Periostin, Eosinophil, Galectin, Allergic inflammation, Neutrophil, Monoclonal antibodies

Background

Severe asthma (SA) is defined as 'asthma which requires treatment with high dose inhaled corticosteroids (ICS) plus a second controller (and/or systemic corticosteroids) to prevent it from becoming 'uncontrolled' or which remains 'uncontrolled' despite this therapy'. This is the European Respiratory Society (ERS)/American Thoracic Society (ATS) definition, utilized across developed countries with general access to inhaled corticosteroid therapy [1, 2]. It is recognized that up to 50 % of patients are not well controlled and 5–10 % of patients suffer from a particularly severe disease that is often refractory to usual treatment [3, 4].

Evidence of any one of the four criteria below, while on current high-dose therapy, identifies the patient as having "severe asthma":

1. Poor symptoms control.

2. Frequent severe exacerbations, defined as two or more bursts of systemic corticosteroids in the previous year.

3. Serious exacerbations, defined as at least one hospitalization, intensive care unit stay or mechanical ventilation in the previous year.

4. Airflow limitation, i.e. forced expiratory volume in 1 s (FEV1), 80 % predicted (in the presence of reduced FEV1/forced vital capacity (FVC) defined as less than the lower limit of normal) following a withhold of both short- and long-acting bronchodilators.

Asthma, and severe asthma in particular, are increasingly considered as heterogeneous diseases, which may respond similarly to therapies. Recently, studies are beginning to identify different phenotypes defined by characteristic clinical manifestations, pathophysiological mechanisms and biomarkers [5].

The first studies performed in asthmatics distinguished subtypes based on inflammatory patterns obtained from bronchoalveolar lavage and endobronchial biopsies. Identifying patients with corticosteroid-naive, mild asthma who exhibited a T-helper (Th)2/Type 2 molecular signature in their epithelial cells, Woodruff et al., began

---
*Correspondence: canonica@unige.it
†Alessandra Chiappori and Laura De Ferrari contributed equally to this work
[1] DIMI-Department of Internal Medicine, Respiratory Diseases and Allergy Clinic, University of Genoa, IRCCS AOU S.Martino-IST, Genoa, Italy
Full list of author information is available at the end of the article

the concept of molecular phenotyping, in which molecular pathways are linked to clinical and physiological characteristics [6].

A more detailed immunopathobiological picture of human SA is therefore emerging as the context of the heterogeneity of the disease, in relation to both inflammation and structural changes [7].

The identification of asthma phenotypes has given a boost to the search for biomarkers to help classifying patients, targeting therapies and predicting different pathological evolution mechanisms of the disease with strong benefits for the affected patients [8].

An ideal biomarker is easy to collect and measure, not invasive nor expensive, and can be used to identify either clinical or treatment response phenotypes, evaluate changes in disease activity, or confirm a diagnosis. This prospect provides the impetus for the research for reliable markers in SA, which are actually under intense study and are hereunder analyzed. In this review we focus the importance and the role of different known and potential biomarkers useful to define the physiopathological and clinical profiles of patients affected by severe asthma.

Neutrophils

Severe asthma is often characterized by neutrophilic inflammation, both in the presence or absence of Th2-induced eosinophilic inflammation [9, 10]. However, the functional role of these cells in disease progression remains unclear. Sputum neutrophil percentages are highly reproducible in patients with moderate to severe asthma, and can be used to assess novel anti-inflammatory therapies: targeting neutrophils has been suggested as a therapeutic option for these patients [11, 12].

Neutrophils recruitment can be mediated by Th17 cells, which are thought to have a role in asthma pathogenesis, especially in patients who do not respond to glucocorticoid therapy and show a decreased improvement in FEV1 and airway hyperresponsiveness (AHR) following treatment [13, 14]. Moreover, it has been demonstrated that, in addition to the specific antigenic components, pollens contain several intrinsic factors able to promote innate immune responses; among them, nicotinamide adenine dinucleotide phosphate oxidase (NADPH) induces the generation of reactive oxygen species (ROS) [15]. This oxidative insult induces an early wave of neutrophil recruitment in the airways and increases significantly ROS-generating activity of these cells [16]. It has been also evidenced that pollen can induce CXCL chemokine synthesis and that neutrophils can be recruited into the airways in a CXCR2-dependent manner [17].

The receptor for advanced glycation end-products (RAGE) is a pattern recognition receptor involved in the response to injury, infection and inflammation.

Perturbations in the RAGE and its soluble forms (sRAGE) balance might be linked to neutrophilic airway inflammation in chronic airways disease [18]. A recent work from Sukkar et al. demonstrated a deficiency in lung and systemic sRAGE, in asthmatic and chronic obstructive pulmonary disease (COPD) patients with neutrophilic airway inflammation. sRAGE might be degraded by neutrophil-derived proteolytic enzymes in subjects with airway neutrophilia and might be identified as a potential biomarker for prognosis or patient management [19].

The metalloproteinase domain 8 (ADAM8) seems also to be involved in facilitating neutrophils migration into tissues [20]. It is highly expressed in bronchial biopsies from moderate and severe asthmatics and its recruitment of both eosinophils and neutrophils into airways tissue suggests a significant role in the pathogenesis of asthma [21–24].

Future therapeutic targets directed at the above mentioned proteins might significantly attenuate asthma symptoms by reducing inflammatory cells, primarily neutrophils, and having few adverse physiological consequences.

Eosinophils

Asthma is also histologically characterized by recruitment of eosinophils into the large airway wall and lumen, along with mucus plugging and epithelium denudation. Being associated with increased transforming growth factor β (TGF-β) expression and reticular basement membrane (RBM) thickness, the amount of these cells might be congruent with symptoms severity, worsened lung function, and near-fatal events [25–27].

The identification of eosinophilic inflammation is of a certain importance due to the severity of attacks which occur to these patients and to the existence of drugs, such as prednisolone, omalizumab and new biological agents, particularly active on this pattern [28].

It is known that Type-2 inflammatory pathways are involved in asthma, and many studies suggest that about 50 % of SA patients present Type-2 inflammation, as measured by eosinophilia or high levels of fractional exhaled nitric oxide (FeNO) [29, 30]. Miranda et al. distinguished early-onset severe asthma patients, characterized by allergen sensitivity, allergic symptoms, eosinophilia and higher serum immunoglobulin E (IgE) levels, and late-onset severe asthma subjects, with lower lung function than early-onset ones, despite a shorter duration of illness and significantly more symptoms if presenting persistent eosinophils at onset [27].

The need to block IgE binding to inflammatory cells and the consequent mediators release cascade concurred to the development of the unique monoclonal antibody approved for patients with severe allergic asthma: omalizumab, a recombinant humanized murine antibody against IgE antibodies. A recent study from our group investigated the effect of long-term anti-IgE treatment on the thickening of the RBM and eosinophil infiltration in bronchial biopsies from patients with severe persistent allergic asthma. Our results showed that a substantial proportion of severe asthmatics reduced the original bronchial RBM thickness and eosinophil infiltration after one-year treatment with anti-IgE, thus emphasizing the possible role of omalizumab in affecting airway remodeling in severe persistent allergic asthma [31]. Up to now, many studies have shown how the anti-IgE treatment in SA patients was effective in modulating airways remodeling and inflammation, as well as in improving lung functions and quality of life (Table 1).

Eosinophils count in induced sputum has long been the method of choice to evaluate eosinophilic lung inflammation and seems to be a reliable biomarker of airway inflammation as well as useful in adjusting corticosteroid treatments in asthma [38–40].

Newby et al. and McGrath et al. by using sputum, identified phenotypes of SA enriched for eosinophilic airway inflammation that might respond to therapies directed toward Th2 immune pathways [41, 42].

Recently, the dose ranging efficacy and safety with mepolizumab (DREAM) study correlated blood eosinophils levels, but not sputum eosinophilia, with response to mepolizumab [43]. These data are supported by many authors who evidenced that sputum eosinophils can not predict treatment response and that increased blood eosinophils are associated with higher risk for exacerbations, maybe owing to interleukin (IL)-5 levels [44, 45]. Following anti-IgE treatment, some studies found decreased blood eosinophils counts [46]. In the EXTRA study, Hanania and colleagues demonstrated that omalizumab efficacy was strongly related to the presence of airways eosinophilic inflammation and more accurately predicted by FeNO and serum periostin rather than IgE levels [47].

It is currently hypothesized that the use of blood eosinophils as biomarkers could help to personalize asthma management in patients with severe allergic asthma.

Active eosinophils recruitment is predominantly exerted by proteins secreted by epithelia, the most potent chemoattractant for these cells being eotaxin-1 (CCL11), that account for 80 % of TGF-ß expression in asthma [48–50]. A recent work evaluated CCL11 levels in bronchoalveolar lavage fluid (BALF), exhaled breath condensate (EBC), blood and sputum and evidenced a

Table 1 Studies on clinical effectiveness of omalizumab in patients with severe asthma

Mediators and parameters	Biologic sample/procedure	Patients	Effects of omalizumab treatment	References
ET-1	EBC	19 severe asthmatics	↓	[32]
FeNO	EB	9/19 omalizumab (+)	↓	
ECP	Blood		↓	
Eosinophils count	Blood		↓	
FEV1	Spirometry		↑	
RANTES/CCL5	EBC	19 severe asthmatics	↓	[33]
FeNO	EB	9/19 omalizumab (+)	↓	
ECP	Blood		↓	
Eosinophils count	Blood		↓	
Eosinophils count	Blood	13 severe sthmatics 13/13 omalizumab (+)	↓	[34]
Quality of life	Questionnaire	26 severe asthmatics	↑	[35]
PEF	Spirometry	26/26 omalizumab (+)	↑	
Unscheduled visits	Clinical data		↓	
Exacerbations	Clinical data		↓	
FeNO	EB		↓	
CalvNO	EB		↓	
Eosinophils count	Sputum		↓	
Airway-wall thickness	CT		↓	
Exacerbations	Clinical data	22 severe asthmatics	↓	[36]
Systemic steroids	Clinical data	22/22 omalizumab (+)	↓	
ACT score	Questionnaire		↑	
Airway-wall thickness	Bronchial biopsies	11 severe asthmatics	↓	[31]
Eosinophils count		11/11 omalizumab (+)	↓	
Bronchial smooth muscle proteins	Bronchial biopsies	8 severe astmatics 8/8 omalizumab (+)	↓	[37]

ET-1 endothelin-1, *FeNO* fractional exhaled nitric oxide, *ECP* eosinophil cationic protein, *FEV1* forced expired volume in 1 s, *EB* exhaled breath, *EBC* exhaled breath condensate, *RANTES/CCL5* regulated on activation, normal T cell expressed and secreted/chemokine (C–C motif) ligand-5, *PEF* peak expiratory flow, *CalvNO* estimated alveolar nitric oxide concentration, *CT* computerized tomography, *ACT* asthma control test.

correlation between this protein in induced sputum and asthma severity [51].

It has also been hypothesized that asthma severity might be linked to a relationship between TGF-ß expression and the presence of submucosal eosinophils. It was evidenced that in bronchial biopsies the majority of eosinophils is TGF-ß1-mRNA positive [25, 52], with a higher extent in SA. Moreover, TGF-ß2 isoforms are expressed by eosinophils in severe allergic asthma where this cytokine promotes fibrotic responses and regulates mucin production [53, 54].

Although still in study and source of debate, the persistent eosinophilic phenotype in adults might be a real candidate for specific therapies thus potentially interfering with the natural history of SA with high exacerbation rates.

Fractional exhaled nitric oxide

Epithelial inducible nitric oxide synthase (NOS) has been shown to be the main determinant of FeNO levels in the respiratory tract [55] due to increased nitric oxide (NO) production by activated bronchial epithelial cells in response to pro-inflammatory stimuli [56]. It is postulated that the decrease in FeNO values seen after steroid treatment might be due to an inhibitory effect of these drugs on inducible NOS activity [55], therefore the measurement of NO concentration in exhaled breath has been standardized for clinical use. It is a quantitative, non-invasive, simple, and safe method to assess airway inflammation, to monitor responsiveness to ICS therapy in adults [57] and to predict asthma control status in childhood [58]. Recently, a retrospective study was performed on 416 asthmatic patients on combined therapy (long-acting β2 agonist and ICS). The authors assessed the correlation between FEV1 and FeNO to ascertain the correct use of FeNO measurement in different asthma phenotypes with regard to disease control, severity, allergy, comorbidity, obesity, age and smoking status. No correlation was found between FeNO levels and asthma severity but it was shown a link to other parameters such as age, gender, history of emergency room visits and atopy [59]. Moreover, cross-sectional study on 100 adult asthmatic patients showed that FeNO levels were correlated primary with asthma control rather than asthma severity, confirming FeNO as reliable biomarker in asthma management [60]. Peirsman et al. performed a randomized controlled trial on 99 children with persistent allergic asthma: patients outcomes were evaluated over a 52-week timeframe and, only in FeNO group, therapeutic approach was guided by FeNO measurements. Results demonstrated that FeNO evaluation diminished asthma exacerbations rate in associated with an increased leukotriene receptor antagonist use and ICS

doses administration [61]. FeNO may also be used as predictor of omalizumab treatment efficacy. Hanania et al. evaluated FeNO, serum periostin and blood eosinophilia as potential biomarkers useful to evaluate effectiveness of anti-IgE treatment on 850 adult persistent SA patients. After 48 weeks of therapy, reduction of exacerbations rate was greater in high versus low subgroup for FeNO levels (53 vs 16 %) [47]. In the Inner-City Anti-IgE therapy of asthma trial, Busse et al. confirmed a clinical benefit from omalizumab treatment in children and adolescents [62]. In a post hoc analysis of the previous study, Sorkeness et al. found that FeNO, together with blood eosinophils and body mass index, can predict omalizumab response [63]. Moreover, preliminary data indicated that elevated FeNO may be indicative of anti-IL-13/IL-4 biological response [64]. However, Haldar et al. showed that FeNO seems to be less closely associated with a response to mepolizumab (anti IL-5) than blood eosinophils count [65].

In SA, the bronchial mucosa is markedly hyperplastic, the epithelium may be susceptible to destruction, flaking and detachment from the RBM. Therefore, FeNO levels can be under-representative [66]. The ERS/ATS Task Force has published a detailed guideline on definition, evaluation and treatment of SA. The Authors defined SA phenotypes giving specific recommendations for the use of diagnostic tools like measurement of FeNO to guide therapy. Elevated FeNO value is considered as a marker of Th2 inflammation and atopy but not an effective biomarker useful in SA management [1].

Exhaled breath condensate

Exhaled breath (EB) is mainly composed by aerosolized, non-volatile particles of airway lining fluid collected from the airways by airflow turbulence, water vapor condensation, inorganic (O_2, N_2), and organic (CO_2) atmospheric volatile water-soluble gases, endogenous and exogenous volatile organic compounds [67]. EBC is the EB that has been condensed, typically by using a commercially available refrigerating device, according to ATS/ERS Guidelines [68]. It is used to investigate the composition of airway fluids and to achieve information about pulmonary alveoli, inflammation, nitrosative and oxidative stress in airways diseases such as COPD [69], asthma [70] and lung cancer [67]. Concerning SA, clinical studies identified chemical and biological characteristics that distinguish EBC of severe asthmatics from those obtained from healthy subjects and mild to moderate asthmatic patients (Fig. 1). Experimental data on EBC pH in SA are contrasting and there are still few studies about it [71, 72]. Eicosanoids as pro-inflammatory Leukotriene B4 (LTB4) and anti-inflammatory Lipoxin A4 (LXA4) are increased in asthmatics versus

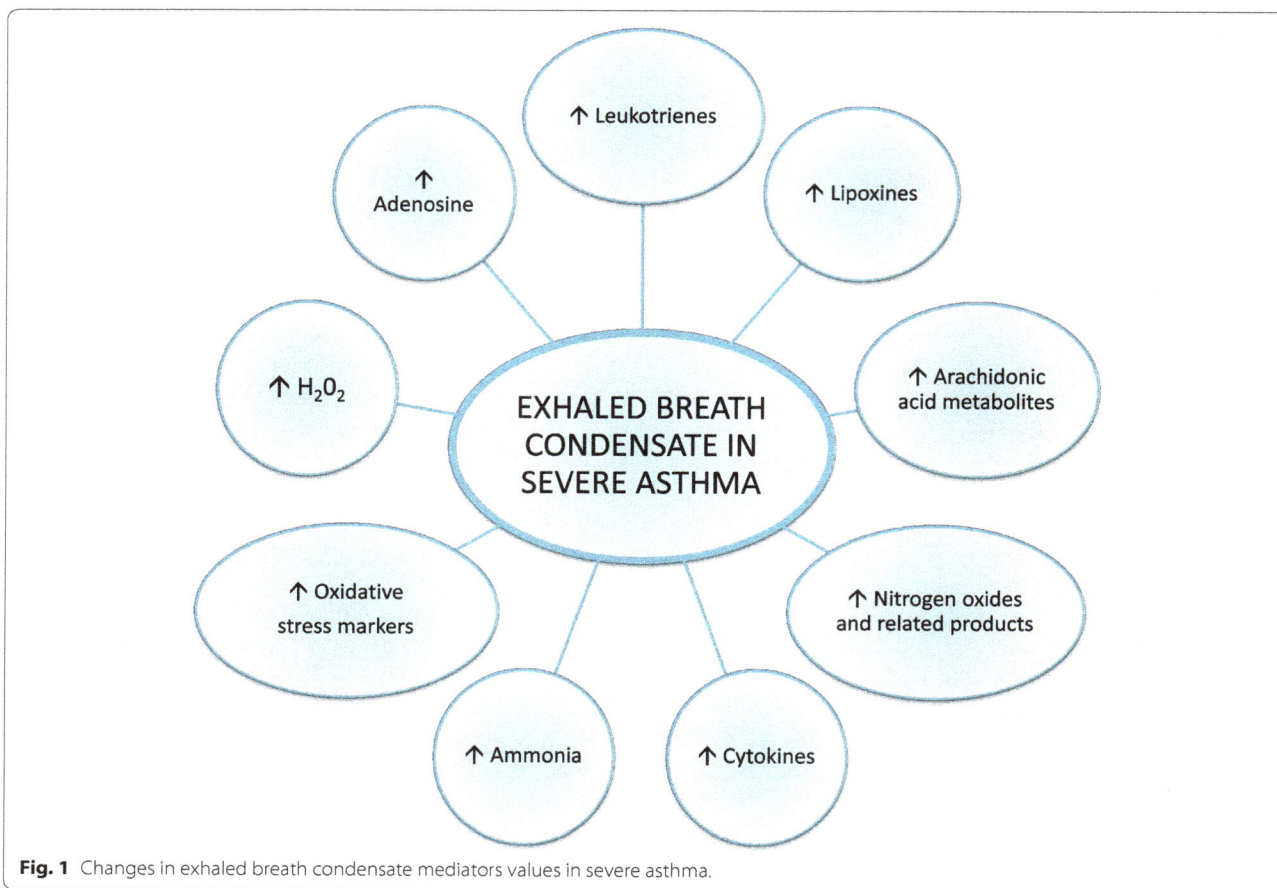

Fig. 1 Changes in exhaled breath condensate mediators values in severe asthma.

healthy subjects and LXA4/LTB4 ratio dramatically decreases in EBC in correlation with asthma severity [73]. Eotaxin-1 was evaluated in blood, EBC, sputum and BALF and was proposed as a tool for assessment of asthma severity [51]. High levels of nitrogen reactive species (NO, NO^{2-}, NO^{3-}) and endogenous ROS (superoxide, hydrogen peroxide, hydroxyl radical) provided evidence for pathologic oxidizing processes in asthma and are indicative of airways oxidative and nitrosative stress [74]. In SA, these pathologic features are exacerbated and correlated to asthma stability and corticosteroid therapy response [75]. Many studies have been published on the use of omics techniques in asthmatic children for the analysis of easy to be collected samples. Using liquid chromatography and mass spectrometry, significant differences useful to distinguish asthma severity between healthy and asthmatic children biochemical profiles were found in urine and in EBC [76–78]. Baraldi et al. proposed the use of metabolomic analysis or breathomic approach of EBC to characterize asthma phenotypes and personalize the therapeutic plan [79]. Fitzpatrick et al. found that SA children showed metabolic differences associated with oxidative

stress-related pathways which may contribute to their corticosteroids refractory state [80]. General recommendations for EBC collection and exhaled biomarkers measurements are available in order to avoid a possible alteration in biomarker concentrations. Despite EBC collection remains a procedure potentially influenced by numerous endogenous and exogenous factors, in present and in future, EBC analysis can turn out as a promising, safe and non-invasive method for monitoring SA patients [68].

Periostin

Periostin is a secreted matricellular protein with a key role in amplification and in persistence of chronic inflammation of allergic diseases [81]. Having the ability to bind fibronectin, tenascin-C, collagen I, III and V, periostin is involved in the process of subepithelial fibrosis in asthma patients [82]. Furthermore, it exerts its biological activity also by binding integrins on cell surfaces and activating intracellular signal pathways [83]. Periostin is induced by IL-4 and IL-13 in bronchial epithelial cells and in lung fibroblasts and its expression is correlated with the RBM thickness [82, 84, 85]. Moreover, this molecule is able to accelerate eosinophils tissue infiltration facilitating their adhesion to extracellular matrix proteins [86]. Serum periostin can be considered a systemic biomarker Th2-high asthma related because it is a signature molecule associated to higher AHR, serum IgE, eosinophilic inflammation, subepithelial fibrosis, compared to Th2-low asthma. It is possible to consider serum periostin a promising biomarker for two main reasons. First of all, this protein easily moves from inflamed tissues to blood circulation so its serum concentrations reflects its local production in lesions induced by Th2-type immune responses [87, 88]. Moreover, its basal serum levels are physiologically relatively low (~50 ng/ml) compared to other extracellular matrix proteins such as fibronectin or vitronectin. Jia et al. in the Bronchoscopic Exploratory Research Study of Biomarkers in Corticosteroid-refractory Asthma (BOBCAT), identified serum periostin as the single best systemic biomarker of airway luminal and tissue eosinophilia in severe, uncontrolled asthmatics. Adopting 25 ng/ml serum periostin as an arbitrary cut-off, eosinophil-low and eosinophil-high patients are effectively differentiated, with a positive predicted value of 93 %. This study evidenced the superiority of serum periostin for predicting sputum and tissue eosinophilia, compared to blood eosinophils, IgE levels, YKL-40 and FeNO [89]. More recently, Kanemitsu et al., in an observational study, found that high serum periostin concentration ($\geq$95 ng/ml) is the unique biomarker, among several serum markers, associated with the greater annual decline in FEV1 (at least 30 ml/year) [90]. In addition to being an encouraging biomarker in predicting responders to traditional ICS therapy, periostin seems to also identify responders to new target treatments [91]. Corren et al. demonstrated that its higher serum levels might predict the response to Th2 target therapy with biologic agents such as anti-IL-13 monoclonal antibody (lebrikizumab). The Authors performed a randomized, double-blind, placebo-controlled study of lebrikizumab in 219 adults with unstable asthma despite ICS treatment. The therapy was associated with increased FEV1 values in patients with high pretreatment levels of serum periostin [92]. Similarly, analyzing the results from the EXTRA study performed with uncontrolled, severe, allergic asthmatics, Hanania et al. found that the high serum periostin group had a greater decreased exacerbation rate after omalizumab treatment compared to low serum periostin group [47]. Finally, in a recently published study, Bobolea et al. investigated the potential role of sputum periostin, more organ-targeted than serum periostin, as a biomarker of SA. The Authors found that sputum periostin levels are associated with persistent airflow limitation and eosinophilic inflammatory phenotype despite high-dose ICS therapy [93].

Taken together, these results show that periostin can be a useful biomarker to apply stratified medicine for SA and to yield better outcomes in asthma management. More evaluations are required to validate and clarify the potential utility of periostin in research and before this measurement can be applied in everyday clinical practice. Future studies should better evaluate this biomarker because it was demonstrated that its high levels could be detected in several conditions associated with increased cellular proliferation, angiogenesis, stress, tissues injury not necessarily dependent on a Th2 immune response, as shown in Table 2. We should also remember that periostin is not specific to asthma or the airway epithelium [81, 109, 123, 124]. These considerations should

Table 2 Overview on periostin as biomarker in different diseases

	References
Allergic and respiratory diseases	
Asthma	[89]
Atopic dermatitis	[94]
IgG4-related sclerosing sialadenitis	[95]
Allergic rhinitis and chronic rhinosinusitis	[96]
Eosinophilic otitis media	[97]
Idiopathic interstitial pneumonias	[98]
Pulmonary fibrosis	[99]
Nasal polyps associated with aspirin-sensitive asthma	[100]
Oncology	
Cholangiocarcinoma	[101, 102]
Ovarian carcinoma	[103, 104]
Colon cancer	[105]
Pancreatic cancer	[106, 107]
Melanoma	[108]
Head and neck cancer	[109]
Glioblastoma	[110]
Breast cancer	[111]
Non-small cell lung carcinoma	[112]
Osteology	
Bone marrow fibrosis	[113]
Fibrous dysplasia	[114]
Other inflammatory diseases	
Systemic sclerosis	[115]
Proliferative diabetic retinopathy	[116]
Psoriasis	[117]
Interstitial renal fibrosis	[118]
Polycystic kidney disease	[119]
Lupus nephritis	[120]
Eosinophilic esophagitis	[86]
Hepatic fibrosis	[121]
Myocardial fibrosis	[122]

lead clinicians to use an integrative approach which links clinical features and molecular mechanisms and should encourage to better investigate analysis of sputum periostin. It will also be necessary to establish and validate cut-off values to define high and low periostin levels. Furthermore, additional carefully designed studies are needed to evaluate if periostin, alone or in combination with other more conventional biomarkers, can be utilized in better redefining current asthma phenotypes and selecting patients for emerging asthma therapeutics targeting Th2 inflammation.

Galectins

Galectins are a family of animal lectins with different cellular and extracellular localizations. These proteins bind the cell-surface and extracellular matrix (ECM) glycans and, thereby, affect a variety of cellular processes and biological activities. To date, 15 galectins having a role in physiological and pathobiological processes like cancer, heart failure, tissue repair and platelets aggregation have been found in mammals [125–128]. Regarding airway diseases, the effects of these proteins on the inflammatory process were analyzed for the first time in murine models. Galectin-9 role is still unclear because it was identified as a possible recruiter of eosinophil granulocytes and promoter of Th2 dominance [129], but also as a IgE binding protein with anti-allergic effects able to prevent acute asthma exacerbations [130, 131].

Another galectin with a demonstrated role in asthma is Galectin-3, the only chimera galectin found in Vertebrates, with biological activities in numerous cellular functions like cellular adhesion, growth, chemoattraction, differentiation, apoptosis and cellular cycle as well as an IgE binding protein activity [132–134]. Evaluation of Galectin-3 expression in deficient and wild-type gal-3 mice with OVA-induced asthma, evidenced that OVA-sensitized gal-3 (−/−) mice developed fewer eosinophils, lower goblet cell metaplasia and significantly less AHR after airway OVA challenge compared to similarly treated gal-3 (+/+) mice [135]. Moreover, studies on Gal-3 gene therapy confirmed how it is possible to reduce eosinophils airway infiltration, AHR and tissue remodeling [136]. The involvement of Galectin-3 in human airways inflammatory process has been ascertained for COPD [137], lung fibrosis [138] and asthma. In asthma, Gal-3 expression seems to be related to the development of a specific inflammatory pattern and biological therapy outcome. Recently, Gao et al. found a significantly reduced sputum Gal-3 in patients with neutrophilic asthma [139]. Moreover, evaluating bronchial biopsies of SA patients treated with omalizumab using proteomic technique, we observed that proteomic profile of bronchial tissue before omalizumab treatment presents a typical pattern indicative of anti-IgE treatment response. Galectin-3 was expressed only in subjects with a positive bronchial morphometric analysis

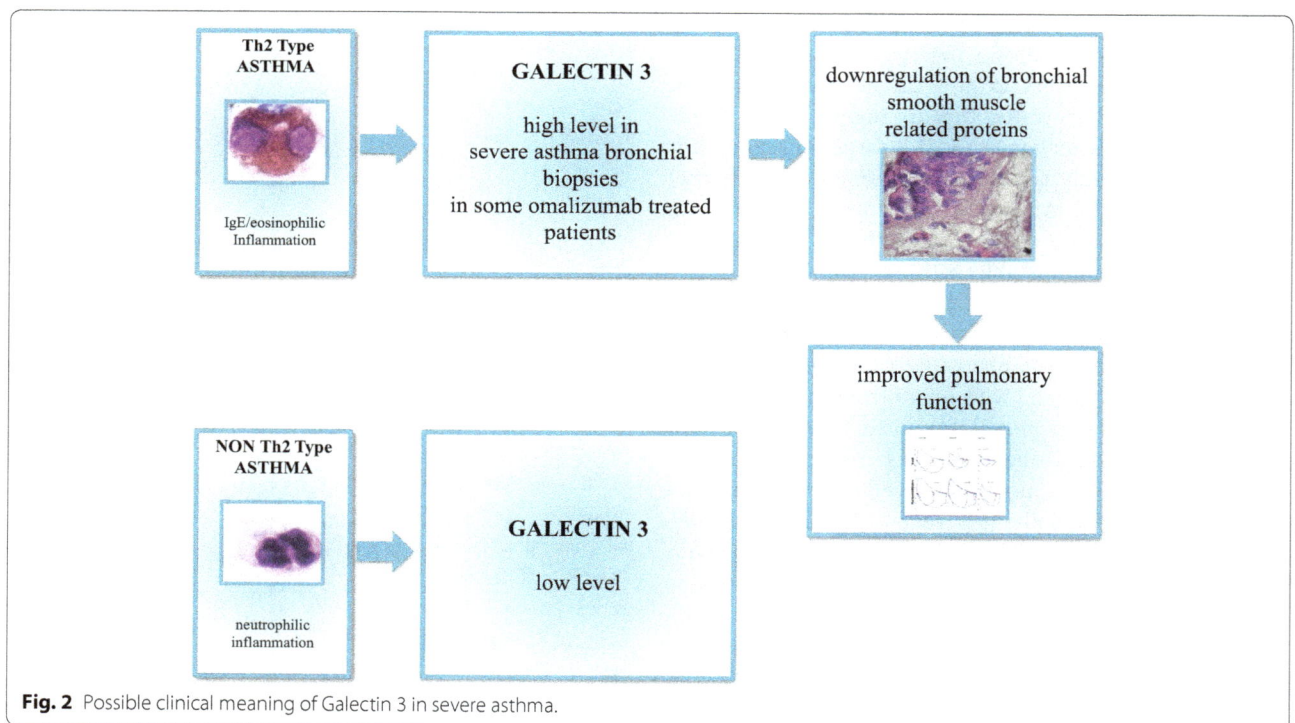

Fig. 2 Possible clinical meaning of Galectin 3 in severe asthma.

response to anti-IgE treatment. In our opinion Galectin-3, having the ability to bind IgE proteins, can be considered a reliable biomarker to predict the modulation of airway remodeling and the improvement of pulmonary function in SA patients before they begin omalizumab therapy (Fig. 2) [37].

Conclusions

The need in finding biomarkers useful to monitor treatment response is evident in clinical practice, however their discovery is made difficulty by the huge number of proteins involved in severe asthma pathogenesis, only a part of which has been cited in this work. Recently, advances have been obtained by data analysis from genomic and proteomic profiling studies but the application of these methods in clinical practice is difficult. One of the main problems is the cost of many techniques, which require specific instrumentation and skills not easy to achieve. Moreover, protein concentrations may change depending on the inflammatory condition of the patient, disease-associated processes and the sample collecting/analysis method. Nonetheless, each of candidate biomarkers is involved in different biological aspects and gives us information that can be largely overlapping. All these reasons make clear that the road to the identification and the daily use of defined biomarkers in SA is still long and winding. Development of novel serum/sputum-based biomarker panels with improved sensitivity and specificity over the ones currently available, will lead to promising future in the diagnosis of SA [140–142]. Accordingly with Gustafson et al., the more suitable reality in clinical practice will be: a definition of different panels composed by different biomarkers leading to the eligibility of the patients to a certain therapeutic treatment [143].

Abbreviations

SA: severe asthma; ICS: inhaled corticosteroids; ERS: European Respiratory Society; ATS: American Thoracic Society; FEV1: forced expiratory volume in 1 second; FVC: forced vital capacity; Th: T helper lymphocyte; AHR: airway hyperresponsiveness; NADPH: nicotinamide adenine dinucleotide phosphate oxidase; ROS: reactive oxygen species; RAGE: receptor for advanced glycation end-products; sRAGE: soluble form of receptor for advanced glycation end-products; COPD: chronic obstructive pulmonary disease; ADAM8: metalloproteinase domain 8; TGF-β: trasforming growth factor β; RBM: reticular basement membrane; FeNO: fractional exhaled nitric oxide; IgE: immunoglobulin E; IL: interleukin; CCL11: eotaxin-1; BALF: bronchoalveolar lavage fluid; EBC: exhaled breath condensate; NOS: nitric oxide synthase; NO: nitric oxide; EB: exhaled breath; LTB4: leukotriene B4; LXA4: lipoxin A4; ECM: extracellular matrix.

Authors' contributions

AC, LDF and CF carried on bibliographic research and took part in the draft of the paper; PM, AMR and GWC contributed to bibliographic research

and reviewed the final manuscript. All authors read and approved the final manuscript.

Author details
[1] DIMI-Department of Internal Medicine, Respiratory Diseases and Allergy Clinic, University of Genoa, IRCCS AOU S.Martino-IST, Genoa, Italy. [2] Institute for Biomedical Technologies, CNR, Segrate, Milan, Italy.

Acknowledgements
This work was partially supported by ARMIA (Associazione Ricerca Malattie Immunologiche ed Allergiche).

References
1. Chung KF, Wenzel SE, Brozek JL, Bush A, Castro M, Sterk PJ et al (2014) International ERS/ATS guidelines on definition, evaluation and treatment of severe asthma. Eur Respir J 43:343–373
2. American Thoracic Society (2000) Proceedings of the ATS workshop on refractory asthma: current understanding, recommendations, and unanswered questions. Am J Respir Crit Care Med 162:2341–2351
3. Moore WC, Bleecker ER, Curran-Everett D, Erzurum SC, Ameredes BT, Bacharier L et al (2007) Characterization of the severe asthma phenotype by the National Heart, Lung, and Blood Institute's Severe Asthma Research Program. J Allergy Clin Immunol 119:405–413
4. Chen H, Blanc PD, Hayden ML, Bleecker ER, Chawla A, Lee JH et al (2008) Assessing productivity loss and activity impairment in severe or difficult-to-treat asthma. Value Health 11:231–239
5. Wenzel SE (2012) Asthma phenotypes: the evolution from clinical to molecular approaches. Nat Med 18:716–725
6. Woodruff PG, Modrek B, Choy DF, Jia G, Abbas AR, Ellwanger A et al (2009) T-helper type 2-driven inflammation defines major subphenptypes of asthma. Am J Respir Crit Care Med 180:388–395
7. Trejo Bittar HE, Yousem SA, Wenzel SE (2015) Pathobiology of severe asthma. Ann Rev Pathol 10:511–545
8. Moore WC, Meyers DA, Wenzel SE, Teague WG, Li H, Li X et al (2010) Identification of asthma phenotypes using cluster analysis in the severe asthma research program. Am J Respir Crit Care Med 181:315–323
9. Jatakanon A, Uasuf C, Maziak W, Lim S, Chung KF, Barnes PJ (1999) Neutrophilic inflammation in severe persistent asthma. Am J Respir Crit Care Med 160:1532–1539
10. Gibson PG, Simpson JL, Saltos N (2001) Heterogeneity of airway inflammation in persistent asthma: evidence of neutrophilic inflammation and increased sputum interleukin-8. Chest 119:1329–1336
11. Rossall MRW, Cadden PA, Molphy SD, Plumb J, Singh D (2014) Repeatability of induced sputum measurements in moderate to severe asthma. Respir Med 108:1566–1568
12. Nair P, Gaga M, Zervas E, Alagha K, Hargreave FE, O'Byrne PM et al (2012) Safety and efficacy of a CXCR2 antagonist in patients with severe asthma and sputum neutrophils: a randomized, placebo-controlled clinical trial. Clin Exp Allergy 42:1097–1103
13. Schleimer RP (2004) Glucocorticoids suppress inflammation but spare innate immune responses in airway epithelium. Proc Am Thorac Soc 1:222–230
14. Barnes PJ, Adcock IM (2009) Glucocorticoid resistance in inflammatory diseases. Lancet 373:1905–1917
15. Hosoki K, Boldogh I, Sur S (2015) Innate responses to pollen allergens. Curr Opin Allergy Clin Immunol 15:79–88
16. Boldogh I, Bacsi A, Choudhury BK, Dharajiya N, Alam R, Hazra TK (2005) ROS generated by pollen NADPH oxidase provide a signal that augments antigen-induced allergic airway inflammation. J Clin Invest 115:2169–2179
17. Hosoki K, Aguilera-Aguirre L, Brasier AR, Kurosky A, Boldogh I, Sur S (2015) Pollen-induced innate recruitment of neutrophils facilitates induction of allergic sensitization and airway inflammation. Am J Respir Cell Mol Biol. doi:10.1165/rcmb.2015-0044OC

18. Sims GP, Rowe DC, Rietdijk ST, Herbst R, Coyle AJ (2010) HMGB1 and RAGE in inflammation and cancer. Ann Rev Immunol 28:367–388

19. Sukkar MB, Wood LG, Tooze M, Simpson JL, McDonald VM, Gibson PG et al (2012) Soluble RAGE is deficient in neutrophilic asthma and COPD. Eur Respir J 39:721–729

20. Gómez-Gaviro M, Domínguez-Luis M, Canchado J, Calafat J, Janssen H, Lara-Pezzi E et al (2007) Expression and regulation of the metalloproteinase ADAM-8 during human neutrophil pathophysiological activation and its catalytic activity on L-selectin shedding. J Immunol 178:8053–8063

21. Johansson MW, Lye MH, Barthel SR, Duffy AK, Annis DS, Mosher DF (2004) Eosinophils adhere to vascular cell adhesion molecule-1 via podosomes. Am J Respir Cell Mol Biol 31:413–422

22. Paulissen G, Rocks N, Quesada-Calvo F, Gosset P, Foidart JM, Noel A et al (2006) Expression of ADAMs and their inhibitors in sputum from patients with asthma. Mol Med 12:171–179

23. Foley SC, Mogas AK, Olivenstein R, Fiset PO, Chakir J, Bourbeau J et al (2007) Increased expression of ADAM-33 and ADAM-8 with disease progression in asthma. J Allergy Clin Immunol 119:863–871

24. Oreo KM, Gibson PG, Simpson JL, Wood LG, McDonald VM, Baines KJ (2013) Sputum ADAM-8 expression in increased in severe asthma and COPD. Clin Exp Allergy 44:342–352

25. Flood-Page P, Menzies-Gow A, Phipps S, Ying S, Wangoo A, Ludwig MS et al (2003) Anti-IL-5 treatment reduces deposition of ECM proteins in the bronchial subepithelial basement membrane of mild atopic asthmatics. J Clin Investig 112:1029–1036

26. Green RH, Brightling CE, Woltmann G, Parker D, Wardlaw AJ, Pavord ID (2002) Analysis of induced sputum in adults with asthma: identification of subgroup with isolated sputum neutrophilia and poor response to inhaled corticosteroids. Thorax 57:875–879

27. Miranda C, Busacker A, Balzar S, Trudeau J, Wenzel SE (2004) Distinguishing severe asthma phenotypes: role of age at onset and eosinophilic inflammation. J Allergy Clin Immunol 113:101–108

28. Hilvering B, Pavord ID (2015) What goes up must come down: biomarkers and novel biologicals in severe asthma. Clin Exp Allergy 45:1162–1169

29. Wenzel SE, Schwartz LB, Langmack EL, Halliday JL, Trudeau JB, Gibbs RL et al (1999) Evidence that severe asthma can be divided pathologically into two inflammatory subtypes with distinct physiologic and clinical characteristics. Am J Respir Crit Care Med 160:1001–1008

30. Dweik RA, Sorkness RL, Wenzel S, Hammel J, Curran-Everett D, Comhair SA et al (2010) Use of exhaled nitric oxide measurement to identify a reactive, at risk phenotype among patients with asthma. Am J Respir Crit Care Med 181:1033–1041

31. Riccio AM, Dal Negro RW, Micheletto C, De Ferrari L, Folli C, Chiappori A et al (2012) Omalizumab modulates bronchial reticular basement membrane thickness and eosinophil infiltration in severe persistent allergic asthma patients. Int J Immunopathol Pharmacol 25:475–484

32. Zietkowski Z, Skiepko R, Tomasiak-Lozowska MM, Bodzenta-Lukaszyk A (2010) Anti-IgE therapy with omalizumab decreases endothelin-1 in exhaled breath condensate of patients with severe persistent allergic asthma. Respiration 80:534–542

33. Zietkowski Z, Skiepko R, Tomasiak-Lozowska MM, Lenczewska D, Bodzenta-Lukaszyk A (2011) RANTES in exhaled breath condensate of patients with severe persistent allergic asthma during omalizumab therapy. Int Arch Allergy Immunol 154:25–32

34. Skiepko R, Ziętkowski Z, Lukaszyk M, Budny W, Skiepko U, Milewski R et al (2014) Changes in blood eosinophilia during omalizumab therapy as a predictor of asthma exacerbation. Postepy Dermatol Alergol 31:305–309

35. Tajiri T, Niimi A, Matsumoto H, Ito I, Oguma T, Otsuka K et al (2014) Comprehensive efficacy of omalizumab for severe refractory asthma: a time-series observational study. Ann Allergy Asthma Immunol 113(470–5):e2

36. Gouder C, West LM, Montefort S (2015) The real-life clinical effects of 52 weeks of omalizumab therapy for severe persistent allergic asthma. Int J Clin Pharm 37:36–43

37. Mauri P, Riccio AM, Rossi R, DiSilvestre D, Benazzi L, DeFerrari L et al (2014) Proteomics of bronchial biopsies: galectin-3 as a predictive biomarker of airway remodelling modulation in omalizumab-treated severe asthma patients. Immunol Lett 162(1 Pt A):2–10

38. Wadsworth S, Sin D, Dorscheid D (2011) Clinical update on the use of biomarkers of airway inflammation in the management of asthma. J Asthma Allergy 4:77–86

39. Eltboli O, Brightling CE (2013) Eosinophils as diagnostic tools in chronic lung disease. Expert Rev Respir Med 7:33–42

40. Szefler SJ, Wenzel S, Brown R, Erzurum SC, Fahy JV, Hamilton RG et al (2012) Asthma outcomes: biomarkers. J Allergy Clin Immunol 129(Suppl):9–23

41. Newby C, Agbetile J, Hargadon B, Monteiro W, Green R, Pavord I et al (2014) Lung function decline and variable airway inflammatory pattern: longitudinal analysis of severe asthma. J Allergy Clin Immunol 134:287–294

42. McGrath KW, Icitovic N, Boushey HA, Lazarus SC, Sutherland ER, Chinchilli VM et al (2012) A large subgroup of mild-to-moderate asthma is persistently noneosinophilic. Am J Respir Crit Care Med 185:612–619

43. Pavord ID, Korn S, Howarth P, Bleecker ER, Buhl R, Keene ON et al (2012) Mepolizumab for severe eosinophilic asthma (DREAM): a multicentre, double-blind, placebo-controlled trial. Lancet 380:651–659

44. Malinovschi A, Fonseca JA, Jacinto T, Alving K, Janson C (2013) Exhaled nitric oxide levels and blood eosinophil counts independently associate with wheeze and asthma events in National Health and Nutrition Examination Survey subjects. J Allergy Clin Immunol 132:821–827

45. Katz LE, Gleich GJ, Hartley BF, Yancey SW, Ortega HG (2014) Blood eosinophil count is a useful biomarker to identify patients with severe eosinophilic asthma. Ann Am Thorac Soc 11:531–536

46. Djukanović R, Wilson SJ, Kraft M, Jarjour NN, Steel M, Chung KF et al (2004) Effects of treatment with anti-immunoglobulin E antibody omalizumab on airway inflammation in allergic asthma. Am J Respir Crit Care Med 170:583–593

47. Hanania NA, Wenzel S, Rosen K, Hsieh HJ, Mosesova S, Choy DF et al (2013) Exploring the effects of Omalizumab in allergic asthma. An analysis of biomarkers in the EXTRA study. Am J Respir Crit Care Med 187:804–811

48. Conroy DM, Williams TJ (2001) Eotaxin and the attraction of eosinophils to the asthmatic lung. Respir Res 2:150–156

49. Zietowski Z, Tomasiek-Lozowska MM, Skiepko R, Zietowska E, Bodzenta-Lukaszyk A (2010) Eotaxin-1 in exhaled breath condensate of stable and unstable asthma patients. Respir Res 11:110

50. Kim CK, Kita H, Callaway Z, Kim HB, Choi J, Fujisawa T et al (2010) The roles of a Th2 cytokine and CC chemokine in children with stable asthma: potential implication in eosinophil degranulation. Pediatr Allergy Immunol 21:e697–e704

51. Wu D, Zhou J, Bi H, Li L, Gao W, Huang M et al (2014) CCL-11 as a potential diagnostic marker for asthma? J Asthma 51:847–854

52. Minshall EM, Leung DY, Martin RJ, Song LY, Cameron L, Ernst P et al (1997) Eosinophil-associated TGF-β1 mRNA expression and airways fibrosis in bronchial asthma. Am J Respir Cell Mol Biol 17:326–333

53. Harrop CA, Gore RB, Evans CM, Thornton DJ, Herrick SE (2013) TGF-ß2 decreases baseline and IL-13-stimulated mucin production by primary human bronchial epithelial cell. Exp Lung Res 39:39–47

54. Al-Alawi M, Hassan T, Chotirmall SH (2014) Transforming growth factor ß and severe asthma: a perfect storm. Respir Med 108:1409–1423

55. Lane C, Knight D, Burgess S, Franklin P, Horak F, Legg J et al (2004) Epithelial inducible nitric oxide synthase activity is the major determinant of nitric oxide concentration in exhaled breath. Thorax 59:757–760

56. Van Den Toorn LM, Overbeek SE, De Jongste JC, Leman K, Hoogsteden HC, Prins JB (2001) Airway inflammation is present during clinical remission of atopic asthma. Am J Respir Crit Care Med 164:2107–2113

57. Dweik RA, Boggs PB, Erzurum SC, Irvin CG, Leigh MW, Lundberg JO et al (2011) on behalf of the American Thoracic Society Committee on Interpretation of Exhaled Nitric Oxide Levels (FeNO) for Clinical Applications. An Official ATS Clinical Practice Guideline: Interpretation of Exhaled Nitric Oxide Levels (FENO) for Clinical Applications. Am J Respir Crit Care Med 184:602–615

58. Yang S, Park J, Lee YK, Kim H, Hahn YS (2015) Association of longitudinal fractional exhaled nitric oxide measurements with asthma control in atopic children. Respir Med 109:572–579

59. Gemicioglu B, Musellim B, Dogan I, Guven K (2014) Fractional exhaled nitric oxide (FeNo) in different asthma phenotypes. Allergy Rhinol 5:157–161

60. Sippel JM, Holden WE, Tilles SA, O'Hollaren M, Cook J, Thukkani N et al (2000) Exhaled nitric oxide levels correlate with measures of disease control in asthma. J Allergy Clin Immunol 106:645–650

61. Peirsman EJ, Carvelli TJ, Hage PY, Hanssens LS, Pattyn L, Raes MM et al (2014) Exhaled nitric oxide in childhood allergic asthma management: a randomised controlled trial. Pediatr Pulmonol 49:624–631

62. Busse WW, Morgan WJ, Gergen PJ, Mitchell HE, Gern JE, Liu AH et al (2011) Randomized trial of omalizumab (anti-IgE) for asthma in inner-city children. N Engl J Med 364:1005–1015

63. Sorkness CA, Wildfire JJ, Calatroni A, Mitchell HE, Busse WW, O'Connor GT et al (2013) Reassessment of omalizumab-dosing strategies and pharmacodynamics in inner-city children and adolescents. J Allergy Clin Immunol Pract 1:163–171

64. Wenzel S, Ford L, Pearlman D, Spector S, Sher L, Skobieranda F et al (2013) Dupilumab in persistent asthma with elevated eosinophil levels. N Engl J Med 368:2455–2466

65. Haldar P, Brightling CE, Hargadon B, Gupta S, Monteiro W, Sousa A et al (2009) Mepolizumab and exacerbations of refractory eosinophilic asthma. N Engl J Med 360:973–984

66. Hamid Q (2003) Gross pathology and hystopatology of asthma. J Allergy Clin Immunol 111:431–432

67. Dent AG, Sutedja TG, Zimmerman PV (2013) Exhaled breath analysis for lung cancer. J Thorac 5:540–550

68. Horváth I, Hunt J, Barnes PJ, Alving K, Antczak A, Baraldi E et al (2005) ATS/ERS Task Force on Exhaled Breath Condensate. Exhaled breath condensate: methodological recommendations and unresolved questions. Eur Respir J 26:523–548

69. Corhay JL, Moermans C, Henket M, Nguyen Dang D, Duysinx B, Louis R (2014) Increased of exhaled breath condensate neutrophil chemotaxis in acute exacerbation of COPD. Respir Res 15:115

70. Schwarz K, Biller H, Windt H, Koch W, Hohlfeld JM (2015) Characterization of exhaled particles from the human lungs in airway obstruction. J Aerosol Med Pulm Drug Deliv 28:52–58

71. Tseliou E, Bessa V, Hillas G, Delimpoura V, Papadaki G, Roussos C et al (2010) Exhaled nitric oxide and exhaled breath condensate pH in severe refractory asthma. Chest 138:107–113

72. Liu L, Teague WG, Erzurum S, Fitzpatrick A, Mantri S, Dweik RA et al (2011) National Heart, Lung, and Blood Institute Severe Asthma Research Program (SARP). Determinants of exhaled breath condensate pH in a large population with asthma. Chest 139:328–336

73. Kazani S, Planaguma A, Ono E, Bonini M, Zahid M, Marigowda G (2013) Exhaled breath condensate eicosanoid levels associate with asthma and its severity. J Allergy Clin Immunol 132:547–553

74. Comhair SA, Erzurum SC (2010) Redox control of asthma: molecular mechanisms and therapeutic opportunities. Antioxid Redox Signal 12:93–124

75. Tomasiak-Lozowska MM, Zietkowski Z, Przeslaw K, Tomasiak M, Skiepko R, Bodzenta-Lukaszyk A (2012) Inflammatory markers and acid-base equilibrium in exhaled breath condensate of stable and unstable asthma patients. Int Arch Allergy Immunol 159:121–129

76. Mattarucchi E, Baraldi E, Guillou C (2012) Metabolomics applied to urine samples in childhood asthma; differentiation between asthma phenotypes and identification of relevant metabolites. Biomed Chromatogr 26:89–94

77. Di Gangi IM, Pirillo P, Carraro S, Gucciardi A, Naturale M, Baraldi E et al (2012) Online trapping and enrichment ultra performance liquid chromatography-tandem mass spectrometry method for sensitive measurement of "arginine-asymmetric dimethylarginine cycle" biomarkers in human exhaled breath condensate. Anal Chim Acta 754:67–74

78. Carraro S, Giordano G, Reniero F, Carpi D, Stocchero M, Sterk PJ et al (2013) Asthma severity in childhood and metabolomic profiling of breath condensate. Allergy 68:110–117

79. Baraldi E, Carraro S, Giordano G, Reniero F, Perilongo G, Zacchello F (2009) Metabolomics: moving towards personalized medicine. Ital J Pediatr 35:30

80. Fitzpatrick AM, Park Y, Brown LA, Jones DP (2014) Children with severe asthma have unique oxidative stress-associated metabolomic profiles. J Allergy Clin Immunol 133:258–261

81. Conway SJ, Izuhara K, Kudo Y, Litvin J, Markwald R, Ouyang G et al (2014) The role of periostin in tissue remodeling across health and disease. Cell Mol Life Sci 71:1279–1288

82. Takayama G, Arima K, Kanaji T, Toda S, Tanaka H, Shoji S et al (2006) Periostin: a novel component of subepithelial fibrosis of bronchial asthma downstream of IL-4 and IL-13 signals. J Allergy Clin Immunol 118:98–104

83. Izuhara K, Arima K, Ohta S, Suzuki S, Inamitsu M, Yamamoto K (2014) Periostin in allergic inflammation. Allergol Int 63:143–151

84. Yuyama N, Davies DE, Akaiwa M, Matsui K, Hamasaki Y, Suminami Y et al (2002) Analysis of novel disease-related genes in bronchial asthma. Cytokine 19:287–296

85. Sidhu SS, Yuan S, Innes AL, Kerr S, Woodruff PG, Hou L et al (2010) Roles of epithelial cell-derived periostin in TFG-beta activation, collagen production, and collagen gel elasticity in asthma. Proc Natl Acad Sci USA 107:14170–14175

86. Blanchard C, Mingler MK, McBride M, Putnam PE, Collins MH, Chang G et al (2008) Periostin facilitated eosinophil tissue infiltration in allergic lung and esophageal responses. Mucosal Immunol 1:289–296

87. Masuoka M, Shiraishi H, Ohta S, Suzuki S, Arima K, Aoki S et al (2012) Periostin promotes chronic allergic inflammation in response to Th2 cytokines. J Clin Invest 122:2590–2600

88. Matsumoto H (2014) Serum periostin: a novel biomarker for asthma management. Allergol Int 63:153–160

89. Jia G, Erickson RW, Choy DF, Mosesova S, Wu LC, Solberg OD et al (2012) Periostin is a systemic biomarker of eosinophilic airway inflammation in asthmatic patients. J Allergy Clin Immunol 130:647–654

90. Kanemitsu Y, Matsumoto H, Izuhara K, Tohda Y, Kita H, Horiguchi T et al (2013) Increased periostin associates with greater airflow limitation in patients receiving inhaled corticosteroids. J Allergy Clin Immunol 132:305–312

91. Parulekar AD, Mustafa AA, Hanania NA (2014) Periostin, a novel biomarker of Th2-driven asthma. Curr Opin Pulm Med 20:60–65

92. Corren J, Lemanske RF, Hanania NA, Korenblat PE, Parsey MV, Arron JR et al (2011) Lebrikizumab treatment in adults with asthma. N Engl J Med 365:1088–1098

93. Bobolea I, Barranco P, Del Pozo V, Romero D, Sanz V, Lopez-Carrasco V et al (2015) Sputum periostin in patients with different severe asthma phenotypes. Allergy. doi:10.1111/all.12580

94. Kou K, Okawa T, Yamaguchi Y, Ono J, Inoue Y, Kohno M et al (2014) Periostin levels correlate with disease severity and chronicity in patients with atopic dermatitis. Br J Dermatol 171:283–291

95. Ohta N, Kurakami K, Ishida A, Furukawa T, Saito F, Kakehata S et al (2012) Clinical and pathological characteristics of IgG4-related sclerosing sialadenitis. Laryngoscope 122:572–577

96. Ishida A, Ohta N, Suzuki Y, Kakehata S, Okubo K, Ikeda H et al (2012) Expression of pendrin and periostin in allergic rhinitis and chronic rhinosinusitis. Allergol Int 61:589–595

97. Nishizawa H, Matsubara A, Nakagawa T, Ohta N, Izuhara K, Shirasaki T et al (2012) The role of periostin in eosinophilic otitis media. Acta Otolaryngol 132:838–844

98. Okamoto M, Hoshino T, Kitasato Y, Sakazaki Y, Kawayama T, Fujimoto K et al (2011) Periostin, a matrix protein, is a novel biomarker for idiopathic interstitial pneumonias. Eur Respir J 37:1119–1127

99. Uchida M, Shiraishi H, Ohta S, Arima K, Taniguchi K, Suzuki S et al (2012) Periostin, a matricellular protein, plays a role in the induction of chemokines in pulmonary fibrosis. Am J Respir Cell Mol Biol 46:677–686

100. Stankovic KM, Goldsztein H, Reh DD, Platt MP, Metson R (2008) Gene expression profiling of nasal polyps associated with chronic sinusitis and aspirin-sensitive asthma. Laryngoscope 118:881–889

101. Fujimoto K, Kawaguchi T, Nakashima O, Ono J, Kawaguchi A, Tonan T et al (2011) Periostin, a matrix protein, has potential as a novel serodiagnostic marker for cholangiocarcinoma. Oncol Rep 25:1211–1216

102. Sirica AE, Almenara JA, Li C (2014) Periostin in intrahepatic cholangiocarcinoma: pathobiological insights and clinical implications. Exp Mol Pathol 97:515–524

103. Zhu M, Fejzo MS, Anderson L, Dering J, Ginther C, Ramos L et al (2010) Periostin promotes ovarian cancer angiogenesis and metastasis. Gynecol Oncol 119:337–344

104. Ryner L, Guan Y, Firestein R, Xiao Y, Choi Y, Rabe C et al (2015) Up-regulation of periostin and reactive stroma is associated with primary chemoresistance and predicts clinical outcomes in epithelial ovarian cancer. Clin Cancer Res. pii: clincanres.3111.2014

105. Xiao ZM, Wang XY, Wang AM (2013) Periostin induces chemoresistance in colon cancer cells through activation of the PI3 K/Akt/survivin pathway. Biotechnol Appl Biochem. doi:10.1002/bab.1193

106. Erkan M, Kleeff J, Gorbachevski A, Reiser C, Mitkus T, Esposito I et al (2007) Periostin creates a tumor-supportive microenvironment in the pancreas by sustaining fibrogenic stellate cell activity. Gastroenterology 132:1447–1464

107. Baril P, Gangeswaran R, Mahon PC, Caulee K, Kocher HM, Harada T et al (2007) Periostin promotes invasiveness and resistance of pancreatic cancer cells to hypoxia-induced cell death: role of the beta4 integrin and the PI3k pathway. Oncogene 26:2082–2094

108. Kotobuki Y, Yang L, Serada S, Tanemura A, Yang F, Nomura S et al (2014) Periostin accelerates human malignant melanoma progression by modifying the melanoma microenviroment. Pigment Cell Melanoma Res 27:630–639

109. Kudo Y, Iizuka S, Yoshida M, Nguyen PT, Siriwardena SB, Tsunematsu T et al (2012) Periostin directly and indirectly promotes tumor lymphangiogenesis of head and neck cancer. PLoS One. doi:10.1371/journal.pone.0044488

110. Zhou W, Ke SQ, Huang Z, Flavahan W, Fang X, Paul J et al (2015) Periostin secreted by glioblastoma stem cells recruits M2 tumor-associated macrophage and promotes malignant growth. Nat Cell Biol 17:170–182

111. Xu D, Xu H, Ren Y, Liu C, Wang X, Zhang H et al (2012) Cancer stem cell-related gene periostin: a novel prognostic marker for breast cancer. PLoS One 7:e46670

112. Takanami I, Abiko T, Koizumi S (2008) Expression of periostin in patients with non-small cell lung cancer: correlation with angiogenesis and lymphangiogenesis. Int J Biol Markers 23:182–186

113. Oku E, Kanaji T, Takata Y, Oshima K, Seki R, Morishige S et al (2008) Periostin and bone marrow fibrosis. Int J Hematol 88:57–63

114. Kashima TG, Nishiyama T, Shimazu K, Shimazaki M, Kii I, Grigoriadis AE et al (2009) Periostin, a novel marker of intramembranous ossification, is expressed in fibrous dysplasia and in c-Fos-overexpressing bone lesions. Hum Pathol 40:226–237

115. Yamaguchi Y, Ono J, Masuoka M, Ohta S, Izuhara K, Ikezawa Z et al (2013) Serum periostin levels are correlated with progressive skin sclerosis on patients with systemic sclerosis. Br J Dermatol 168:717–725

116. Ishikawa K, Yoshida S, Nakao S, Nakama T, Kita T, Asato R et al (2014) Periostin promotes the generation of fibrous membranes in proliferative vitreoretinopathy. FASEB J 28:131–142

117. Arima K, Ohta S, Takagi A, Shiraishi H, Masuoka M, Ontsuka K et al (2015) Periostin contributes to epidermal hyperplasia in psoriasis common to atopic dermatitis. Allergol Int 64:41–48

118. Sen K, Lindermeyer MT, Gaspert A, Eichinger F, Neusser MA, Kretzler M et al (2011) Periostin is induced in glomerular injury and expressed de novo in interstitial renal fibrosis. Am J Pathol 179:1756–1767

119. Bible E (2014) Polycystic kidney disease: Periostin is involved in cell proliferation and interstitial fibrosis in polycystic kidney disease. Nat Rev Nephrol 10:66

120. Wantanasiri P, Satirapoj B, Charoenpitakchai M, Aramwit P (2015) Periostin: a novel tissue biomarker correlates with chronicity index and renal function in lupus nephritis patients. Lupus. pii:0961203314566634

121. Huang Y, Liu W, Xiao H, Maitikabili A, Lin Q, Wu T et al (2015) Matricellular protein periostin contributes to hepatic inflammation and fibrosis. Am J Pathol 185:786–797

122. Zhao S, Wu H, Xia W, Chen X, Zhu S, Zhang S et al (2014) Periostin expression is upregulated and associated with myocardical fibrosis in human failing hearts. J Cardiol 63:373–378

123. Nair P, Kraft M (2012) Serum periostin as a marker of Th2-dependent eosinophilic airway inflammation. J Allergy Clin Immunol 130:655–656

124. Ruan K, Bao S, Ouyang G (2009) The multifaceted role of periostin in tumorigenesis. Cell Mol Life Sci 66:2219–2230

125. Ebrahim AH, Alalawi Z, Mirandola L, Rakhshanda R, Dahlbeck S, Nguyen D et al (2014) Galectins in cancer: carcinogenesis, diagnosis and therapy. Ann Transl Med 2:88

126. Meijers WC, Januzzi JL, DeFilippi C, Adourian AS, Shah SJ, van Veldhuisen DJ et al (2014) Elevated plasma galectin-3 is associated with near-term rehospitalization in heart failure: a pooled analysis of 3 clinical trials. Am Heart J 167:853–860

127. Panjwani N (2014) Role of galectins in re-epithelialization of wounds. Ann Transl Med 2:89

128. Schattner M (2014) Platelets and galectins. Ann Transl Med 2:85

129. Sziksz E, Kozma GT, Pállinger E, Komlósi ZI, Adori C, Kovács L et al (2010) Galectin-9 in allergic airway inflammation and hyper-responsiveness in mice. Int Arch Allergy Immunol 151:308–317

130. Niki T, Tsutsui S, Hirose S, Aradono S, Sugimoto Y, Takeshita K et al (2009) Galectin-9 is a high affinity IgE-binding lectin with anti-allergic effect by blocking IgE-antigen complex formation. J Biol Chem 284:32344–32352

131. Katoh S, Shimizu H, Obase Y, Oomizu S, Niki T, Ikeda M et al (2013) Preventive effect of galectin-9 on double-stranded RNA-induced airway hyperresponsiveness in an exacerbation model of mite antigen-induced asthma in mice. Exp Lung Res 39:453–462

132. Di Lella S, Sundblad V, Cerliani JP, Guardia CM, Estrin DA, Vasta GR et al (2011) When galectins recognize glycans: from biochemistry to physiology and back again. Biochemistry 50:7842–7857

133. Newlaczyl AU, Yu LG (2011) Galectin-3 a jack-of-all-trades in cancer. Cancer Lett 313:123–128

134. Hsu DK, Zuberi RI, Liu FT (1992) Biochemical and biophysical characterization of human recombinant IgE-binding protein, an S-type animal lectin. J Biol Chem 267:14167–14174

135. Zuberi RI, Hsu DK, Kalayci O, Chen HY, Sheldon HK, Yu L et al (2004) Critical role for galectin-3 in airway inflammation and bronchial hyperresponsiveness in a murine model of asthma. Am J Pathol 165:2045–2053

136. López E, del Pozo V, Miguel T, Sastre B, Seoane C, Civantos E et al (2006) Inhibition of chronic airway inflammation and remodeling by galectin-3 gene therapy in a murine model. J Immunol 176:1943–1950

137. Pilette C, Colinet B, Kiss R, André S, Kaltner H, Gabius HJ (2007) Increased galectin-3 expression and intra-epithelial neutrophils in small airways in severe COPD. Eur Respir J 29:914–922

138. Nishi Y, Sano H, Kawashima T, Okada T, Kuroda T, Kikkawa K et al (2007) Role of galectin-3 in human pulmonary fibrosis. Allergol Int 56:57–65

139. Gao P, Gibson PG, Baines KJ, Yang I, Upham JW, Reynolds PN et al (2015) Anti-inflammatory deficiencies in neutrophilic asthma: reduced galectin-3 and IL-1RA/IL-1β. Respir Res 16:5

140. Baines KJ, Simpson JL, Wood LG, Scott RJ, Fibbens NL, Powell H et al (2014) Sputum gene expression signature of 6 biomarkers discriminates asthma inflammatory phenotypes. J Allergy Clin Immunol 133:997–1007

141. George BJ, Reif DM, Gallagher JE, Williams-DeVane CR, Heidenfelder BL, Hudgens EE et al (2015) Data-driven asthma endotypes defined from blood biomarker and gene expression data. PLoS One 10:e0117445

142. Christenson SA, Steiling K, van den Berge M, Hijazi K, Hiemstra PS, Postma DS et al (2015) Asthma-COPD overlap. Clinical relevance of genomic signatures of type 2 inflammation in chronic obstructive pulmonary disease. Am J Respir Crit Care Med 191:758–766

143. Gustafsson M, Nestor CE, Zhang H, Barabási AL, Baranzini S, Brunak S et al (2014) Modules, networks and systems medicine for understanding disease and aiding diagnosis. Genome Med 6:82

7

Pharmacoeconomics of sublingual immunotherapy with the 5-grass pollen tablets for seasonal allergic rhinitis

Carlo Lombardi[1], Valerie Melli[2]* ⓘ, Cristoforo Incorvaia[3] and Erminia Ridolo[2]

Abstract

Allergic rhinitis has a very high burden regarding both direct and indirect costs. This makes essential in the management of AR to reduce the clinical severity of the disease and thus to lessen its costs. This particularly concerns allergen immunotherapy (AIT), that, based on its immunological action on the causes of allergy, extends its benefit also after discontinuation of the treatment. From the pharmacoeconomic point of view, any treatment must be evaluated according to its cost-effectiveness, that is, the ratio between the cost of the intervention and its effect. A favorable cost-benefit ratio for AIT was defined, starting from the first studies in the 1990s on subcutaneous immunotherapy (SCIT) in AR patients, that highlighted a clear advantage on costs over the treatment with symptomatic drugs. Such outcome was confirmed also for sublingual immunotherapy (SLIT), that has also the advantage on SCIT to be free of the cost of the injections. Here we review the available literature on pharmacoeconomic data for SLIT with the 5-grass pollen tablets.

Keywords: Allergic rhinitis, Pharmacoeconomics, Cost-effectiveness, Allergen immunotherapy, Sublingual immunotherapy

Background

The steadily increasing prevalence of allergic disorders, including allergic rhinitis (AR), asthma, and atopic dermatitis, with global figures currently corresponding to more than 20% of the general population [1–4] results in a relevant individual and social economic burden. For example, concerning AR, in a retrospective analysis performed in the 2000s using data from a US health plan covering about 15 million patients, the mean total costs per year related to rhinitis were $657 per patient, the primary contributor being outpatient visits [5]. The economic burden includes direct costs, that are related to drug treatment and visits at physician office, and indirect costs, that are associated to reduced/missed work productivity [6]. In the late 1990s the cost for AR in the US were estimated in $4.5 billion for direct and $3.4 billion for indirect costs, respectively, [7] and by 2005 total expenditures to treat AR reached $11.2 billion [8]. In Europe, a study conducted in 2003 found a mean annual cost of €1089 for child/adolescents and €1543 per adults, respectively, with predominance of indirect costs in adults (about 50%) compared with children (6%), in whom however the estimate did not include school absences [9]. A probabilistic cost of illness study in Italy estimated a global economic burden associated with respiratory allergies and their main co-morbidities of €7.33 billion (95% CI: €5.99–€8.82). A percentage of 27.5% was associated with indirect costs and 72.5% with direct costs [10]. A very recent study from UK on 1000 adults patients with seasonal AR demonstrated that limiting the assessment to absenteeism (on average, 4 days/year) a cost of £1.14 billion/year was estimated [11]. Pharmacoeconomics is the scientific discipline that analyzes the value of different drug therapies, serving to guide the optimal allocation of healthcare resource by standardized and scientifically solid methods [12]. From the pharmacoeconomic point of view, any drug treatment

*Correspondence: valerie.melli@gmail.com
[2] Department of Clinical & Experimental Medicine, University of Parma, Via Gramsci 14, Parma, Italy
Full list of author information is available at the end of the article

must be evaluated according to its cost-effectiveness, the cost referring to the resource expenditure for the intervention, that is usually measured in pecuniary terms [13]. For example, in AR first generation antihistamines may impair mental performances (due to their sedating effects) more than in untreated patients [14] and thus rise indirect cost. By a global therapeutic approach to AR, any preventive strategy that is aimed at reducing the severity of the rhinitis is likely to lessen its costs, and this particularly concerns allergen immunotherapy (AIT).

Cost effectiveness of allergen immunotherapy

Allergen immunotherapy is aimed at reducing the symptoms of allergy by increasing the tolerance to the administered allergen and modifying the natural history of the allergic disease [15]. The first pharmaco-economic studies were conducted in the 1990s in patients treated with subcutaneous immunotherapy (SCIT). Their results, that are summarized in Table 1, were favorable, showing significant reductions of direct and indirect costs. The cost saving reaches its maximum when SCIT is stopped after the recommended 3 years of treatment and continues to work due to the persistent modification of the immunological response to the specific allergen. This was apparent in a study on patients from Italy with AR and asthma induced by sensitization to *Parietaria* pollen, who underwent 3 years of SCIT by a *Parietaria judaica* extract or with symptomatic drugs [19]. The patient were evaluated before SCIT initiation and then each year for a period of 6 years during the pollen period of *Parietaria* by measuring the nose, eye, and lung symptom scores, also registering by diary cards the drug consumption. The data obtained showed a significant difference in favor of SCIT plus drug treatment vs. only drug treatment. The cost reduction was about 15% at the 2nd year and 48% at the 3rd year, when a high statistical significance was detected. This was then maintained until the 6th year, i.e. 3 years after discontinuing SCIT, when the reduction of cost was 80%, with a net saving

corresponding to €623 per year for each patient at the final evaluation.

On the other hand, a recent study showed that the cost-saving may also occur early. In fact, a retrospective analysis based on Florida Medicaid claims estimated the mean 18-month health care cost of 4967 patients with newly diagnosed AR who were treated for the first time with SCIT compared with 19,278 control subjects treated only with drugs [24]. In SCIT-treated patients a mean 18-month total health care cost of $6637 was calculated, compared with $10,644 in controls (38% lower in SCIT-treated, P < 0.0001). Significant savings were detected within 3 months from starting SCIT, with no significant difference between the savings observed in SCIT-treated adults and SCIT-treated children ($4397 vs. $3965). The fact that the more recently introduced sublingual immunotherapy (SLIT) is performed by patients at home and thus is free of the cost of injections suggests that the cost-effectiveness of SLIT may be even better than SCIT.

Studies on sublingual immunotherapy

The first study, that involved one Allergy center in Italy, evaluated the cost effectiveness of SLIT in pediatric patients with respiratory allergy [25]. A group of 135 children with AR and asthma was studied, the data concerned 1-year prior to receive SLIT and 3-year after starting SLIT. The outcome measures were the number of disease exacerbations, visits, and missed nursery or school days, including direct and indirect costs. Forty-six patients had perennial allergy and 89 had seasonal allergy. All outcome measures showed a considerable reduction during SLIT compared to the previous 1-year period. The annual cost/patient averaged to €2672 before starting SLIT and to €629/year during SLIT, with comparable results for allergen subgroups. These findings suggested that SLIT was able to reduce the global cost of AR. Such outcome was confirmed in a number of subsequent studies, that were reviewed in 2008 by Berto et al. [26] In particular, a study performed in patients with AR from

Table 1 Studies on pharmacoeconomics of subcutaneous immunotherapy

Author (year)	Patients	Allergen	Study duration (years)	Results
Buchner (1995) [16]	Adults	Pollen, mites	10	−54% costs for symptomatic treatment
Schadlich (2000) [17]	Adults	Pollen, mites	10	€332-608 saving per patient
Petersen (2005) [18]	Adults	Pollen	4	€203 saving per patient
Ariano (2006) [19]	Adults	Pollen	6	48% money saving at year 4
Omnes (2007) [20]	Adults & children	Pollen, mites	6	€1327 saving per patient for pollen, €393 for mites
Hankin (2008) [21]	Children	Pollen, mites	1.5	€308 6-month saving per patient
Hankin (2010) [22]	Children	Pollen, mites	1.5	−34% total healthcare cost per patient
Wang (2011) [23]	Adults	Pollen, mites	1.5	−41% total healthcare cost per patient

Czech Republic compared directly the treatment with the two forms of AIT (SCIT and SLIT) and only drug treatment for 3 years. The mean direct cost per patient was estimated in €482 for SCIT and €416 for SLIT, a SLIT-treated patient paying more than a SCIT-treated patient for allergen extracts (€72 vs. €55) but paying less for out-of-pocket costs (€176 vs. €255). The figure of direct and indirect costs over the 3-year treatment was €1004 for SCIT and €684 for SLIT [27].

Studies on the 5-grass pollen tablets

The 5-grass pollen tablets, that contain pollen extracts from Pooideae family (*Anthoxanthum odoratum, Poa pratensis, Dactylis glomerata, Phleum pratense,* and *Lolium perenne*) were approved and registered, based on regulatory large trials that fulfilled all requirements by the European Medicine Agency (EMA) in Europe and Food and Drug Administration (FDA) in the US [28–30]. The 5-grass pollens tablets were accepted for full reimbursement by the Agenzia Italiana del Farmaco (AIFA) [31], with the indication for AR and/or conjunctivitis treatment in adult or pediatric patients (over 5 years) with severe symptoms, by a pre-co-seasonal course of administration. The first study on the cost-effectiveness of 5-grass tablets was conducted by Ruggeri et al., based on post hoc analysis of the VO34.04 and VO53.06 trials [28, 29]. The economic data from the perspective of Italian third-party payer, as well as a societal perspective based on the costs related to the losses of productivity were analyzed [32]. Medication effectiveness was assessed using as main outcome parameter the Quality Adjusted Life Years (QALYs), that is a multi-attribute scale generating a single numeric index of health-related Quality of life (Qol) of patients ranging from 0 (death) to 1 (perfect health). A decision tree modeling the likely outcomes and costs for adults and children with a low, medium, and high score of allergic symptoms was used. Compared to placebo, the 5-grass tablet treatment resulted in 0.127 QALYs in patients with moderate allergic symptoms and in 0.143 QALYs in patients with severe symptoms. The 5-grass pollen tablet treatment had a cost of €1024/QALY for patients with moderate symptoms and €1035/QALY for those with severe symptoms. The authors concluded that, based on the cost-effectiveness for adult patients with moderate to severe AR, the 5-grass tablet should be carefully considered when choosing the management strategy for AR [32]. An investigation conducted in Germany on the outcomes, costs and cost-effectiveness compared the 5-grass tablets to the one-grass tablet and the one-grass extract for subcutaneous injection, using as control the drug treatment alone for grass pollen-induced AR. A Markov model was used to assess the costs and outcomes of a 3-year treatment for a period of

9 years, estimating the treatment efficacy by an indirect comparison of published clinical trials on grass pollen immunotherapy with placebo. The analysis included both public and private health insurance payments. Outcomes were reported as QALYs and symptom-free days. The 5-grass tablet had a predicted cost-utility ratio vs. drug treatment of €14,728 per QALY, with incremental costs corresponding to €1356 and incremental QALYs to 0.092. SLIT with the 5-grass tablet was the prevailing strategy compared to one-grass tablet and SCIT, with incremental costs estimated in −€1142 and −€54 and incremental QALYs estimated in 0.015 and 0.027, respectively. Even though the indirect comparison involving several steps to assess the treatment effects was a limitation, the study suggested that the 5-grass tablet was cost-effective compared to one-grass tablet and injective immunotherapy [33]. In a recent study, the same authors compared, by reviewing the literature and performing meta-analysis and cost-effectiveness analysis the effects and costs of the 5-grass tablet vs. a mix of allergoids for SCIT in grass pollen allergic rhinoconjunctivitis. As for the previous study, a Markov model with a 9 year time length was used to assess the costs and effects of a 3-year-long treatment. Drug acquisition and medical costs, estimates for use of the resources, persistence of AIT and asthma occurrence were obtained from published sources. The analysis was performed from the payer's perspective in Germany, that includes payments of NHS and additional payments by insurants. A cost-utility ratio of the 5-grass tablet vs. the mix of injectable allergoids of €12,593 per QALY was observed, with predicted incremental costs and QALYs corresponding to €458 and 0.036, respectively. The probability of the 5-grass tablet to be the most cost-effective treatment option was estimated in 76% at a willingness-to-pay threshold of €20,000. These data confirmed the cost-effectiveness of the 5-grass tablet also over SCIT with a mix of allergoids [34].

Conclusions

In times when a rigid control of expenditures for NHSs is needed, the cost-effectiveness of medical treatments is of paramount importance. Among treatment options for AR, AIT (that includes SCIT and SLIT) has exclusive features, that include the ability to alter the natural history of allergy and to extend its effectiveness, differently from drug treatment, to several years after discontinuing the therapy. A growing bulk of data indicates that SCIT and SLIT may be very advantageous to the healthcare systems [35–38]. However, the pharmacoeconomic advantage demonstrated in optimally performed studies needs to be confirmed by real-life experiences. In fact, in the latest years data showing a poor adherence to long-term SLIT, with a minority of patients completing the recommended 3 years of treatment duration, [39] makes unlikely that the cost effectiveness is achieved when SLIT is abandoned before reaching a duration able to extend the benefit on symptoms and use of drugs over time. This issue needs to be considered by all specialists concerned in this treatment.

Abbreviations

AR: allergic rhinitis; AIT: allergen immunotherapy; SCIT: subcutaneous immunotherapy; SLIT: sublingual immunotherapy; EMA: European Medicine Agency; FDA: Food and Drug Administration; AIFA: Agenzia Italiana del Farmaco; QALYs: Quality Adjusted Life Years; QoL: quality of life; AS: allergic symptoms; NHS: National Health System.

Authors' contributions

CI and CL wrote and coordinated the draft of the manuscript. VM and ER carried out the bibliographic search, contributed to the draft of the manuscript and made substantial contribution to the revision of the article. All authors read and approved the final manuscript.

Author details

[1] Allergy and Pneumology Departmental Unit, Fondazione Poliambulanza Hospital, Brescia, Italy. [2] Department of Clinical & Experimental Medicine, University of Parma, Via Gramsci 14, Parma, Italy. [3] Pulmonary Rehabilitation, Centro Specialistico Gaetano Pini/CTO, Milan, Italy.

References

1. The International Study of Asthma and Allergies in Childhood (ISAAC). Steering Committee. Worldwide variation in prevalence of symptoms of asthma, allergic rhino conjunctivitis, and atopic eczema. Lancet. 1998;351:1225–32.
2. Sly RM. Changing prevalence of allergic rhinitis and asthma. Ann Allergy Asthma Immunol. 1999;82:233–48.
3. Upton MN, McConnachie A, McSharry C, et al. Intergenerational 20 year trends in the prevalence of asthma and hay fever in adults: the Midspan family study survey of parents and offspring. BMJ. 2000;321:88–92.
4. Linneberg A, Nielsen NH, Madsen F, et al. Increasing prevalence of specific IgE to aeroallergens in an adult population: two cross-sectional studies 8 years apart; the Copenhagen Allergy Study. J Allergy Clin Immunol. 2000;106:247–52.
5. Dalal AA, Stanford R, Henry H, et al. Economic burden of rhinitis in managed care: a retrospective claims data analysis. Ann Allergy Asthma Immunol. 2008;101:23–9.
6. Reed SD, Lee TA, McCrory DC. The economic burden of allergic rhinitis. Pharmacoeconomics. 2004;22:345–61.
7. Mackowiak JI. The health and economic impact of rhinitis. Am J Manag Care. 1997;3:S8–18.
8. Medical expenditure panel survey. Statistical brief #204: allergic rhinitis: trends in use and expenditures, 2000 and 2005. 2008. http://www.meps. ahrq.gov/mepsweb/data_files/publications/st204/stat204.pdf.
9. Schramm B, Ehlken B, Smala A, et al. Cost of illness of atopic asthma and seasonal allergic rhinitis in Germany: 1-year retrospective study. Eur Respir J. 2003;21:116–22.
10. Marcellusi A, Viti R, Incorvaia C, et al. Direct and indirect costs associated with respiratory allergic diseases in Italy. A probabilistic cost of illness study. Recenti Prog Med. 2015;106:517–27.
11. Price D, Scadding G, Ryan D, et al. The hidden burden of adult allergy rhinitis: UK healthcare resource utilisation survey. Clin Transl Allergy. 2015;5:39.
12. Arnold RJG, Ekins S. Time for cooperation in health economics among the modelling community. Pharmacoeconomics. 2010;28:609–13.
13. Bleichrodt H, Quiggin J. Life-cycle preferences over consumption and health: when is cost-effectiveness analysis equivalent to cost-benefit analysis? J Health Econ. 1999;18:681–708.
14. Vuurman EF, van Veggel LM, Uitenwijk MM, et al. Seasonal allergic rhinitis and antihistamine effect on children's learning. Ann Allergy. 1993;71:121–6.
15. Bousquet J, Lockey RF, Malling HJ. WHO Position Paper. Allergen immunotherapy: therapeutic vaccines for allergic diseases. Allergy. 1998;53(Suppl 44):4–30.
16. Buchner K, Siepe M. Nutzen der Hyposensibilierung unter wirtschaftlichen Aspekten. Allergo J. 1995;4:156–63.
17. Schadlich PK, Brecht JG. Economic evaluation of specific immunotherapy versus symptomatic treatment of allergic rhinitis in Germany. Pharmacoeconomics. 2000;17:37–52.
18. Petersen KD, Gyrd-Hansen D, Dahl R. Health-economic analyses of subcutaneous specific immunotherapy for grass pollen and mite allergy. Allergol Immunopathol. 2005;33:296–302.
19. Ariano R, Berto P, Tracci D, et al. Pharmacoeconomics of allergen immunotherapy compared with symptomatic drug treatment in patients with allergic rhinitis and asthma. Allergy Asthma Proc. 2006;27:159–63.
20. Omnes LF, Bousquet J, Scheinmann P, et al. Pharmacoeconomic assessment of specific immunotherapy versus current symptomatic treatment for allergic rhinitis and asthma in France. Eur Ann Allergy Clin Immunol. 2007;39:148–56.
21. Hankin C, Cox L, Lang D, et al. Allergy immunotherapy among Medicaid-enrolled children with allergic rhinitis: patterns of care, resource use, and costs. J Allergy Clin Immunol. 2008;121:227–32.
22. Hankin C, Cox L, Lang D, et al. Allergen immunotherapy and health care cost benefits for children with allergic rhinitis: a large-scale, retrospective, matched cohort study. Ann Allergy Asthma Immunol. 2010;104:79–85.
23. Wang Z, Hankin CS, Cox L, Bronstone A. Allergen immunotherapy significantly reduces healthcare costs among US adults with allergic rhinitis: a retrospective matched cohort study jointly funded by the AAAAI and ACAAI. J Allergy Clin Immunol. 2011;127(2):150.
24. Hankin CS, Cox L, Bronstone A, et al. Allergy immunotherapy: reduced health care costs in adults and children with allergic rhinitis. J Allergy Clin Immunol. 2013;131:1084–91.
25. Berto P, Bassi M, Incorvaia C, et al. Cost effectiveness of sublingual immunotherapy in children with allergic rhinitis and asthma. Eur Ann Allergy Clin Immunol. 2005;37:303–8.
26. Berto P, Frati F, Incorvaia C. Economic studies of immunotherapy: a review. Curr Opin Allergy Clin Immunol. 2008;8:585–9.
27. Podladnikova J, Krcmova I, Vlcek J. Economic evaluation of sublingual vs. subcutaneous allergen immunotherapy. Ann Allergy Asthma Immunol. 2008;100:482–9.
28. Didier A, Malling HJ, Worm M, et al. Optimal dose, effectiveness, and safety of once-daily sublingual immunotherapy with a 5-grass pollen tablet for seasonal allergic rhinitis. J Allergy Clin Immunol. 2007;120:1338–45.
29. Didier A, Worm M, Horak F, et al. Sustained-3-year effectiveness of pre- and co-seasonal 5-grass pollen sublingual immunotherapy tablets in patients with grass pollen-induced rhinoconjunctivitis. J Allergy Clin Immunol. 2011;128:559–66.
30. Cox LS, Casale TB, Nayak AS, et al. Clinical efficacy of 300IR 5-grass pollen sublingual tablet in a US study: the importance of allergen-specific serum IgE. J Allergy Clin Immunol. 2012;130:1327–34.
31. Ciprandi G. A major step forward for sublingual immunotherapy: the quality of 5-grass pollen tablets is recognized also in Italy. J Asthma Allergy. 2015;8:25–7.
32. Ruggeri M, Oradei M, Frati F, Puccinelli P, et al. Economic evaluation of 5-grass pollen tablets versus placebo in the treatment of allergic rhinitis in adults. Clin Drug Investig. 2013;33:343–9.
33. Westerhout KY, Verheggen BG, Schreder CH, et al. Cost effectiveness analysis of immunotherapy in patients with grass pollen allergic rhinoconjunctivitis in Germany. J Med Econ. 2012;15:906–17.
34. Verheggen BG, Westerhout KY, Schreder CH, et al. Health economic comparison of SLIT allergen and SCIT allergoid immunotherapy in patients with seasonal grass-allergic rhinoconjunctivitis in Germany. Clin Transl Allergy. 2015;5:1.
35. Bachert C, Noergaard Andreasen J. Cost-effectiveness of immunotherapy in the treatment of seasonal allergic rhinitis: identifying product-specific parameters of relevance for health care decision-makers and clinicians. Int Arch Allergy Immunol. 2015;168:213–7.

36. French C, Seiberling K. Comparative costs of subcutaneous and sublingual immunotherapy. Curr Opin Otolaryngol Head Neck Surg. 2015;23:226–9.

37. Cox L. Allergy immunotherapy in reducing healthcare cost. Curr Opin Otolaryngol Head Neck Surg. 2015;23:247–54.

38. Rønborg S, Johnsen CR, Theilgaard S, et al. Cost-minimization analysis of sublingual immunotherapy versus subcutaneous immunotherapy for house dust mite respiratory allergic disease in Denmark. J Med Econ. 2016;19:735–41.

39. Incorvaia C, Mauro M, Leo G, et al. Adherence to sublingual immunotherapy. Curr Allergy Asthma Rep. 2016;16:12.

8

Quality of life in patients with food allergy

Darío Antolín-Amérigo[1]*, Luis Manso[2], Marco Caminati[3], Belén de la Hoz Caballer[4], Inmaculada Cerecedo[5], Alfonso Muriel[6], Mercedes Rodríguez-Rodríguez[1], José Barbarroja-Escudero[1], María José Sánchez-González[1], Beatriz Huertas-Barbudo[2] and Melchor Alvarez-Mon[1]

Abstract

Food allergy has increased in developed countries and can have a dramatic effect on quality of life, so as to provoke fatal reactions. We aimed to outline the socioeconomic impact that food allergy exerts in this kind of patients by performing a complete review of the literature and also describing the factors that may influence, to a greater extent, the quality of life of patients with food allergy and analyzing the different questionnaires available. Hitherto, strict avoidance of the culprit food(s) and use of emergency medications are the pillars to manage this condition. Promising approaches such as specific oral or epicutaneous immunotherapy and the use of monoclonal antibodies are progressively being investigated worldwide. However, even that an increasing number of centers fulfill those approaches, they are not fully implemented enough in clinical practice. The mean annual cost of health care has been estimated in international dollars (I$) 2016 for food-allergic adults and I$1089 for controls, a difference of I$927 (95 % confidence interval I$324–I$1530). A similar result was found for adults in each country, and for children, and interestingly, it was not sensitive to baseline demographic differences. Cost was significantly related to severity of illness in cases in nine countries. The constant threat of exposure, need for vigilance and expectation of outcome can have a tremendous impact on quality of life. Several studies have analyzed the impact of food allergy on health-related quality of life (HRQL) in adults and children in different countries. There have been described different factors that could modify HRQL in food allergic patients, the most important of them are perceived disease severity, age of the patient, peanut or soy allergy, country of origin and having allergy to two or more foods. Over the last few years, several different specific Quality of Life questionnaires for food allergic patients have been developed and translated to different languages and cultures. It is important to perform lingual and cultural translations of existent questionnaires in order to ensure its suitability in a specific region or country with its own socioeconomic reality and culture. Tools aimed at assessing the impact of food allergy on HRQL should be always part of the diagnostic work up, in order to provide a complete basal assessment, to highlight target of intervention as well as to evaluate the effectiveness of interventions designed to cure food allergy. HRQL may be the only meaningful outcome measure available for food allergy measuring this continuous burden.

Keywords: Quality of life, Food allergy, Questionnaire, Specific questionnaire, Health-related quality of life (HRQL), Anaphylaxis

Background

Food allergy (FA) has increased in developed countries and can have a dramatic effect on quality of life, so as to provoke fatal reactions [1–4]. We aimed to outline the socioeconomic impact that food allergy exerts in this kind of patients, by performing a complete review of the literature and also describing the factors that may influence, to a greater extent, the quality of life (QoL) of patients with food allergy. Moreover, the impairment in QoL may differ depending on the age, and as several specific questionnaires have been developed, we sought to describe into detail the different questionnaires available

*Correspondence: dario.antolin@gmail.com
[1] Servicio de Enfermedades del Sistema Inmune-Alergia, Hospital Universitario Príncipe de Asturias. Departamento de Medicina y Especialidades Médicas, Universidad de Alcalá, Carretera de Alcalá-Meco s/n, 28085 Alcalá de Henares, Madrid, Spain
Full list of author information is available at the end of the article

(Tables 1, 2, 3). Besides, as the terminology used with regards QoL is concrete and presumably complex, we wanted to clarify it, providing succinct definitions, for the sake of clarity (Table 4).

Hitherto, strict avoidance of the culprit food(s) and the use of emergency medications are the pillars to manage this condition [3, 5]. Promising approaches such as specific oral or epicutaneous immunotherapy and the use of monoclonal antibodies are progressively being investigated worldwide. However, even that an increasing number of centers fulfill those approaches, they are not fully implemented enough in clinical practice.

The fact that neither the time of onset nor the intensity of the reaction is predictable can significantly influence QoL. Likewise, uncertainty when reading the ingredients and trace elements included in the food labelling on packaged food products may be bothersome for food allergic patients and their relatives [6]. The constant threat of exposure, need for vigilance and expectation of outcome can have a tremendous impact on their QoL [7, 8]. Several studies have analyzed the impact of FA on health-related quality of life (HRQL) in adults and children in different countries [7–11] (Tables 1, 2).

Review
Quality of life in children with food allergy
One of the most important issues about QoL in FA is to describe different predictors that shall contribute to modify HRQL. Identification of these predictors which have potential to decrease the patients' HRQL could improve allergic patients by means of implementing adequate and specific approaches. [11] (Table 3).

In addition, we have to mention that a proven diagnosis of FA does not seem to be an independent predictor of HRQL, when compared to self-reported or perceived FA [11]. Although, HRQL in caregivers is heterogeneous and worse in those that are not followed-up at a FA referral clinic, in a tertiary center [12]. It has been stated that parents report a lower impact on HRQL than their allergic children (considering a similar perception of the allergy severity) [13]. In this line, it has been observed that, caregivers without food-allergic children may have different coping strategies than caregivers with FA children, revealing the importance of providing specific FA education to caregivers [14].

An elegant multicenter, multinational study describes several predictors of health-related QoL in European children [15]. Perceived disease severity, having a peanut or soy allergy, and the country of origin should be considered as contributors of the variance in HRQL (Table 3). Likewise, children with more than two food allergies had lower values of QoL scores compared with those with one or two food allergies [16]. Additionally, it has been observed that older children, the ones with severe systemic reactions, or those with mothers or siblings also affected by allergies, as well as girls, and children with multiple food allergies showed worse QoL scores [17].

Oral immunotherapy for different foods has been found to result in HRQL improvement, at least in participants with peanut or cow milk allergy [18, 19]. It has also been observed in a study comprising food-allergic children, where multiple-oral immunotherapies led to improvement in caregiver HRQL [20].

HRQL in food-allergic patients should be measured to have a global assessment of these patients, and for this reason specific questionnaires have been developed in recent times (Tables 1, 2), to be completed by parents [21, 22], but some of them also by children [23, 24]. These questionnaires should be short and easy to complete, to become both a useful and a suitable tool for evaluation of patients with food allergy.

One of the most used food allergy-related QoL questionnaires in children is probably the *Food Allergy Quality of Life Questionnaire (FAQLQ)*, which was developed and validated in Europe as a part of the EuroPrevall Project. These questionnaires include versions for children from 0 to 18 years old and for their parents [25]. But there are also other questionnaires that could be employed, for example the *Food Allergy Quality of Life–Parental Burden (FAQL-PB) Questionnaire* [26] developed in the US or the *Food Allergy Self-Efficacy scale for Parents (FASE-P)* that have been proved to be useful to identify areas where parents have less confidence in managing their child's FA [22]. All these questionnaires have demonstrated good internal consistency (measured as Cronbach's α), as well as good correlation with other generic and FA QoL questionnaires (Table 4).

It is important to perform lingual and cultural translations of existent questionnaires in order to ensure their suitability in a specific region or country, with its own socioeconomic reality and culture [27–29].

Briefly, for children there are general food questionnaire items that impair QoL to a greater extent, namely, "able to eat fewer products" and "always be alert as to what you are eating", included in Allergen Avoidance and Dietary Restrictions domain; and the item "change of ingredients of a product" related with Risk of Accidental Exposure domain. The *FAQLQ-PF* showed that psychosocial impact in food-allergic children exerted a severe impact of on HRQL, due to the anxiety about food issues and the risk of a potential reaction [21] (Table 1).

Quality of Life in Teenagers with Food Allergy
It is estimated that around 2 % of adolescents suffer from FA [30]. In healthy individuals the adolescence is a very critical time, characterized by accelerated growth

Table 1 Children/adolescents food allergy specific QoL questionnaires

Questionnaire	#Items	Domains/covered issues	Age	Completed by	Result	Reliability	Validity	Patients included in development	References
Food allergy quality of life-parental burden (FAQL-PB)	17	Family, school and social events, time employed to prepare foods, physical and mental state	0–17	Parents	parents whose children had multiple (>2) food allergies were more affected than parents whose children had fewer allergies	Internal consistency (test–retest)	Internal: inter-item correlations; external: criterion validity, construct, content	Yes	Cohen et al., USA [26]
Food allergy impact scale (FAIS)	32	Family and social events, field trips, parties, sleepovers and playing at friends' houses	0–18	Parents	Daily family life (Meal preparation and family social activities)	Internal consistency (test–retest)	Internal: not proven; external: content, face validity	Yes	Bollinger et al., USA [55]
Food allergy parent questionnaire (FAPQ)	18	Parental anxiety/distress, psychosocial impact of allergies, parental coping/ competence, and family support	0–18	Parents	Greater number of food allergies, positive history of anaphylaxis: higher scores on the anxiety/distress and psychosocial impact subscales. Internal consistency good for the anxiety/distress and psychosocial impact subscales	Internal consistency (test–retest)	Internal: factor analysis; external: face-validity, content	No	LeBovidge et al., USA [56]
Child health questionnaire parental form–28 (CHQ-PF 28)	28	Issues related to children, parents and family	9	Parents	Lower scores for physical functioning and role/social limitations	Not proven	Not proven	Yes	Östblom et al., Sweden [57]
Food allergy self-efficacy scale for parents (FASE-P)	21	Managing Social activities precaution and prevention. Allergic treatment food allergen identification seeking information about food allergy	0–18	Parents	Poorer self-efficacy was related to egg and milk allergy; self-efficacy was not related to severity of allergy	Internal consistency	External: discriminative, face-validity, construct, convergent	Yes	Knibb et al., UK [22]
Pediatric allergic disease quality of life questionnaire (PADQLQ)	26	Practical problems, symptoms, emotional problems	6–16	Children	A potentially useful outcome measure in the evaluation of systemic treatments in children with multisystem allergic disease	Internal consistency	Internal: inter item-correlations; external: construct, longitudinal	Yes	Roberts et al., UK [58]

Table 1 continued

Questionnaire	#Items	Domains/covered issues	Age	Completed by	Result	Reliability	Validity	Patients included in development	References
Food allergy quality of life questionnaire-parent form (FAQLQ-PF)	30	Emotional impact; food-related anxiety; dietary and social restrictions	0–12	Parents	Domains and total score improved significantly at pos-challenge time-points for pre-challenge and post-challenge. Poorer quality of life at baseline increased the odds by over 2.0 of no improvement in HRQL scores 6-month time-point	Internal consistency (test–retest)	Internal: inter-item correlations, factor analysis, ceiling/floor effect; external: face-validity, content, convergent/discriminative, construct	Yes	DunnGalvin et al., Ireland [21]
Food allergy quality of life question-naire-child form (FAQLQ-CF)	24	Allergen avoidance and dietary restrictions; emotional impact; risk of accidental exposure;	8–12	Children	Discriminated between children who differed in number of food allergies (>2 food allergies) vs. < or = 2 food allergies	Internal consistency (test–retest)	Internal: inter-item correlations; external: face-validity, content, convergent/discriminative, construct	Yes	Flokstra-de Blok et al., The Netherlands [24]
Food allergy quality of life question-naire-teenager form (FAQLQ-TF)	23	Allergen avoidance and dietary restrictions; emotional impact; risk of accidental exposure;	13–17	Children	Discriminated between children who differed in number of food allergies (>2 food allergies) vs. < or = 2 food allergies	Internal consistency (test–retest)	Internal: inter-item correlations; external: face-validity, content, convergent/discriminative, construct	Yes	Flokstra-Blok et al., The Netherlands [23]
Food allergy quality of life assessment tool for adolescents (FAQL-teen)	17	Impact of food allergy-related limitations, perception of food allergy as a burden; fear for allergic reactions; disappointment for carrying the adrenaline auto-injector	13–19	Children	Areas most troubling included limitations on social activities, not being able to eat what others were eating, and limited choice of restaurants	Internal consistency	External: face-validity, discriminative, Cross-sectional construct validity	Yes	Resnick et al., USA [39]
You and your food allergy	34	Social well-being and independence, support, day-to-day activities, family relations and emotional well-being	13–18	Children	Discriminates by disease severity	Internal consistency (test–retest)	Internal: inter-item correlations; external: convergent/discriminative, construct	Yes	MacKenzie et al., UK [40]

Table 2 Adult food allergy specific questionnaires

Questionnaire	#Items	Domains	Age	Completed by	Result	Reliability	Validity	Patients included in development	References
Food allergy quality of life questionnaire-adult form (FAQLQ-AF)	29	Allergen avoidance and dietary restrictions; emotional impact; risk of accidental exposure; Food allergy related health	≥18	Adults	Discriminated between patients who differ in severity of symptoms (anaphylaxis vs no anaphylaxis), and number of food allergies (>3 food allergies vs < or = 3 food)	Internal consistency (test–retest)	Internal: correlations interitem. External: face, content, convergent/discriminative, construct	Yes	Flokstra-de Blok et al., The Netherlands [41]
Food allergy quality of life questionnaire-adult form spanish version (FAQLQ-AF)	29	Allergen avoidance and dietary restrictions; emotional impact; risk of accidental exposure; food allergy related health	≥18	Adults	>3 foods = greater impact on QoL excellent internal consistency (Cronbach α, 0.95). S-FAQLQ-AF domains also had excellent internal consistency: α = 0.93 for allergen avoidance-dietary restrictions; α = 0.83 for emotional impact; α = 0.85 for risk of accidental exposure, and α = 0.66 for food allergy related health	Internal consistency (test–retest)	Internal: correlations inter-items. External: face, content, convergent/discriminative, construct	Yes	Antolin-Amerigo et al., Spain [42]
Food allergy quality of life questionnaire-adult form swedish version (FAQLQ-AF)	29	Allergen avoidance and dietary restrictions; emotional impact; risk of accidental exposure; food allergy related health	≥18	Adults	O gender differences Allergen avoidance and Dietary Restrictions (AADR) highest HRQL) number of food items to avoid did not influence QoL	Internal consistency (test–retest)	Internal: correlations interitem. External: face, content, convergent/discriminative, construct	Yes	Jansson SA et al., Sweden [59]

Table 3 Factors with statistical significance that affect QoL in Fa

#	Factor	Article	Reference
1	Constant vigilance in the avoidance of specific foods to prevent an allergic reaction	Carrard et al.	[60]
2	Management of an acute reaction	Carrard et al.	[60]
3	Experience of anaphylaxis has a limited impact in QoL	Saleh-Langenberg et al.	[15, 36]
4	Allergies to fish and milk in adults and peanuts and soy in children caused greater HRQL impairment as compared to other foods	Saleh-Langenberg et al.	[15, 36]
5	Performing food challenge improved QoL irrespective of the outcome of the challenge (waines after 6 months in allergic patients)	Soller et al.	[49]
6	Perceived disease severity	Saleh-Langenberg et al.	[15, 36]
7	Country of origin	Saleh-Langenberg et al.	[15, 36]
8	Children >2 allergies	Sicherer et al.	[3]
9	Older children and those with mother or siblings affected by allergies	Wassenberg et al.	[17]
10	Oral induction of Tolerance (OIT) with peanut or cow milk: improves QoL	Factor JM et al., Carraro S et al.	[18, 19]

and tremendous physiological, neurocognitive and emotional changes. In this context, chronic diseases like FA can have an even higher impact on the individual's development and future wellbeing. Social isolation, depression, difficulties in school performance and leisure activities have been reported by food allergic adolescents as a result of their disease, along with the fear of allergic reactions [31–33]. On the other side, it is well known that a kind of incorrect belief of lack of risk leads teenagers to underestimate the severity of FA, as they think they will not die from any cause. It might result in risk-taking behaviours that can increase the risk of dying from FA [32, 34]. One of the major consequences is the reluctance to carry an epinephrine auto-injector, because the treatment is considered burdensome or simply not needed [35, 36]. According to recent data, the perceived burden of treatment is not directly associated with the overall HRQL, disease severity or trait anxiety, but it does significantly affect the non-compliance attitude towards epinephrine auto-injector and food restrictions [36]. Furthermore, a significant disagreement on health-related quality of life, mainly associated with adolescents' rather than parents' perceptions and characteristics, has been highlighted between parents and affected teenagers. Parents may not recognize the social impact of food restrictions or annoyance at having to carry self-injectable adrenaline [31, 37].

Up to now three tools for assessing HRQL in food allergic adolescents have been validated and can be used as reliable tool in daily clinical practice (Table 1).

It has been observed that UK and US teenagers, but not the Dutch ones, consider of primary importance the impact of FA on their social activities. US adolescents perceive their FA as a burden to others, but UK and Dutch teenagers do not confirm it. Dutch adolescents only experience the risk of accidental exposure as a concern. Support in managing FA is highly considered by UK teenagers but it does not appear to be the case for the Dutch and US ones [23, 38–40]. For these reasons the development of country-specific tools for assessing FA-related QoL should be one of the priorities in the FA management.

Quality of life in adults with food allergy

Studies on food-allergic adult patients assessing QoL are scarce [41, 42] and the impact could be influenced by the fact that patients who have sought for medical help could have a worse QoL than those who have not actively looked for medical assessment [42, 43] (Table 2).

The *Food Allergy Quality of Life Questionnaire-Adult Form* (FAQLQ-AF) showed that uncertainty and anxiety seem to account for the greatest impact on HRQL in European food-allergic adults [7, 41, 42] (Table 2). Notwithstanding, both uncertainty and anxiety decreased in patients who underwent a double-blinded, placebo-controlled food challenge in the Netherlands [44].

The FAQLQ-AF is available for adults and was developed and validated in the context of the EuroPrevall Project, a multicenter European FA research project which objectives include analyzing the impact of food allergies on quality of life. It is currently available in several European languages [7–9, 41, 42] (Table 2).

Construct validity of the FAQLQ-AF was assessed in patients from eight European countries, resulting as strong to very strong (Fig. 1). Moreover, internal consistency was excellent in all eight countries. A very interesting finding was that participants from eight European countries did not have comparable HRQL (as measured with total FAQLQ-AF scores). This result reinforces the value of the instrument, as it proves its sensitivity for differences in HRQL between populations with different socio-economic backgrounds [7] (Table 2).

Table 4 QoL terminology [38, 41]

Concept	Definition	Concept	Definition
Reliability	Extent to which the questionnaire is repeatable and consistently produces the same results	Validity	Degree to which the questionnaire measures what it is intended to measure
Internal consistency	How well the items of a questionnaire relate to each other and to the total questionnaire. It is most commonly evaluated by Cronbach's alpha. An alpha $\geq$0.70 indicates good internal consistency	Internal validity	Internal structure of the questionnaires and is usually evaluated by factor analysis, inter-items correlations and floor and ceiling effects
Test–retest	Reproducibility of the questionnaire over time. The questionnaire is completed on two occasions by the same patients in whom no change in the condition has taken place. It is most commonly evaluated by the intraclass correlation coefficient (ICC). An ICC $\geq$0.70 indicates good test–retest reliability	External validity	Relationship between the questionnaire and an external criterion (e.g. other measures of the same or different dimensions of health), and the most common types are face, content, convergent/discriminant and construct validity
		Face validity	Determined by expert opinion as to whether the questionnaire seems to measure HRQL related to the disease in question. Least rigorous form of validity. Type of external validity
		Content validity	Based on subjective assessment of the extent to which a questionnaire represents all dimensions of a construct. Type of external validity
		Convergent/discriminant validity	Assessed by calculating the correlation between the questionnaire and measures of similar or dissimilar constructs. Type of external validity
		Construct validity	Ascertained by calculating the correlation between the questionnaire and an independent measure, which reflects the severity of the disease in question. Type of external validity

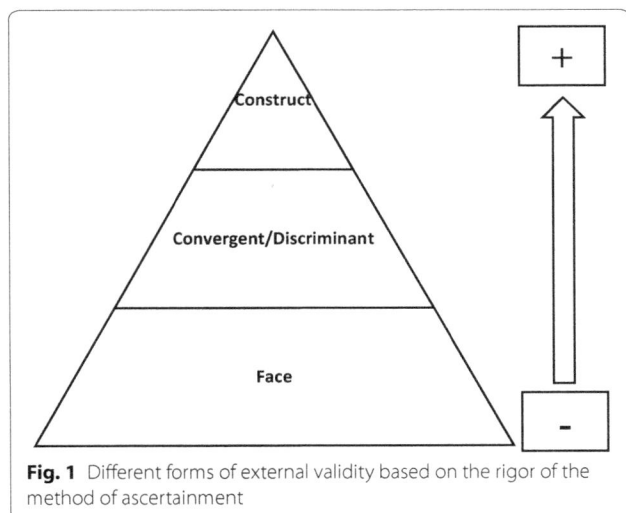

Fig. 1 Different forms of external validity based on the rigor of the method of ascertainment

In addition, studies have found significant differences in HRQL between countries, even when corrected for differences in perceived disease severity [15]. To unveil this aspect, *Saleh-Langenberg* et al. recruited a total of 648 European food-allergic patients (404 adults, 244 children) whom completed an age-specific questionnaire package including descriptive questions. Unexpectedly, the authors found that both for adults and children neither experiencing anaphylaxis nor being prescribed an epinephrine auto-injector (EAI) contributed to impairment of HRQL [15]. On the other hand, previous studies have shown that both confirmed and perceived FA impair equally HRQL [45].

The culture and traditions of eating might vary among different countries [42, 46], consequently, the impact of FA on quality of life shall diverge. Another important outcome was that forty-seven percent of all participants who reported anaphylaxis and who were diagnosed by a health care professional were not prescribed an epinephrine auto-injector, which corroborates previous findings about the suboptimal management of acute food-allergic reactions by both patients and physicians [47].

Other authors have suggested that as individual's age, they probably become more aware of the severity of symptoms and may take into account the threatening effect of FA [42].

The healthcare cost in terms of FA has been investigated, in an elegant patient-based cost study. It has been reported that adults with 'possible' food allergy visited health professionals, on average, 11.17 (SD = 16.14) times per year compared with 7.11 (SD = 12.80) visits per year reported by controls. Similarly, children with 'possible' FA visited health professionals 10.75 times per

year (SD = 13.23) compared with 6.56 (SD = 9.78) visits per year reported by controls. Consequently, food-allergic individuals had higher health care costs than controls. The mean annual cost of health care was international dollars (I$) 2016 for food-allergic adults and I$1089 for controls, a difference of I$927 (95 % confidence interval I$324–I$1530). A similar result was found for adults in each country, and for children, and interestingly, it was not sensitive to baseline demographic differences. Cost was significantly related to severity of illness in cases in nine countries [48].

In another study, QoL in adults with peanut allergy was compared with other disease groups. In contrast to children, the former group was observed to have better QoL than rheumatologic patients [45].

In addition, in a large population survey performed in Canada, individuals of low education and new Canadians self-reported fewer allergies, which may be due to genetics, environment, lack of appropriate health care, or lack of awareness of allergies, which could eventually reduce self-report [49].

Just to underline the impact that FA exerts in food-allergic patients, access to a 24-h telephone hotline specifically designed for this kind of patients in Ireland, significantly improved the measured QoL, and continued to do so for 6 months after the study time, even just two out of the 24 patients actually used it [50].

Moreover, some studies have shown the long-term positive effect food challenges yield on QoL. Unpredictably, this positive effect was not conditioned by the outcome of food challenges [51, 52].

Conclusions

FA is suffered by patients but also by their relatives, friends and acquaintances [16, 26, 53] (Tables 1, 2). There have been described different factors that could modify HRQL in food allergic patients, considering as the most influential: perceived disease severity, age of the patient, peanut or soy allergy, country of origin and having allergy to two or more foods. Nevertheless, further studies are necessary to elucidate all these predictors and to achieve a good HRQL in food-allergic patients.

Over the last few years, several different specific QoL questionnaires for food-allergic patients have been developed and translated to different languages and cultures (Fig. 1). Tools designed to assess the impact of FA on HRQL should be always part of the diagnostic work up, in order to provide a complete basal assessment, to highlight target of intervention as well as to evaluate the effectiveness of interventions designed to cure FA [54–60]. HRQL may be the only meaningful outcome measure suitable and available for FA, measuring this continuous burden.

Authors' contributions

All the authors have collaborated in searching the bibliography and writing the manuscript. All authors read and approved the final manuscript.

Author details

[1] Servicio de Enfermedades del Sistema Inmune-Alergia, Hospital Universitario Príncipe de Asturias. Departamento de Medicina y Especialidades Médicas, Universidad de Alcalá, Carretera de Alcalá-Meco s/n, 28085 Alcalá de Henares, Madrid, Spain. [2] Hospital del Sureste. Arganda del Rey, Unidad de Alergia, Madrid, Spain. [3] Allergy Unit, Verona University and General Hospital, Verona, Italy. [4] Servicio de Alergia, Hospital Universitario Ramón y Cajal, IRYCIS, Madrid, Spain. [5] Servicio de Alergia, Hospital Universitario Clínico San Carlos, Madrid, Spain. [6] Unidad de Bioestadística Clínica, Hospital Universitario Ramón y Cajal, IRYCIS, Madrid, Spain.

Acknowledgements

This work was partially supported by a grant from Comunidad de Madrid S2010/BMD-2502 MITIC and also FIS PI11/02758 and EUROPREVALL FP6–CT-2005-514000.

References

1. Vieths S, Reese G, Ballmer-Weber BK, Beyer K, Burney P, Fernandez-Rivas M, et al. The serum bank of EuroPrevall—the prevalence, cost and basis of food allergy across Europe. Food Chem Toxicol. 2008;46(Suppl 1):12–4.
2. Muraro A, Roberts G, Worm M, Bilo MB, Brockow K, Fernandez Rivas M, Santos AF, Zolkipli ZQ, Bellou A, Beyer K, Bindslev-Jensen C, Cardona V, Clark AT, Demoly P, Dubois AE, DunnGalvin A, Eigenmann P, Halken S, Harada L, Lack G, Jutel M, Niggemann B, Rueff F, Timmermans F, Vlieg-Boerstra BJ, Werfel T, Dhami S, Panesar S, Akdis CA, Sheikh A, EAACI Food Allergy and Anaphylaxis Guidelines Group. Anaphylaxis: guidelines from the European academy of allergy and clinical immunology. Allergy. 2014;69:1026–45.
3. Sicherer SH. Epidemiology of food allergy. J Allergy Clin Immunol. 2011;127:594–602.
4. Ben-Shoshan M, Turnbull E, Clarke A. Food allergy: temporal trends and determinants. Curr Allergy Asthma Rep. 2012;12:346–72.
5. Fernandez Rivas M. Food allergy in alergologica-2005. J Investig Allergol Clin Immunol. 2009;19(Suppl 2):37–44.
6. Barnett J, Leftwich J, Muncer K, Grimshaw K, Shepherd R, Raats MM, et al. How do peanut and nut-allergic consumers use information on the packaging to avoid allergens? Allergy. 2011;66:969–78.
7. Goossens NJ, Flokstra-de Blok BM, van der Meulen GN, Arnlind MH, Asero R, Barreales L, et al. Health-related quality of life in food-allergic adults from eight European countries. Ann Allergy Asthma Immunol. 2014;113(63–8):e1.
8. de Blok BM, Vlieg-Boerstra BJ, Oude Elberink JN, Duiverman EJ, DunnGalvin A, Hourihane JO, et al. A framework for measuring the social impact of food allergy across Europe: a EuroPrevall state of the art paper. Allergy. 2007;62:733–7.
9. Flokstra-de Blok BMJ, van der Velde JL, Vlieg-Boerstra BJ, Oude Elberink JNG, DunnGalvin A, Hourihane JO, et al. Health-related quality of life of food allergic patients measured with generic and disease-specific questionnaires. Allergy. 2010;65:1031–8.
10. Flokstra-de Blok BMJ, Dubois AEJ, Vlieg-Boerstra BJ, Oude Elberink NG, Raat H, DunnGalvin A, et al. Health-related quality of life of food allergic patients: comparison with the general population and other diseases. Allergy. 2010;65:238–44.
11. Venter C, Sommer I, Moonesinghe H, Grundy J, Glasbey G, Patil V, et al. Health-Related Quality of Life in children with perceived and diagnosed food hypersensitivity. Pediatr Allergy Immunol. 2015;26:126–32 **(Epub ahead of print)**.
12. Ward C, Greenhawt M. Differences in caregiver food allergy quality of life between a tertiary care, specialty clinic, and a caregiver reported food allergic populations. J Allergy Clin Immunol Pract. 2015;. doi:10.1016/j.jaip.2015.07.023.
13. van der Velde JL, Flokstra-de Blok BM, Dunngalvin A, Hourihane JO, Duiverman EJ, Dubois AE. Parents report better health-related quality of life for their food-allergic children than children themselves. Clin Exp Allergy. 2011;41:1431–9.
14. Yamamoto-Hanada K, Futamura M, Takahashi O, Narita M, Kobayashi F, Ohya Y. Caregivers of children with no food allergy-their experiences and perception of food allergy. Pediatr Allergy Immunol. 2015;26:614–7.
15. Saleh-Langenberg J, Goossens NJ, Flokstra-de Blok BM, Kollen BJ, van der Meulen GN, Le TM, Knulst AC, et al. Predictors of health-related quality of life of European food-allergic patients. Allergy. 2015;70:616–24.
16. Sicherer SH, Noone SA, Muñoz-Furlong A. The impact of childhood food allergy on quality of life. Ann Allergy Asthma Immunol. 2001;87:461–4.
17. Wassenberg J, Cochard MM, Dunngalvin A, Ballabeni P, Flokstra-de Blok BM, Newman CJ, et al. Parent perceived quality of life is age-dependent in children with food allergy. Pediatr Allergy Immunol. 2012;23:412–9.
18. Factor JM, Mendelson L, Lee J, Nouman G, Lester MR. Effect of oral immunotherapy to peanut on food-specific quality of life. Ann Allergy Asthma Immunol. 2012;109:348–52.
19. Carraro S, Frigo AC, Perin M, Stefani S, Cardarelli C, Bozzetto S, et al. Impact of oral immunotherapy on quality of life in children with cow milk allergy: a pilot study. Int J Immunopathol Pharmacol. 2012;25:793–8.
20. Otani IM, Bégin P, Kearney C, Dominguez TL, Mehrotra A, Bacal LR, et al. Multiple-allergen oral immunotherapy improves quality of life in caregivers of food-allergic pediatric subjects. Allergy Asthma Clin Immunol. 2014;10:25.
21. DunnGalvin A, Cullinane C, Daly DA, Flokstra-de Blok BM, Dubois AE, Hourihane JO. Longitudinal validity and responsiveness of the Food allergy quality of life questionnaire—Parent Form in children 0–12 years following positive and negative food challenges. Clin Exp Allergy. 2010;40:476–85.
22. Knibb RC, Barnes C, Stalker C. Parental confidence in managing food allergy—development and validation of the food allergy self-efficacy scale for parents (FASE-P). Clin Exp Allergy. 2015;45:1681–9.
23. Flokstra-de Blok BM, DunnGalvin A, Vlieg-Boerstra BJ, Oude Elberink JN, Duiverman EJ, Hourihane JO, et al. Development and validation of the self-administered Food allergy quality of life questionnaire for adolescents. J Allergy Clin Immunol. 2008;122:139–44.
24. Flokstra-de Blok BM, DunnGalvin A, Vlieg-Boerstra BJ, Oude Elberink JN, Duiverman EJ, Hourihane JO, et al. Development and validation of a self-administered food allergy quality of life questionnaire for children. Clin Exp Allergy. 2009;39:127–37.
25. Flokstra-de Blok BM, Dubois AE. Quality of life measures for food allergy. Clin Exp Allergy. 2012;42:1014–20.
26. Cohen BL, Noone S, Muñoz-Furlong A, Sicherer SH. Development of a questionnaire to measure quality of life in families with a child with food allergy. J Allergy Clin Immunol. 2004;114:1159–63.
27. Teixeira IP, Novais Ide P, Pinto Rde M, Cheik NC. Cultural adaptation and validation of the KINDL questionnaire in Brazil for adolescents between 12 and 16 years of age. Rev Bras Epidemiol. 2012;15:845–57.
28. Chen YM, He LP, Mai JC, Hao YT, Xiong LH, Chen WQ, et al. Validity and reliability of pediatric quality of life inventory version 4.0 generic core scales in Chinese children and adolescents. Zhonghua Liu Xing Bing Xue Za Zhi. 2008;29:560–3.
29. Rajmil L, Serra-Sutton V, Fernandez-Lopez JA, Berra S, Aymerich M, Cieza A, et al. The Spanish version of the German health-related quality of life questionnaire for children and adolescents: the Kindl. An Pediatr (Barc). 2004;60:514–21.
30. Pereira B, Venter C, Grundy J, Clayton CB, Arshad HS, Dean T. Prevalence of sensitization to food allergens, reported adverse reactions to foods, food avoidance, and food hypersensitivity among teenagers. J Allergy Clin Immunol. 2005;116:884–92.
31. Cummings AJ, Knibb RC, King RM, Lucas JS. The psychosocial impact of food allergy and food hypersensitivity in children, adolescents and their families: a review. Allergy. 2010;65:933–45.
32. MacKenzie H, Roberts G, van Laar D, Dean T. Teenagers' experiences of living with food hypersensitivity: a qualitative study. Pediatr Allergy Immunol. 2010;21:595–602.

33. Sommer I, Mackenzie H, Venter C, Dean T. An exploratory investigation of food choice behavior of teenagers with and without food allergies. Ann Allergy Asthma Immunol. 2014;112:446–52.

34. Monks H, Gowland MH, Mackenzie H, Erlewyn-Lajeunesse M, King R, Lucas JS, et al. How do teenagers manage their food allergies? Clin Exp Allergy. 2010;40:1533–40.

35. Flokstra-de Blok BM, Doriene van Ginkel C, Roerdink EM, Kroeze MA, Stel AA, van der Meulen GN, et al. Extremely low prevalence of epinephrine auto injectors in high-risk food-allergic adolescents in Dutch high schools. Pediatr Allergy Immunol. 2011;22:374–7.

36. Saleh-Langenberg J, Flokstra-de Blok BM, Goossens NJ, Kemna JC, van der Velde JL, Dubois AE. The compliance and burden of treatment with the epinephrine auto-injector in food-allergic adolescents. Pediatr Allergy Immunol. 2015 Aug 13. [Epub ahead of print].

37. van der Velde JL, Flokstra-de Blok BM, Hamp A, Knibb RC, Duiverman EJ, Dubois AE. Adolescent-parent disagreement on health-related quality of life of food-allergic adolescents: who makes the difference? Allergy. 2011;66:1580–9.

38. Salvilla SA, Dubois AE, Flokstra-de Blok BM, et al. Disease-specific health related quality of life instruments for IgE-mediated food allergy. Allergy. 2014;69:834e84.

39. Resnick ES, Pieretti MM, Maloney J, Noone S, Muñoz-Furlong A, Sicherer SH. Development of a questionnaire to measure quality of life in adolescents with food allergy: the FAQL-teen. Ann Allergy Asthma Immunol. 2010;105:364–8.

40. Mackenzie H, Roberts G, Van Laar D, Dean T. A new quality of life scale for teenagers with food hypersensitivity. Pediatr Allergy Immunol. 2012;23:404–11.

41. Flokstra-de Blok BM, van der Meulen GN, DunnGalvin A, Vlieg-Boerstra BJ, Oude Elberink JN, Duiverman EJ, et al. Development and validation of the food allergy quality of life questionnaire—adult form. Allergy. 2009;64:1209–17.

42. Antolin-Amerigo D, Cerecedo Carballo I, Muriel A, Fernández-Rivas M, Diéguez Pastor M, Flokstra-de Blok B, et al. Validation of the Spanish version of the food allergy quality of life questionnaire-adult form (S-FAQLQ-AF). J Investig Allergol Clin Immunol. 2015;25:270–5.

43. Lange L. Quality of life in the setting of anaphylaxis and food allergy. Allergo J Int. 2014;23:252–60.

44. van der Velde JL, Flokstra-de Blok BM, de Groot H, Oude-Elberink JN, Kerkhof M, Duiverman EJ, et al. Food allergy-related quality of life after double-blind, placebo-controlled food challenges in adults, adolescents, and children. J Allergy Clin Immunol. 2012;130(5):1136–1143e2.

45. Primeau MN, Kagan R, Joseph L, Lim H, Dufresne C, Duffy C, et al. The psychological burden of peanut allergy as perceived by adults with peanut allergy and the parents of peanutallergic children. Clin Exp Allergy. 2000;30:1135–43.

46. Goossens NJ, Flokstra-de Blok BM, Vlieg-Boerstra BJ, Duiverman EJ, Weiss CC, Furlong TJ, et al. Online version of the food allergy quality of life questionnaire-adult form: validity, feasibility and cross-cultural comparison. Clin Exp Allergy. 2011;41:574–81.

47. Le TM, van Hoffen E, Pasmans SG, Bruijnzeel-Koomen CA, Knulst AC. Sub-optimal management of acute food-allergic reactions by patients, emergency departments and general practitioners. Allergy. 2009;64:1227–8.

48. Fox M, Mugford M, Voordouw J, Cornelisse-Vermaat J, Antonides G, de la Hoz Caballer B, et al. Health sector costs of self-reported food allergy in Europe: a patient-based cost of illness study. Eur J Public Health. 2013;23:757–62.

49. Soller L, Ben-Shoshan M, Harrington DW, Knoll M, Fragapane J, Joseph L, et al. Prevalence and predictors of food allergy in Canada: a focus on vulnerable populations. J Allergy Clin Immunol Pract. 2015;3:42–9.

50. Kelleher MM, Dunngalvin A, Sheikh A, Cullinane C, Fitzsimons J, Hourihane JO. Twenty four-hour helpline Access to expert management advice for food-allergy-triggered anaphylaxis in infants, children and young people: a pragmatic, randomized controlled trial. Allergy. 2013;68:1598–604.

51. van der Velde JL, Flokstra-de Blok BM, de Groot H, Oude-Elberink JN, Kerkhof M, Duiverman EJ, et al. Food allergy related quality of life after double-blind, placebo-controlled food challenges in adults, adolescents, and children. J Allergy Clin Immunol. 2012;130:1136–43.

52. Knibb RC, Ibrahim NF, Stiefel G, Petley R, Cummings AJ, King RM, et al. The psychological impact of diagnostic food challenges to confirm the resolution of peanut or tree nut allergy. Clin Exp Allergy. 2012;42:451–9.

53. Marklund B, Ahlstedt S, Nordström G. Health-related quality of life among adolescents with allergy-like conditions—with emphasis on food hypersensitivity. Health Qual Life Outcomes. 2004;2:65.

54. Muraro A, Dubois AE, DunnGalvin A, Hourihane JO, de Jong NW, Meyer R, Panesar SS, Roberts G, Salvilla S, Sheikh A, Worth A, Flokstra-de Blok BM, European Academy of Allergy and Clinical Immunology. EAACI food allergy and anaphylaxis guidelines. food allergy health-related quality of life measures. Allergy. 2014;69:845–53.

55. Bollinger M, Dahlquist L, Mudd K, Sonntag C, Dillinger L, McKenna K. The impact of food allergy on the daily activities of children and their families. Ann Allergy Asthma Immunol. 2006;96:415–21.

56. Lebovidge JS, Stone KD, Twarog FJ, Raiselis SW, Kalish LA, Bailey EP, Schneider LC. Development of a preliminary questionnaire to assess parental response to children's food allergies. Ann Allergy Asthma Immunol. 2006;96:472–7.

57. Ostblom E, Egmar AC, Gardulf A, Lilja G, Wickman M. The impact of food hypersensitivity reported in 9-year-old children by their parents on health-related quality of life. Allergy. 2008;63:211–8.

58. Roberts G, Hurley C, Lack G. Development of a quality-of-life assessment for the allergic child or teenager with multisystem allergic disease. J Allergy Clin Immunol. 2003;111:491–7.

59. Jansson SA, Heibert-Arnlind M, Middelveld RJ, Bengtsson UJ, Sundqvist AC, Kallström-Bengtsson I. Health-related quality of life, assessed with a disease-specific questionnaire, in Swedish adults suffering from well-diagnosed food allergy to staple foods. Clin Transl Allergy. 2013;3:21.

60. Carrard A, Rizzuti D, Sokollik C. Update on food allergy. Allergy. 2015;70(12):1511–20.

Sensitization to secretoglobin and lipocalins in a group of young children with risk of developing respiratory allergy

Mizuho Nagao[1], Magnus P. Borres[2,3], Mayumi Sugimoto[1], Carl Johan Petersson[2], Satoshi Nakayama[4], Yu Kuwabara[5], Sawako Masuda[6], Patrik Dykiel[2] and Takao Fujisawa[1*]

Abstract

Background: Multiple sensitizations in early age have been reported to be a risk for development of asthma. This study evaluates the emergence and evolution of IgE to aeroallergens among a cohort of children with physician-diagnosed atopic dermatitis and/or showing food allergy symptoms and to examine the relation to asthma development.

Methods: Three-hundred and four children (median age 13.4 months at entry) with food allergy symptoms and/or atopic dermatitis without asthma at inclusion were analysed for IgE antibodies against food-, indoor- and outdoor-allergens and pet allergen components and correlated to the individuals' outcome on asthma inception.

Results: At 2 years of follow-up, physician-diagnosed asthma was 19.7% (n = 49) and asthma diagnosed any time was 24% (n = 67). History of persistent cough and asthma of father, combination of milk- and wheat-allergy symptoms and dual sensitization to house dust mite and Japanese cedar were independent risk factors for asthma. Sensitization to dog was the most prevalent inhalant allergen at entry. Asthma children had a higher proportion of sensitization to dog, cat and horse allergens at entry compared with non-asthma children. Being sensitized to both food, house dust mite and pet allergens was strongly associated with asthma (p = 0.0006). Component resolved diagnosis for dog and cat allergens showed that IgE antibodies to Can f 1 and Fel d 1 was common even at very young age.

Conclusions: Early sensitization to inhalant allergens increases the risk of developing asthma as well as having milk and wheat allergy symptoms. Sensitization to dog, was common at an early age despite dog ownership. Sensitization to secretoglobin and lipocalins and less to serum albumins explained the pet sensitization.

Keywords: Asthma, Allergy, Children, Molecular allergy diagnostics, Pet allergen components, Component resolved diagnosis, Food allergy, Secretoglobin, Lipocalin, Sensitization

Background

The combination of atopic dermatitis and food allergy in young children reflect a strong risk for the development of asthma-like disease [1]. Symptomatic food allergy is especially associated with asthma among children with multiple or severe allergies [2]. Approximately one half of children with moderate to severe atopic dermatitis will have clinically relevant IgE antibodies to food allergens [3]. As atopic children grow older, the majority of allergen-specific IgE antibodies are directed against inhalant sources [4]. Sensitization to multiple allergens along with high IgE antibodies levels are features of severe atopic dermatitis in childhood. The knowledge that children with atopic dermatitis are at risk of developing asthma is poorly understood in general among health care providers. This is partially due to the fact that there is a wide variability in asthma development, 10–25%, in the risk estimate in longitudinal studies. A better recognition of the children at highest risk of developing asthma among the group of individuals with atopic dermatitis and food allergy is therefore needed.

*Correspondence: fujisawa@mie-m.hosp.go.jp
[1] Allergy Center and Department of Clinical Research, Mie National Hospital, IDD, Tsu, Mie, Japan
Full list of author information is available at the end of the article

At present, the identification of a child at high risk might not be possible with certainty. Current research points to some indicators including family history, history of asthma and allergies, early and severe sensitization to some food antigens and to aeroallergens and early viral infection associated with wheeze and adverse environmental exposures [5].

An atopic history of early life seems to be one of the key factors to identify an individual's risk of persistent asthma. Illi et al. reported a cumulative prevalence of atopic dermatitis in the first 2 years of life of 21.5% among a general population of children [6]. When associated with allergic sensitization, atopic dermatitis was a good predictor of asthma at school age: the risk was not seen with atopic dermatitis in the absence of sensitization. Sensitization to hen's egg seems to convey the greatest risk.

Birth cohorts in Europe, USA and Australia show that early sensitization and severe sensitization are risk factors for persistence of asthma [7–9]. Little is known about the timing and pattern of sensitization to individual aeroallergen in relation to the development of asthma in children with atopic dermatitis and food allergy. Sensitisation to animal and dust mite allergens are each a risk factor for the development of asthma. There seems to be a higher probability of wheeze for cat versus mite at a given IgE value among preschool children [10]. In the same study, summing IgE levels for mite, cat and dog at age 3 strengthened the risk for wheeze at age 5. Wisniewski et al. were not able to verify that multisensitization increase the risk for asthma [11]. Stoltz et al. have examined specific patterns of allergic sensitization in early childhood in relation to the risk of developing asthma and rhinitis [12]. They found that at 1 year of age only IgE antibodies to cat and dog were significantly associated with having asthma at age 6. Konradsen et al. have in a recent review stated that the prevalence of allergy to furry animal has been increasing in later years and allergy to cats, dogs or both is considered a major risk factor for the development of asthma and rhinitis [13].

We hypothesised that early onset of sensitization to aeroallergen in children with atopic dermatitis and/or showing food allergy symptoms beginning within the first years of life is important in order to identify those at most risk of developing asthma.

The aim of this study was to evaluate the emergence and evolution of IgE antibodies to aeroallergens among a cohort of children with physician-diagnosed atopic dermatitis and/or showing food allergy symptoms and to examine the relation to asthma development during a 2-year follow up.

Methods

This study was based on children who participated in the IRAM (Impact of Rhinitis on Atopic March; UMIN000004157) cohort. The study was a prospective five visit study during 2 years. Beside medical history, children were also recorded for atopic dermatitis, allergic rhinitis, parents' allergy/asthma and smoking history and age, gender, height and weight. Inclusion criteria for this study were confirmed atopic dermatitis and/or suspicion of food allergy. Suspicion of food allergy was based on clinical history of food-induced symptoms and corresponding sensitization to the food. In uncertain cases oral food challenges were added to determine allergy to the food in question following the procedure for food allergy diagnosis in the EAACI and Japanese guidelines [14]. As oral food challenges were not done in all children, the term "food allergy symptom" will be used instead of "food allergy" throughout this study combining the groups of children with confirmed food allergy and of children with suspicion of food allergy, respectively. The diagnosis of atopic dermatitis was made by the study physicians based on the criteria by Hanifin and Rajka [15]. Blood samples were taken for specific IgE antibody determinations (Table 1). Physician diagnosis of asthma, (at each visit), was based on the Japanese Paediatric Guideline for the treatment and management of bronchial asthma [16]. A previously known diagnosis of asthma was criteria for exclusion.

The informed consent was signed by a legal guardian and the protocol was reviewed and approved by the ethics committee in Mie National Hospital, Japan.

Serum samples were analysed for IgE antibodies using the ImmunoCAP® system according to the manufacturer's guidelines (Phadia AB, Uppsala, Sweden).

Statistical analyses were performed using the SAS® 9.3 (SAS Institute Inc., Cary, USA) and R 3.2.3 (R Foundation for Statistical Computing, Vienna, Austria,). All tests were two-sided and using significance level of 5%. The Chi square test or, when appropriate, Fischer's exact test were used to compare proportions. The Mann–Whitney test was used to compare specific IgE levels at entry and after 2 year follow up. The effect of demographic variables, medical history and sensitisation to allergen components were jointly investigated using a logistic regression model.

Results

Number of patients and prevalence figures are presented in Table 1. The average number of allergens that a child was sensitized against was at entry 3.0 (SD 2.4; range 0–13) and after 2 years, 5.1 (3.2; 0–13). Amongst the

Table 1 Number of patients and prevalence figures

Number of children (entry/1 year/2 years)	304/270/242		
Physician diagnosed	Number of children (%)		
Atopic dermatitis (at entry)	210 (71)		
Having symptoms for			
Food allergy (at entry)	259 (88)		
Egg allergy (at entry)	232 (79)		
Milk allergy (at entry)	128 (44)		
Wheat allergy (at entry)	75 (26)		
History of prolonged cough	62 (21)		
Patients by sex (missing # = 2)	Girls	Boys	
	106 (36)	193 (64)	
Bronchial asthma (after 2 year)	49 (20)		
Bronchial asthma (anytime during follow up)	67 (~24)		
Age in month (at entry)/(sdv)	13.4/(5.5)		
Pet ownership (at entry)	Dog: 28 (9)	Cat: 4 (1)	Dog and cat: 31 (10)
Pet ownership (any time)	Dog: 38 (13)	Cat: 11 (4)	Dog and cat: 42 (14)

	Sensitization		
	Prevalence and 95% CI %[a] and total # tested (>0.35 kU$_A$/L)		
	Entry (n = 304)	1 year (n = 270)	2 years (n = 242)
Allergen extracts			
m3 Aspergillus	3.6 (1.8–6.4)	4.4 (2.3–7.6)	9.9 (6.5–14.3)
m6 Alternaria	1.3 (0.4–3.3)	1.5 (0.4–3.7)	5.0 (2.6–8.5)
g3 Orchard grass	4.3 (2.3–7.2)	15.2 (11.1–20.0)	27.7 (22.2–33.8)
t24 Japanese cypress	3.0 (1.4–5.6)	12.6 (8.9–17.2)	32.8 (26.9–39.1)
f1 Egg white	86.2 (81.8–89.9)	83.7 (78.8–87.9)	85.1 (80.0–89.4)
f2 Milk	54.6 (29.5–40.5)	56.3 (50.2–62.3)	57.0 (50.5–63.3)
f4 Wheat	44.4 (38.7–50.2)	45.2 (39.1–51.3)	50.4 (43.9–56.9)
e1 Cat	18.8 (14.5–23.6)	25.2 (20.1–30.8)	33.5 (27.6–39.8)
e3 Horse d	6.3 (3.7–9.9)[a]	5.4 (3.0–9.0)[b]	7.4 (4.4–11.6)[c]
e5 Dog d	36.8 (31.4–42.5)	44.4 (38.4–50.6)	47.1 (40.7–53.6)
w1 Comm ragw	4.6 (2.6–7.6)	17.4 (13.1–22.5)	26.0 (20.6–32.0)
t17 Japanese cedar	3.9 (2.1–6.8)	24.4 (19.4–30.0)	51.7 (45.2–58.1)
d1 D.pteronyssinus	30.6 (25.5–36.1)	57.8 (51.6–63.7)	74.8 (68.8–80.1)

	Prevalence and 95% CI %[a] and total # tested (>0.1 kUA/L)		
Allergen components			
Bos d 6	(Milk)	22.7 (18.1–27.8)	25.6 (20.5–31.2)	24.0 (18.7–29.9)
Can f 1	(Dog)	18.4 (14.2–23.2)	20.7 (16.1–26.1)	26.4 (21.0–32.5)
Can f 2		7,6 (4.9–11.1)	11.5 (7.9–15.9)	14.5 (10.3–19.5)
Can f 3		9.5 (6.5–13.4)	12.2 (8.6–16.7)	12.8 (8.9–17.7)
Can f 5		8.2 (5.4–11.9)	10.0 (6.7–14.2)	12.0 (8.2–16.8)
Fel d 1	(Cat)	13.2 (9.6–17.5)	16.3 (12.1–21.3)	25.2 (19.9–31.2)
Fel d 2		8.6 (5.7–12.3)	12.2 (8.6–16.7)	12.0 (8.2–16.8)
Fel d 4		9.9 (6.8–13.8)	9.3 (6.1–13.4)	15.7 (11.4–20.9)
Equ c 1	(Horse)	7.6 (4.9–11.1)[a]	8.5 (5.5–12.5)[b]	10.7 (7.2–15.3)[c]

[a] n = 271

[b] n = 257

[c] n = 230

children that were diagnosed with bronchial asthma anytime during the course of the study (n = 67), the corresponding figure at entry was 3.8 (2.8; 0–13) whilst in the group of children (n = 236) that did not develop asthma the mean number of positive allergens was 2.8 (2.2; 0–13) (p = 0.019). Corresponding figures after 2 years were 6.2 (3.4; 0–13) and 4.7 (3.1; 0–13) respectively (p = 0.025). At entry, among the children diagnosed with asthma 6% were not sensitized to any of the tested allergens, 16% were monosensitized, 30% were sensitized to two up to a maximum of three allergens and 48% to more than three allergens. Corresponding numbers for the non-asthma group were 11, 20, 39 and 30% respectively.

Forty-nine out of the 67 (73%) children that were diagnosed with asthma anytime during the 24 months follow-up time period had an asthma diagnosis at the last visit.

Asthma were significantly associated with persistent cough (OR 3.7, 95% CI 1.75–7.80), asthma of father (2.39, 1.14–5.04) and milk allergy symptoms (2.48, 1.22–5.05), when using >0.1 kU_A/L as cut-off. When using >0.34 kU_A/L as cut-off, house dust mites in addition to the same factors as mentioned above were associated with higher risk of asthma diagnosis (Table 2).

Having a combination of milk and wheat allergy symptoms and house dust mite and cedar pollen sensitization had a likelihood of 38 and 45% respectively of being diagnosed with asthma anytime during follow-up (Table 3). Children with wheat allergic symptoms did not differ in their sensitization pattern at entry or at 2 year follow up compared to children with no wheat allergy symptoms. The results from the logistic regression were in line with

this finding as sensitisation to Japanese cedar and wheat allergy symptoms were associated with increased probability of asthma diagnosis during follow-up, although they did not reach statistical significance (Table 2).

Children diagnosed with asthma at follow up were significantly more likely to be multi-sensitized to animals compared to the non-asthmatic children at entry (Fig. 1). Thirty-three percent of the asthma children were sensitized to two or more animals compared to 15% of the non-asthmatic children.

Sensitization to three different groups of allergens, pets, house dust mite and food, was analysed one by one or in combination in respect to asthma prevalence. Being sensitized to pet allergens and to house dust mite allergen independently of each other was associated with asthma (Fig. 2). Sensitization to all three groups in their combination was strongly associated with asthma (p = 0.0006).

Two hundred and ten children had atopic dermatitis at entry and 35 children were diagnosed with asthma at 2 years follow up. Totally 48 children were diagnosed with asthma anytime during the study. Mean number of positive allergens among these were 6.3 and 5.7 respectively. Corresponding figures in the non-asthmatic groups were 5.0 and 4.0 respectively. An increased risk of developing asthma (odds ratio = 1.22, CI 1.03–1.45, p = 0.02) was observed with increased number of positive allergens amongst the AD children.

Ninety-six percent (189/196) of the dog sensitized individuals had complete data set for measurements of IgE to Can f 1, Can f 2, Can f 3 and Can f 5 at entry. Overall sensitization to least one of these components was

Table 2 For each variable—likelihood of being diagnosed with asthma

Parameter	>0.1 kUA/L			>0.35 kUA/L		
	Odds ratio	95% CI	p value	Odds ratio	95% CI	p value
Asthma of father	2.39	1.14–5.04	*0.022*	2.19	1.04–4.63	*0.039*
Atopic dermatitis	1.32	0.64–2.73	0.459	1.23	0.59–2.56	0.581
Cat dander sensitivity	0.64	0.27–1.51	0.307	1.11	0.46–2.67	0.813
Dog dander sensitivity	1.00	0.41–2.43	0.995	0.79	0.35–1.78	0.573
Egg allergy symptoms	0.79	0.34–1.85	0.586	0.80	0.34–1.86	0.604
HDM sensitivity	1.81	0.84–3.93	0.131	2.45	1.15–5.22	*0.021*
Hist. of pneum./bronch.	2.06	0.57–7.43	0.267	1.91	0.53–6.96	0.324
Horse dander sensitivity	1.11	0.41–3.00	0.833	0.55	0.14–2.19	0.392
Milk allergy symptoms	2.48	1.22–5.05	*0.013*	2.52	1.26–5.05	*0.009*
Persistent cough	3.69	1.75–7.80	*0.001*	3.66	1.73–7.76	*0.001*
Smoking in family	1.04	0.53–2.04	0.915	1.04	0.53–2.07	0.900
T17 sensitivity	1.88	0.74–4.76	0.184	2.22	0.53–9.31	0.276
Wheat allergy sympt.	1.60	0.76–3.37	0.215	1.70	0.81–3.55	0.158
Milk wheat al. sympt	3.97	1.47–10.68	*0.003*	4.29	1.60–11.47	*0.002*
HDM and t17 sens.	3.41	1.16–9.96	*0.013*	5.43	1.18–24.96	*0.015*

Odds ratio with 95% confidence interval and p value. Shown for cut-off s: ≥0.1 and ≥0.35 kUA/L respectively

Italic values are statictically significant (p < 0.05)

Table 3 Distribution of patients diagnosed with asthma in groups of patients with (A) milk and wheat allergy symptoms (yes or no) and (B) in groups of patients sensitized or not sensitized to house mite and cedar pollen (yes or no)

Symptoms of			
Milk allergy	Wheat allergy	Number of patients: asthma/total	% Diagnosed with asthma
A			
N	N	24/137	17.5
N	Y	5/28	17.9
Y	N	19/81	23.5
Y	Y	18/47	38.3
H. dust mite	Cedar	Number of patients: asthma/total	% Diagnosed with asthma
B			
N	N	36/210	17.1
N	Y	1/1	(100.0)
Y	N	25/82	30.5
Y	Y	5/11	45.5

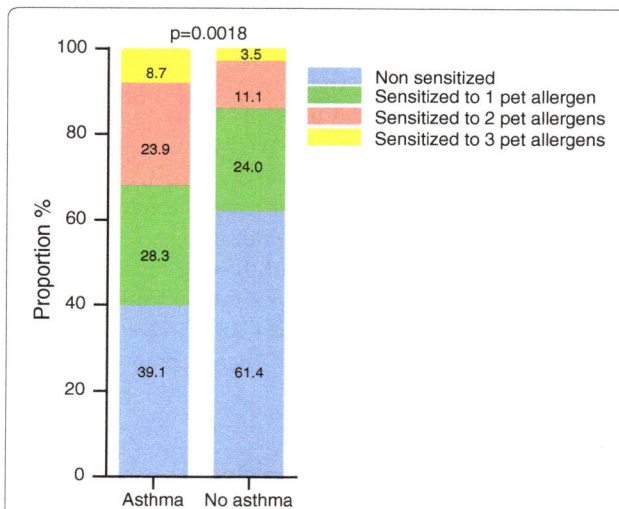

Fig. 1 Proportional distribution of allergen sensitizations at study entry to cat and/or dog and/or horse in patients with and without current asthma

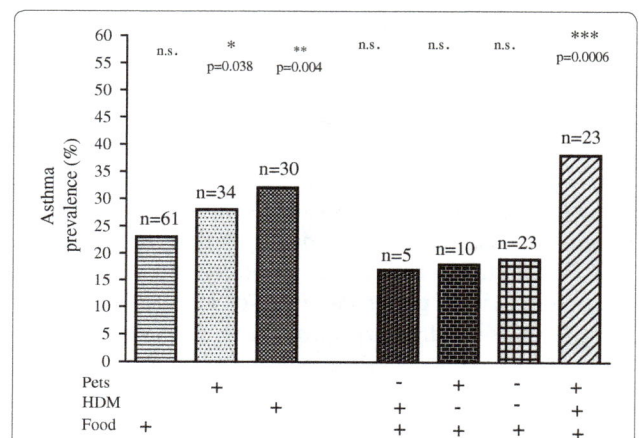

Fig. 2 Asthma prevalence in relation to sensitization to pets, HDM and food allergens. p Values were calculated when compared with the group without any sensitization, *n.s.* not significant. Not shown: Pets(+)HDM(−)Food(−), Pets(−)HDM(+)Food(−) and Pets(+) HDM(+)Food(−) because of too few number of observations in these combinations

37% (n = 69). Sensitization was highest for the lipocalins Can f 1/Can f 2 (30%, n = 56) followed by Can f 3 (15%, n = 29) and Can f 5 (13%, n = 25) (Fig. 3a). Fifteen percent were sensitized to at least two dog components whilst 7% were sensitized to all three components. Corresponding figures at 2 year follow up from 151 children with complete data set showed an overall sensitization to at least one component was 52% (n = 78). The most prevalent sensitization was found for Can f 1/Can f 2 (46%, n = 69) followed by Can f 3 (21%, n = 31) and Can f 5 (19%, n = 29) (Fig. 3b). At 2 year follow up, 23% were sensitized to at least two dog components whilst

11% were sensitized to all three components. Thirty-five (71%) of the asthma children were dog sensitized at entry. All these 35 children had complete data set for the dog components and 23 (47%) of them were positive to at least one of these components. In the group of non-asthmatic children after 2 years followed up 119 children were dog sensitized (62%) and 115 of them had complete data set. Fifty (29%) children were positive to at least one of the dog components.

Ninety-four percent (102/108) of the cat sensitized children had complete data set for cat components Fel d 1, Fel d 2 and Fel d 4 (cut-off = 0.1 kU_A/L). Overall

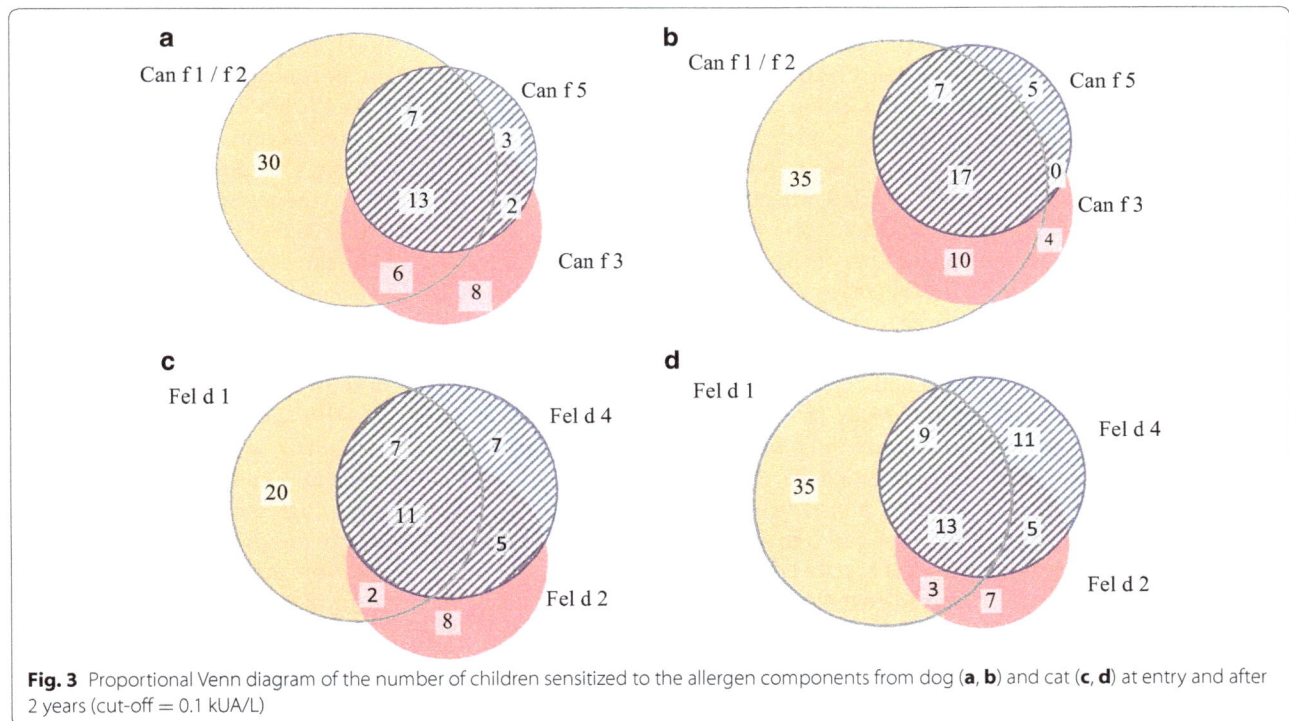

Fig. 3 Proportional Venn diagram of the number of children sensitized to the allergen components from dog (**a**, **b**) and cat (**c**, **d**) at entry and after 2 years (cut-off = 0.1 kUA/L)

sensitization to at least one of these components was 59% (n = 69). Sensitization to Fel d 1 was found to be most prevalent (39%, n = 30) followed by Fel d 4 (29%, n = 26) and Fel d 2 (25%, n = 26) (Fig. 3c). Twenty-five percent were sensitized to at least two cat components whilst 11% were sensitized to all three components. Corresponding figures after 2 years follow up from 115 children with complete data set showed an overall sensitization to at least one of the components of 72%. Sensitization to Fel d 1 was most prevalent (52%, n = 60) followed by Fel d 4 (33%, n = 38) and Fel d 2 (24%, n = 28) (Fig. 3d). Here, 26% were sensitized to at least two cat components whilst 11% were sensitized to all three components. In the group of the 49 children that eventually were diagnosed with asthma 31 (63%) were cat sensitized. All these 31 children had complete data set and 19 (61%) were found to be positive to at least one of the components. Forty-three percent (84/193) of the non-asthmatic children were cat sensitized after 2 years followed up and they all had complete data set. In this group 64 (76%) of the children were positive to at least one of these components.

Discussion

In this study we examined predictors of asthma among children with atopic dermatitis and/or food allergy symptoms. We found that being sensitized to both house dust mite and cedar pollen or having both milk and wheat allergy symptoms were associated with asthma

development during a 2 year follow up. A high proportion were sensitized to dogs and cats and mainly due to sensitization to secretoglobin and lipocalins and less due to serum albumins.

Sensitization to cat and dog components per se were not better predictors of asthma development than sensitization to cat and dog whole allergens. However, Wisniewski et al. found that both Fel d 1 and Fel d 4 were identified as predictors of wheeze among cat sensitized children with atopic dermatitis [11]. One explanation to the different findings could be differences in age in the two study population. Median age in the American study was 7.5 years compared to the median age of 1.5 year in our study [11]. This means that the asthma diagnosis will be based on a much shorter observational period compared to the study of Wisniewski et al.

Having milk and wheat allergy symptoms in combination was associated with increased risk of asthma diagnosis during the follow up. Eighty-eight percent of the included children had food allergy symptoms and 47 of them had this milk- and wheat allergy symptoms combination, of which 40% developed asthma within 2 years. In comparison, out of the children with a single milk or wheat allergy symptom 23 and 18% developed asthma respectively. We know from the literature that especially egg but also milk sensitization are associated with development of IgE to respiratory allergens [17–19]. Few prospective studies have studied the impact of wheat allergy/

sensitization on asthma development. Illi et al. showed that early atopic sensitization played a major role for the prognosis of atopic dermatitis and sensitization to wheat showed the strongest association. The group with early atopic dermatitis and wheeze showed sensitization to wheat, cat, mite, soy and birch. Nilsson et al. found that 72% of children with a challenge verified wheat allergy had or have had milk allergy and 75% reported asthma symptoms pointing to a relationship between milk- and wheat-allergy with asthma [20]. The reason why symptoms for egg allergy did not single out as a risk factor for asthma in our study is probably due to that most of the children included in the study had egg allergic symptoms at entry. We observed in our study that sensitization to HDM, pets and food was higher in children with asthma compared with the non-asthmatics. Furthermore we could see that there was a higher prevalence of sensitization to these allergen groups in children with AD than in the non-AD children (79 vs 21%, data not shown). Wisniewski et al. [11] also reported that the prevalence of sensitization to these allergens increased considerable in AD-children less than 2 years of age up to 15 years of age. Even though the follow up period in our study period was limited to 24 months, from 1 year of age to the age of around 3 years we could also observed a clear increase in the sensitization prevalence for many of these allergens. However, the short follow up period and the young age of the children in our study limits the possibility to compare our study results with other longitudinal studies with long follow up periods.

Typical symptom patterns are important for the establishment of an asthma diagnosis. These include recurrent episodes of cough, wheeze, difficulty in breathing, chest tightness, and respiratory infections [21]. We found in our population that persistent cough was strongly associated with development of asthma. Cough is the most common cause for new visits in childhood ambulatory care and it is important to remember that this symptom is not pathognomonic for asthma and may occur as a result of several different conditions. Ongoing attempts are being made to simplify prediction tools for identifying children with wheeze or cough who are at risk for asthma. Pescatore et al. provided a simple, low-cost and non-invasive questionnaire based method to predict the risk of later asthma in symptomatic preschool children [22]. However, we do need objective biomarkers for diagnosing asthma in young children as cough and other symptoms may occur as a result of several different respiratory conditions. Being sensitized to both house dust mite and cedar pollen increased the risk significantly of developing asthma during the follow up period. A limitation of the study is that this finding is based on only eleven children sensitized at this early age and this finding has to be verified by others.

The high sensitization prevalence for dog was a surprise and no equivalent data has been found in the literature. This is surprisingly high as only 19% of the children were exposed to dog at home. One possible explanation is cross-reactions between bovine and pet albumins. However, Bos d 6 was positive in 23% of the children but Fel d 2 and Can f 3 were only positive in 9 and 8% respectively. This explanation could be partially true as we could document that monosensitisation to pet albumins decreased significantly over the study period, which might be an effect of development of milk tolerance. Instead the most likely explanation is that the majority of the animal sensitized individuals are genuinely sensitized to the secretoglobin (Fel d 1) and lipocalin (Can f 1). Eighteen percent were positive to the major dog component Can f 1 and 13% to Fel d 1, the major cat component already at entry. We have no similar data to compare this with but the picture looks very different from pet component pattern in older children. Bjerg et al. performed a population-based study of animal component sensitization, asthma and rhinitis in schoolchildren and found that 32% were sensitized to dog and 30% to cat [23]. Furthermore, only 5 and 4 of the children that developed asthma were sensitized to Can f 3 and Fel d 2 respectively, which gives a total different sensitization pattern to animal components. Simpson et al. have described patterns of IgE responses to multiple allergen components using latent variable modelling in association with different clinical symptoms [24]. They found that sensitization to the group with component from domestic pets was strongly associated with asthma. Uriatre and Sastre were able to associate IgE sensitization to the different animal molecules with asthma severity [25]. We could not verify this finding but found that if sensitized to two or more animals at an early age, you are more likely to develop asthma. This seems to be even more likely if you are also sensitized to house dust mite and food on the same time. However, our observation period was only 2 years, which is a drawback if studying asthma development in childhood.

Conclusions

We conclude that early sensitization to inhalant allergens increase the risk of developing asthma as well as having milk and wheat allergy symptoms. The most common inhalant allergens causing sensitisation was dog allergen, but prevalence and concentration remained stable over the 2 year follow up compared to house dust mite and cedar pollen. The dog and cat sensitisation was mainly explained by sensitisation to major allergens and not cross reactions to serum albumin.

Abbreviations

Specific IgE: specific immunoglobulin E; SD: standard deviation; OR: odds ratios; kUA/L: kilo units (arbitrary) per litre; AD: atopic dermatitis.

Authors' contributions

TF and MN conceived the idea and designed this study. MN, MS, and YK collected the data and CJP, SN, and PD performed the statistical analyses. CJP and MPB drafted the manuscript and all co-authors gave input and agreed to the final submitted version. All authors read and approved the final manuscript.

Author details

[1] Allergy Center and Department of Clinical Research, Mie National Hospital, IDD, Tsu, Mie, Japan. [2] Thermo Fisher Scientific, Uppsala, Sweden. [3] Department of Women's and Children's Health, Uppsala University, Uppsala, Sweden. [4] Thermo Fisher Scientific, Uppsala, Tokyo, Japan. [5] Department of Pediatrics, Mie National Hospital, Tsu, Mie, Japan. [6] Department of Otorhinolaryngology, Mie National Hospital, Tsu, Mie, Japan.

Acknowledgements

The authors would like to thank Mr. Yoshiki Segawa at Institute for Clinical Research, Mie National Hospital for his excellent technical assistance and Dr. Yuji Tohda at Department of Respiratory Medicine and Allergology, Kinki University School of Medicine for his general support for the study.

The authors would also like to thank the IRAM study investigators who actively participated in the study: Dr. Satoko Usui (Department of Otorhinolaryngology, Mie National Hospital), Dr. Ogura Kanae (Department of Pediatrics, Kyoto Yawata Hospital), Drs. Yutaka Suehiro and Yukiko Hiraguchi and Yuko Ebishima and Saeko Shimodera (Department of Pediatrics, Osaka Prefectual Medical Center for Respiratory and Allergic Deseases), Drs. Makoto Kameda and Yuri Takaoka and Tomoki Nishikido and Hiroko Yajima and Mineko Ikeoka (Department of Pediatrics, Osaka Prefectual Medical Center for Respiratory and Allergic Deseases), Drs. Hideo Ogura and Yukiko Ogura (Department of Pediatrics, Kochi National Hospital), Dr. Gyokei Murakami (Murakami Pediatric & Allergy Clinic), Drs. Toshimi Nakamura and Yoko Yamashita (Department of Pediatrics, Kanazawa Medical University Hospital), Dr. Yoko Kawasaki (Hotarugawa Clinic), Drs. Taku Oishi and Hiroaki Hisakawa and Akihiko Hisakawa and Hiroshi Wakiguchi (Department of Pediatrics, Kochi University), Dr. Hiroyasu Okahata (Department of Pediatrics, Kure Kyousai Hospital), Drs. Ikuo Okafuji and Shigeta Shimizu (Kobe City Medical Center General Hospital), Drs. Naomi Kondo and Eiko Matsui and Kazuo Kubota (Department of Pediatrics, Gifu University Hospital), Dr. Yutaka Morisawa (Kera Child & Allergy Clinic), Dr. Mitsuhiko Nambu (Department of Pediatrics, Tenri Hospital), Dr. Miki Takao (Department of Pediatrics, Takashige Memorial Hospital), Dr. Yoshinori Matsuwaki (Department of Otorhinolaryngology, Ota General Hospital), Drs. Yuichi Adachi and Toshiko Itazawa (Department of Pediatrics, Toyama University), Dr. Youichi Onoue (Onoue Pediatric Clinic), Dr Osamu Higuchi (Department of Pediatrics, Kurobe City Hospital), Dr. Yoko Adachi (Department of Pediatrics, Takaoka Minami Hospital), Dr. Akihiko Terada (Terada Kid's Allergy & Asthma Clinic), Dr. Yoko Osawa (Department of Otorhinolaryngology, Tannan Regional Medical Center), Dr. Rentaro Abumi (Abumi Clinic), Drs. Tatsuya Fuchizawa and Junko Yamamoto (Saiseikai Takaoka Hospital), Drs. Motokazu Nakabayashi and Masaharu Kasei (Department of Pediatrics, Kouseiren Takaoka Hospital), Drs. Takanori Abe and Mayumi Sugimoto (Department of Pediatrics, Japanese Red Cross Kochi Hospital), Dr. Hisashi Kondo (Kondo Pediatrics Clinic), Drs. Akiko Toga and Nobuyuki Doichi (Department of Pediatrics, Fukui-ken Saiseikai Hospital).

Competing interests

Takao Fujisawa and Mizuho Nagao received lecture fees from Thermo Fisher Scientific, Siemens Healthcare Diagnostics, MSD KK, Glaxo SmithKline, and Kyorin Pharmaceutical. Magnus P Borres, Carl Johan Petersson, Satoshi Nakayama and Patrik Dykiel are employed by ThermoFisher Scientific, Uppsala, Sweden. All other authors have declared they have no competing interests.

Funding

This study was supported, in part, by unconditional grant from Kyorin Pharmaceutical Inc.

References

1. Laan MP, Baert MR, Bijl AM, Vredendaal AE, De Waard-van der Spek FB, Oranje AP, Savelkoul HF, Neijens HJ. Markers for early sensitization and inflammation in relation to clinical manifestations of atopic disease up to 2 years of age in 133 high-risk children. Clin Exp Allergy. 2000;30:944–53.
2. Schroeder A, Kumar R, Pongracic JA, Sullivan CL, Caruso DM, Costello J, Meyer KE, Vucic Y, Gupta R, Kim JS, Fuleihan R, Wang X. Food allergy is associated with an increased risk of asthma. Clin Exp Allergy. 2009;39:261–70.
3. Eigenmann PA, Calza AM. Diagnosis of IgE-mediated food allergy among Swiss children with atopic dermatitis. Pediatr Allergy Immunol. 2000;11:95–100.
4. Fiocchi A, Pecora V, Petersson CJ, Dahdah L, Borres MP, Amengual MJ, Huss-Marp J, Mazzina O, Di Girolamo F. Sensitization pattern to inhalant and food allergens in symptomatic children at first evaluation. Ital J Pediatr. 2015;41:96.
5. Sly PD, Boner AL, Bjorksten B, Bush A, Custovic A, Eigenmann PA, Gern JE, Gerritsen J, Hamelmann E, Helms PJ, Lemanske RF, Martinez F, Pedersen S, Renz H, Sampson H, von Mutius E, Wahn U, Holt PG. Early identification of atopy in the prediction of persistent asthma in children. Lancet. 2008;372:1100–6.
6. Illi S, von Mutius E, Lau S, Nickel R, Gruber C, Niggemann B, Wahn U, Multicenter Allergy Study G. The natural course of atopic dermatitis from birth to age 7 years and the association with asthma. J Allergy Clin Immunol. 2004;113:925–31.
7. Peat JK, Salome CM, Woolcock AJ. Longitudinal changes in atopy during a 4-year period: relation to bronchial hyperresponsiveness and respiratory symptoms in a population sample of Australian schoolchildren. J Allergy Clin Immunol. 1990;85:65–74.
8. Rhodes HL, Thomas P, Sporik R, Holgate ST, Cogswell JJ. A birth cohort study of subjects at risk of atopy: twenty-two-year follow-up of wheeze and atopic status. Am J Respir Crit Care Med. 2002;165:176–80.
9. Sherrill D, Stein R, Kurzius-Spencer M, Martinez F. On early sensitization to allergens and development of respiratory symptoms. Clin Exp Allergy. 1999;29:905–11.
10. Simpson A, Soderstrom L, Ahlstedt S, Murray CS, Woodcock A, Custovic A. IgE antibody quantification and the probability of wheeze in preschool children. J Allergy Clin Immunol. 2005;116:744–9.
11. Wisniewski JA, Agrawal R, Minnicozzi S, Xin W, Patrie J, Heymann PW, Workman L, Platts-Mills TA, Song TW, Moloney M, Woodfolk JA. Sensitization to food and inhalant allergens in relation to age and wheeze among children with atopic dermatitis. Clin Exp Allergy. 2013;43:1160–70.
12. Stoltz DJ, Jackson DJ, Evans MD, Gangnon RE, Tisler CJ, Gern JE, Lemanske RF Jr. Specific patterns of allergic sensitization in early childhood and asthma & rhinitis risk. Clin Exp Allergy. 2013;43:233–41.
13. Konradsen JR, Fujisawa T, van Hage M, Hedlin G, Hilger C, Kleine-Tebbe J, Matsui EC, Roberts G, Ronmark E, Platts-Mills TA. Allergy to furry animals: new insights, diagnostic approaches, and challenges. J Allergy Clin Immunol. 2015;135:616–25.
14. Urisu A, Ebisawa M, Ito K, Aihara Y, Ito S, Mayumi M, Kohno Y, Kondo N. Japanese guideline for food allergy 2014. Allergol Int. 2014;63:399–419.
15. Hanifin JM, Rajka G. Diagnostic features of atopic dermatitis. Acta Derm Venereol Suppl (Stockh). 1980;92:44–7.
16. Hamasaki Y, Kohno Y, Ebisawa M, Kondo N, Nishima S, Nishimuta T, Morikawa A, Aihara Y, Akasawa A, Adachi Y, Arakawa H, Ikebe T, Ichikawa K, Inoue T, Iwata T, Urisu A, Ohya Y, Okada K, Odajima H, Katsunuma T, Kameda M, Kurihara K, Sakamoto T, Shimojo N, Suehiro Y, Tokuyama K, Nambu M, Fujisawa T, Matsui T, Matsubara T, Mayumi M, Mochizuki H, Yamaguchi K, Yoshihara S. Japanese pediatric guideline for the treatment and management of bronchial asthma 2012. Pediatr Int. 2014;56:441–50.
17. Illi S, von Mutius E, Lau S, Niggemann B, Gruber C, Wahn U, Multicentre Allergy Study G. Perennial allergen sensitisation early in life and chronic asthma in children: a birth cohort study. Lancet. 2006;368:763–70.
18. Lowe AJ, Abramson MJ, Hosking CS, Carlin JB, Bennett CM, Dharmage SC, Hill DJ. The temporal sequence of allergic sensitization and onset of infantile eczema. Clin Exp Allergy. 2007;37:536–42.

19. Lowe AJ, Hosking CS, Bennett CM, Carlin JB, Abramson MJ, Hill DJ, Dharmage SC. Skin prick test can identify eczematous infants at risk of asthma and allergic rhinitis. Clin Exp Allergy. 2007;37:1624–31.

20. Nilsson N, Sjolander S, Baar A, Berthold M, Pahr S, Vrtala S, Valenta R, Morita E, Hedlin G, Borres MP, Nilsson C. Wheat allergy in children evaluated with challenge and IgE antibodies to wheat components. Pediatr Allergy Immunol. 2015;26:119–25.

21. Papadopoulos NG, Arakawa H, Carlsen KH, Custovic A, Gern J, Lemanske R, Le Souef P, Makela M, Roberts G, Wong G, Zar H, Akdis CA, Bacharier LB, Baraldi E, van Bever HP, de Blic J, Boner A, Burks W, Casale TB, Castro-Rodriguez JA, Chen YZ, El-Gamal YM, Everard ML, Frischer T, Geller M, Gereda J, Goh DY, Guilbert TW, Hedlin G, Heymann PW, Hong SJ, Hossny EM, Huang JL, Jackson DJ, de Jongste JC, Kalayci O, Ait-Khaled N, Kling S, Kuna P, Lau S, Ledford DK, Lee SI, Liu AH, Lockey RF, Lodrup-Carlsen K, Lotvall J, Morikawa A, Nieto A, Paramesh H, Pawankar R, Pohunek P, Pongracic J, Price D, Robertson C, Rosario N, Rossenwasser LJ, Sly PD, Stein R, Stick S, Szefler S, Taussig LM, Valovirta E, Vichyanond P, Wallace D, Weinberg E, Wennergren G, Wildhaber J, Zeiger RS. International consensus on (ICON) pediatric asthma. Allergy. 2012;67:976–97.

22. Pescatore AM, Dogaru CM, Duembgen L, Silverman M, Gaillard EA, Spycher BD, Kuehni CE. A simple asthma prediction tool for preschool children with wheeze or cough. J Allergy Clin Immunol. 2014;133(111–8):e1–13.

23. Bjerg A, Winberg A, Berthold M, Mattsson L, Borres MP, Ronmark E. A population-based study of animal component sensitization, asthma, and rhinitis in schoolchildren. Pediatr Allergy Immunol. 2015;26:557–63.

24. Simpson A, Lazic N, Belgrave DC, Johnson P, Bishop C, Mills C, Custovic A. Patterns of IgE responses to multiple allergen components and clinical symptoms at age 11 years. J Allergy Clin Immunol. 2015;136:1224–31.

25. Uriarte SA, Sastre J. Clinical relevance of molecular diagnosis in pet allergy. Allergy. 2016;71:1066–8.

Skin microbiota of first cousins affected by psoriasis and atopic dermatitis

Lorenzo Drago[1,2]*, Roberta De Grandi[2], Gianfranco Altomare[3,4], Paolo Pigatto[3,4], Oliviero Rossi[5] and Marco Toscano[1]

Abstract

Background: Psoriasis and atopic dermatitis (AD) are chronic inflammatory skin diseases, which negatively influence the quality of life. In the last years, several evidences highlighted the pivotal role of skin bacteria in worsening the symptomatology of AD and psoriasis. In the present study we evaluated the skin microbiota composition in accurately selected subjects affected by (AD) and psoriasis.

Methods: Three first cousins were chosen for the study according to strict selection of criteria. One subject was affected by moderate AD, one had psoriasis and the last one was included as healthy control. Two lesional skin samples and two non-lesional skin samples (for AD and psoriatic subjects) from an area of 2 cm^2 behind the left ear were withdrawn by mean of a curette. For the healthy control, two skin samples from an area of 2 cm^2 behind the left ear were withdrawn by mean of a curette. DNA was extracted and sequencing was completed on the Ion Torrent PGM platform. Culturing of *Staphylococcus aureus* from skin samples was also performed.

Results: The psoriatic subject showed a decrease in *Firmicutes* abundance and an increase in *Proteobacteria* abundance. Moreover, an increase in *Streptococcaceae, Rhodobacteraceae, Campylobacteraceae* and *Moraxellaceae* has been observed in psoriatic subject, if compared with AD individual and control. Finally, AD individual showed a larger abundance of *S. aureus* than psoriatic and healthy subjects. Moreover, the microbiota composition of non-lesional skin samples belonging to AD and psoriatic individuals was very similar to the bacterial composition of skin sample belonging to the healthy control.

Conclusion: Significant differences between the skin microbiota of psoriatic individual and healthy and AD subjects were observed.

Keywords: Psoriasis, Atopic dermatitis, Metagenomics, Skin microbiota

Background

The largest organ of human body is the skin, which plays a pivotal role in protecting the host from pathogenic infections and penetration of harmful agents [1]. Before birth, the skin is completely sterile but after birth it is colonized by environmental microbes that are in homeostasis with the host [2, 3]. Moreover, after a vaginal delivery, fecal and vaginal microbes belonging to the mother's bacterial microflora also colonize the skin of infants. The microbial community living on the human skin is called skin microbiota, and it is constituted by over 100 distinct species of bacteria [4]. Generally, we find four dominant phyla of bacteria colonizing the skin: *Actinobacteria, Proteobacteria, Firmicutes* and *Bacteroidetes* [5]. Several evidences exist about the pivotal role of bacteria in the development and persistence of atopic dermatitis (AD), a chronic itchy, inflammatory skin condition, very common in childhood. AD is considered to be a multifactorial disease, in which environmental and genetic factors contribute to its pathogenesis [1]. The incidence of AD has increased significantly in the last decades worldwide,

*Correspondence: lorenzo.drago@unimi.it
[1] Clinical Chemistry and Microbiology Laboratory, IRCCS Galeazzi Orthopaedic Institute, Via R. Galeazzi 4, 20164 Milan, Italy
Full list of author information is available at the end of the article

Oliviero Rossi is the member of the Executive Committee of the Italian Society of Allergy Asthma and Immunology (SIAAIC)

leading the scientific community to hypothesize that the change in the lifestyle and nutrition may be involved in the development of aforementioned disease [5–7]. In the majority of individuals affected by AD, *Staphylococcus aureus* was found on the skin lesions. Furthermore, also the skin commensal *Staphylococcus epidermidis* has been observed to be increased with clinical disease activity, while bacteria belonging to the genera *Streptococcus*, *Propionibacterium* and *Corynebacterium* were increased only after a pharmacological therapy [8]. The skin microbiota dysbiosis may lead to a lack of immune system stimulation, together with an imbalance of type 1 T helper cells (T_H1) and type 2 cells (T_H2) activity, which might be involved in worsening of AD symptoms [9].

Psoriasis, instead, is a common inflammatory disease affecting 2–5 % of the population in industrialized countries. The disease is characterized by cutaneous inflammation and keratinocyte hyperproliferation, and it is often linked to severe complications, such as psoriatic arthritis [1]. Psoriasis has been hypothesized to result from a lack of immune tolerance to the skin microbiota in genetically predisposed individuals [10]. The aforementioned skin disease forms lesions on body often associated with beta-hemolytic streptococcal infection, where streptococcal superantigen leads T cell stimulation and expansion in the skin [11]. Several evidences highlighted the association between psoriasis and skin microbiota dysbiosis, underlying the relative abundance of *Corynebacterium*, *Propionibacterium*, *Staphylococcus* and *Streptococcus* in psoriasis plaques [12].

To date, the specific role of the skin microbiota in psoriasis and AD is still unknown, and it is unclear if the changes observed in the skin bacterial composition of individuals affected by psoriasis and AD are a cause or a consequence of alteration of the skin barrier, following the pathogenesis of aforementioned skin diseases. Certainly, the skin microbiota interacts with the host organism by producing several metabolites, which modulate cutaneous pro- and anti-inflammatory responses [13]. The current study used a next generation sequencing (NGS) approach to determine if some differences in the skin microbiota composition occur between individuals affected by psoriasis and AD, compared with a healthy control.

Methods

Study population

Three male first cousins aged 50 ± 3 years were chosen for the present study, according to specific and strict characteristics shared by all of them (Table 1). All subjects followed a diet rich in bifidogenic factors that promoted the growth of beneficial bacteria, such as bifidobacteria, and poor in allergenic foods that could worsening the

symptomatology of psoriasis and atopic dermatitis. In particular, food containing vitamin A (peppers, carrots, spinach, basil, pumpkin), vitamin C (orange, lemon, and kiwi), folic acid (legumes, cereals, lettuce, asparagus), zinc (figs, sunflower seeds, potatoes) and omega-3 (fish) were allowed. In contrast, strawberries are often associated to allergies, in particular to atopic dermatitis, while tomato may lead to bowel dysfunction and it is not recommended for atopic subjects. Therefore, these foods were excluded from the diet of subjects enrolled in the study. Moreover, shellfish, cheese, fatty foods and red meat were not recommended (Table 1).

The selection criteria were chosen in agreement with dermatologists of the Clinical Dermatology Unit of IRCCS Galeazzi Orthopaedic Institute in Milan, Italy, where the study was conducted. One subject was affected by moderate AD, one had psoriasis and the last one was included as healthy control. The inclusion criteria for atopic dermatitis were moderate AD according to Hanifin and Rajka [14], with predominant rough and fissured skin as well as pruritus for at least 2 months. The inclusion criteria for psoriasis, instead, were the presence of psoriatic erythematous patches and the evaluation of psoriasis area and severity index (PASI) score, a tool used for the measurement of psoriasis severity. In particular, the PASI score of psoriatic subject enrolled in the study was 20.0, while the SCORAD for the AD subject was 32.46, underlying the presence of a moderate psoriasis and a moderate AD, respectively. Furthermore, subjects affected by psoriasis and AD had no concomitant diseases and both healthy and psoriatic individual had no any history of atopic dermatitis in childhood. The primary exclusion factors were the presence of chronic dermatosis such as seborrheic dermatitis, contact dermatitis, nummular eczema, ichthyosis, an immunodeficiency or any other immunological disorder, scabies, cutaneous fungal infection, HIV-associated skin disorders, malignant diseases, T-cell lymphoma, Letterer-Siwe disease, progressive systemic diseases, serious internal diseases (e.g., serious decompensated diseases of the heart, liver, and/or kidneys, or diabetes mellitus). The study was conducted according to ICH guidelines for Good Clinical Practice. All procedures followed were in accordance with the Declaration of Helsinki of 1975, as revised in 2000 and 2008. The study was approved by the Ethic Committee and Scientific Direction of the IRCCS Galeazzi Orthopaedic Institute. Subjects enrolled in the study provided verbal informed consent, which was carefully recorded in the study worksheets, to participate in the present study. Two lesional skin samples from a damaged area of 2 cm^2 behind the left ear were withdrawn by mean of a curette from AD and psoriatic subjects. Moreover, two non-lesional skin samples were taken from the

Table 1 Subjects' selection criteria

Subjects' characteristics	
Sex	Male
Age	50–53 years old
Subjects relationship	All individuals were first cousins
Diet	A Mediterranean diet was followed for 1 month before the day sampling. Pollen- and allergen- associated food, such as apple, hazelnut, celery, strawberries, shellfish and read meat were excluded from diet. Furthermore, milk intake was not recommended. Foods and beverages allowed were: bread, potatoes, vegetables, fresh fruit, meat and meat products, fish and fish products, eggs, edible fat, coffee, tea and soft drinks
Lifestyle	All individuals lived in the same neighborhood. No sport or daily exercises were practiced during the study period. No travel or excursion were carried out for at least 1 month before the day of sampling
Occupation	All subjects had a sedentary office work
Sexual activity	No sexual activity for 2 weeks before the day of sampling
Clothing	All individuals used only cotton clothes for all the study period
Pharmacological therapy	No antibiotic therapy was administered for at least 1 month before the day of sampling and they were not subjected to any kind of pharmacological therapy
Probiotic therapy	No probiotic therapy was administered for at least 1 month before the day of sampling
Personal care	All subjects used Cetaphil, a free-preservatives soap, once a day for 1 month before the day of sampling. Cetaphil is an oil-in-water petrolatum-based cream used to treat dry skin and often recommended for the management of AD. Moreover, no skin perfume or cream was used during the study
Others	No allergy to food, dust, pollen, grasses and drugs was present The subjects enrolled in the study shared no genetic diseases All subjects had not pets and/or contacts with any kind of animals All individuals were nonsmokers and not subjected to passive smoking The day of sampling took place the same day for all subjects enrolled in the study. The study was conducted during the winter season, in order to avoid excessive sweating

same area from AD and psoriatic individuals and used as internal control. For the healthy control, instead, two skin samples from an area of 2 cm² behind the left ear were withdrawn by mean of a curette. Samples were placed in sterile Petri dishes (one dish for each subject's sample) and stored at 4 °C until analysis. Of the two samples, one was used for metagenomics, and the other for cultural analysis. None of the individuals enrolled in the study was currently receiving specific therapy for psoriasis and AD (i.e. methotrexate, tacrolimus or pimecrolimus). No additional drugs (i.e. corticosteroids, anti-histamines) were used by subjects enrolled in the study. In particular, during the month before the day of sampling, the psoriatic individual was subjected to specific clinical investigations, such as screening for latent tuberculosis and rheumatoid arthritis, to determine the appropriate systemic therapy to be administered after the sampling. During this period, psoriatic individual could use lanolin, a skin protector, if necessary. The study was carried out after obtaining informed consent from all subjects, and in line with the guidelines for experimental studies on humans applicable within our Institute.

DNA extraction
Total DNA was extracted from skin samples using the Genomic DNA Mini Kit (Tissue) following the manufacturer's instructions (Geneaid, Italy). The protocol included an initial mechanical disruption step with a micropestle, followed by an enzymatic lysis incubation for 30 min at 60 °C.

16S rRNA gene amplification
Partial 16S rRNA gene sequences were amplified from extracted DNA using the 16S Metagenomics Kit (Life Technologies, Italy) that is designed for rapid analysis of polybacterial samples using Ion Torrent sequencing technology. The kit includes two primer sets that selectively amplify the corresponding hypervariable regions of the 16S region in bacteria: primer set V2–4–8 and primer set V3–6, 7–9. The PCR conditions used were 10 min at 95 °C, 30 cycles of 30 s at 95 °C, 30 s at 58 °C and 20 s at 72 °C, followed by 10 min at 72 °C. Amplification was carried out by using a SimpliAmp thermal cycler (Life Technologies, Italy). The integrity of the PCR amplicons was analyzed by electrophoresis on 2 % agarose gel.

Ion torrent PGM sequencing of 16S rRNA gene-based amplicons
The PCR products derived from amplification of specific 16S rRNA gene hypervariable regions were purified by a purification step involving the Agencourt AMPure XP DNA purification beads (Beckman Coulter

Genomics, Germany) in order to remove primer dimers. From the concentration and the average size of each amplicon, the amount of DNA fragments per microliter was calculated and libraries created by using the Ion Plus fragment Library kit (Life Technologies, Italy). Barcodes were also added to each sample, using the Ion Xpress Barcode Adapters 1–16 kit (Life Technologies, Italy). Emulsion PCR was carried out using the Ion OneTouch TM 400 Template Kit (Life Technologies, Italy). Sequencing of the amplicon libraries was carried out on a 318 chip using the Ion Torrent Personal Genome Machine (PGM) system and employing the Ion PGM Hi-Q kit (Life Technologies, Italy) according to the supplier's instructions. After sequencing, the individual sequence reads were filtered by the PGM software to remove low quality and polyclonal sequences. Sequences matching the PGM 3' adaptor were also automatically trimmed. 16 rRNA sequences were then analyzed by Ion Reporter Software, which comprises a suite of bioinformatics tools that streamline and simplify analysis of semiconductor-based sequencing data. The 16S rRNA workflow module in Ion Reporter Software was able to classify individual reads combining a Basic Local Alignment Search Tool (BLAST) alignment to the curated Greengenes database, which contains more than 400,000 records, with a BLAST alignment to the premium curated MicroSEQ ID database, a high-quality library of full-length 16S rRNA sequences. The final output of Ion Reporter Software was the identification of microorganisms and their abundance in the sample.

Quantification of *Staphylococcus aureus* by means of cultivable method

Skin samples were transferred to 1.5 ml tubes and one ml of normal sterile solution (NaCl 9 g/l) was added. After homogenization to a homogeneous solution, samples were serially diluted in saline and appropriate dilutions were plated onto Mannitol Salt Agar (MSA), a selective medium for the growth of *Staphylococcus* spp, and incubated in aerobiosis for 48 h at 37 °C. All colonies of different morphology were identified according to: growth on selective medium, Gram staining, colony and cell morphology and the catalase and oxidase tests. The identification of *S. aureus* was performed by mean of RAPID Staph assay (Thermofisher, Italy). Finally, the percentage of occurrence of *S. aureus* in skin samples was calculated as follow:% *S. aureus* = [mean of CFU/cm^2 (*S. aureus*)]/ [mean of log10 CFU/cm^2 (total staphylococci)] × 100.

Statistics

Differences in *S. aureus* counts between the three individuals were evaluated by means of Student t test.

Results

Metagenomics analysis of skin microbiota in AD and psoriatic individuals and in healthy control

Figures 1, 2 and 3 represent the comparison between the cutaneous microbiota of damaged skin from AD and psoriatic individuals and the skin of healthy control. Comparing lesional skin samples from AD and psoriatic subjects to the skin sample of healthy control, the most prevalent phyla detected in all subjects included *Firmicutes*, *Bacteroidetes*, *Proteobacteria* and *Actinobacteria*. Subject affected by psoriasis showed a decrease in *Firmicutes* abundance and an increase in *Proteobacteria* abundance, if compared with AD patient and healthy individual (Fig. 1). A prevalence of *Proteobacteria* and *Bacteroidetes* over other phyla has been observed in psoriatic individual (Fig. 1). At family level, subject affected by psoriasis showed an increase in *Streptococcaceae*, *Rhodobacteraceae*, *Campylobacteraceae*, and *Moraxellaceae* if compared with control and AD patient (Fig. 2). However, even if psoriatic subject had a larger amount of *Rhodobacteriaceae*, a minor diversity in the family composition has been detected (Fig. 3). Indeed, in this subject the most abundant genus was *Parococcus* (i.e. >90 % of total *Rhodobacteraceae* total reads) while in healthy and atopic individuals also *Rhodobacter* and *Haematobacter* were found in skin microbiota (Fig. 3). Furthermore, psoriatic patient showed a decrease in *Staphylococcaceae* and *Propionibacteriaceae* abundance if compared with AD and healthy individual (Fig. 2). In particular, the total skin microbiota of psoriatic individual showed a decrease in *Propionibacterium acnes* abundance (i.e. <2 % of total reads), while in AD and healthy subject *P. acnes* was more abundant (i.e. >10 % of total reads). *Lactobacillaceae* were the population that contributed in the minor proportion to the overall skin microbiota (i.e. <0.5 % of total reads). Interestingly, no differences between the skin microbiota composition of AD patient and healthy control has been observed (Figs. 1, 2). Comparing non-lesional skin samples from AD and psoriatic subjects to the skin sample of healthy control, we did not observed any differences in the skin microbiota composition; indeed, bacterial phyla (Fig. 4a) and family (Fig. 4b) composition in AD and psoriatic individuals was very similar to that observed in healthy subject. Furthermore, in non-lesional skin samples of AD and psoriatic individuals we observed a similar composition at genus level among the *Rhodobacteraceae* family, if compared with the healthy control (Fig. 4c).

Quantification of *S. aureus* in skin samples

Patient affected by AD showed the larger abundance of *S. aureus* (Fig. 5a), with a frequency of 73 % of *S. aureus* on the total staphylococci load found on skin sample. By

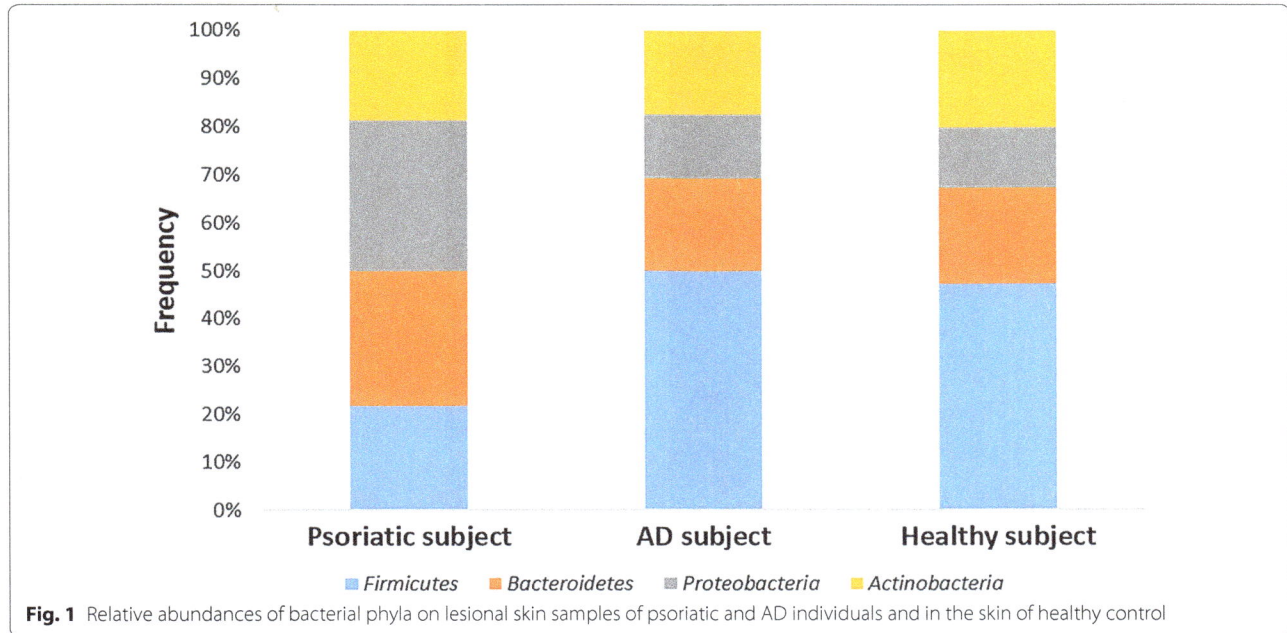

Fig. 1 Relative abundances of bacterial phyla on lesional skin samples of psoriatic and AD individuals and in the skin of healthy control

contrast, psoriatic individual had only a 2 % of *S. aureus* on his skin, while healthy control showed a frequency of 18 % (Fig. 5a). Moreover, no differences in *S. aureus* frequency were observed between non-lesional skin samples of AD and psoriatic subjects and healthy control (Fig. 5b).

Discussion

This is the first study in which the skin microbiota of AD and psoriatic selected individuals subjected to the same lifestyle and environment factors has been compared. Indeed, we evaluated the skin microbiota of much selected subjects affected by psoriasis and AD, compared with the microbiota of a healthy related control. In particular, we analyzed samples from the area behind the left ear, evaluating the microbiota associated to this specific anatomical district. One of the main factor that seem to be involved in the development of allergic diseases is the mode of delivery; indeed, cesarean section has been observed to be associated with a moderately risk of allergic rhinitis, asthma and hospitalization for asthma [15]. One hypothesis concerns the composition of the gut microbiota, which is established early in childhood. Vaginal delivery leads to the first colonization of infant gut with maternal vaginal and fecal bacteria, while cesarean babies are deprived of this natural exposure and present a different gut microbiota [15]. The first steps of infant gut colonization play a pivotal role in normal tolerance induction, as well as in the development and homeostasis of the immune system.

Therefore, cesarean delivery may lead to an increased susceptibility to atopic conditions. Interestingly, all subjects enrolled in the present study were born by vaginal delivery and no correlations with the development of AD and psoriasis can be suggested. However, significant differences have been detected in the abundance of several bacterial family in subjects enrolled in the study. *Propionibacteriaceae*, indeed, showed a different distribution among the three groups analyzed, as AD and healthy individuals had a larger abundance of aforementioned bacterial family and its major human species *Propionibacterium acnes*, if compared with the subject affected by psoriasis. *P. acnes* are dominant microorganisms in normal skin [16–19], and a decrease in the number of these microbes could be a reflection of disordered ecological niches that become inhospitable to these microorganisms, and probably play a pivotal role in the pathogenesis of psoriasis or could be involved in the disease worsening [17]. *P. acnes* could have a beneficial and protective role on the human organism, and in particular, at skin level, by mean of its immunomodulatory action in signaling human cells [18, 19]. It has been hypothesized that *P. acnes* could protect the human skin from the action of several pathogenic bacteria, and its decrease could lead to a reduction of the protective skin barrier [17]. However, to date it is not clear if the decrease observed in *P. acnes* abundance is a consequence of the inflammatory state of psoriasis, or if this reduction is involved in the pathogenesis of the aforementioned disease.

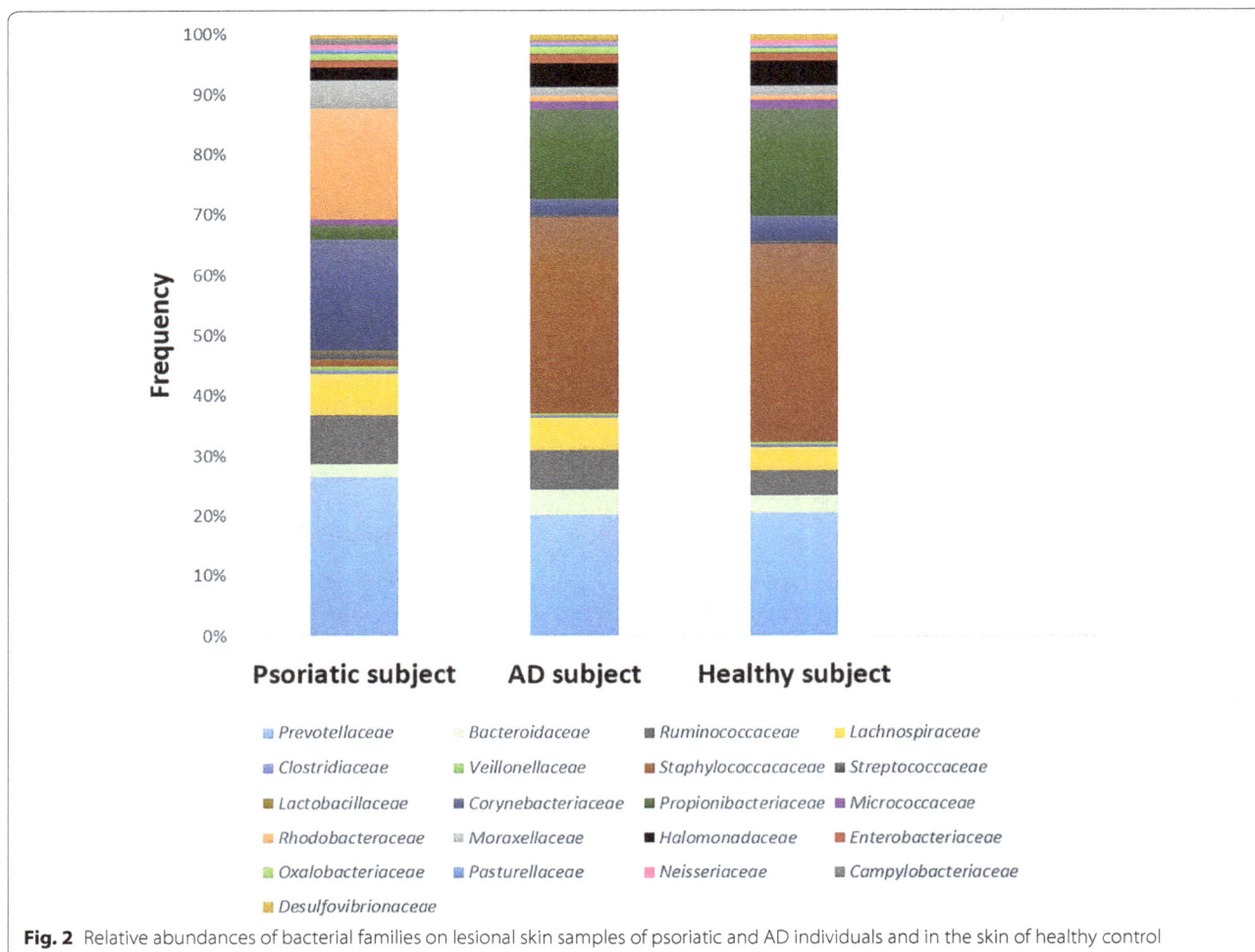

Fig. 2 Relative abundances of bacterial families on lesional skin samples of psoriatic and AD individuals and in the skin of healthy control

An increase in *Streptococcaceae* has been observed in psoriatic subject, confirming data of previous works, in which the presence of *Streptococcus* spp was linked to the pathogenesis of psoriasis [20, 21]. *Streptococcaceae* are highly relevant among the environmental factors that are involved in the development of psoriasis [21]. Different mechanisms, such as molecular mimicry, superantigens and the ability of streptococci for intracellular uptake and persistence in skin cells, may be involved in the pathogenesis of the disease. Furthermore, the skin microbiota associated to the subject with psoriasis showed a larger abundance of *Rhodobacteraceae*, in comparison to that of healthy and AD individual. Interestingly, a minor bacterial diversity has been observed in psoriatic sample, as *Paracoccus* was the predominant bacterial family detected. At the contrary, *Rhodobacter* and *Haematobacter* represented a significant part of the skin microbiota of AD and healthy subjects. *Rhodobacter* spp are able to produce a molecule, named lycogen, structurally similar to lycopene, which can acts as anti-inflammatory agent

and as inhibitor of melanogenesis. This molecule is able to prevent the down-regulation of procollagen I and inhibit elevated production of NFκB, a transcription factor involved in cellular stress, which were elicited by UV-light exposure [22–24]. The absence of *Rhodobacteraceae* among the skin microbiota observed in psoriatic individual could be linked to the reduction of the physiological skin barrier integrity that is involved in the symptomatology and etiopathology of psoriasis.

Finally, our results did not underline a difference between the microbiota composition of AD individual and the healthy control, except for the higher frequency of occurrence of *S. aureus* in AD subject, even if a high abundance of *Staphylococcaceae* has been detected in both groups of individuals. Several evidences exist about the mainly role of *S. aureus* in the pathogenesis of AD [25–27]. In particular, the skin of AD subjects has been observed to be more frequently colonized by *S. aureus* if compared to that of healthy control. This microorganism is able to increase the skin inflammation by mean

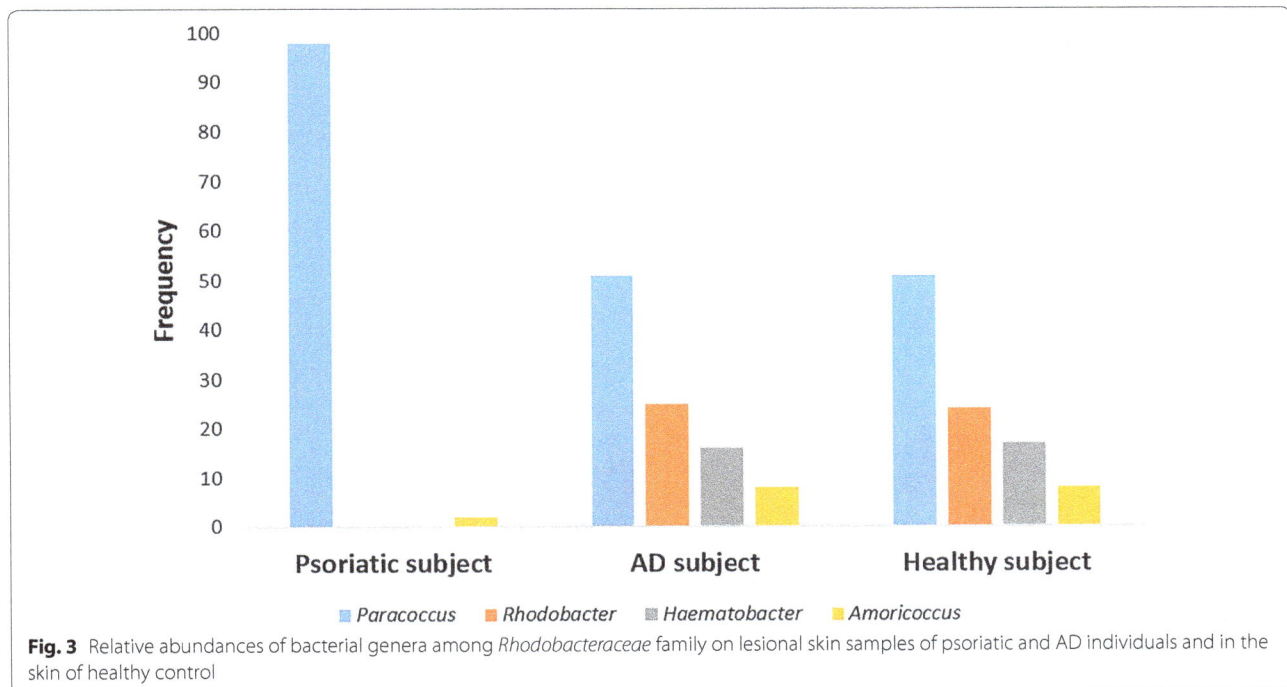

Fig. 3 Relative abundances of bacterial genera among *Rhodobacteraceae* family on lesional skin samples of psoriatic and AD individuals and in the skin of healthy control

of specific toxins which act as superantigens and, as a consequence, they may induce monocytes and lymphocytes activation, increasing also the production of several pro-inflammatory cytokines [28, 29]. Interestingly, as the severity of AD lesions increased, also the load of *S. aureus* has been observed to become higher. Probably, the high abundance of *S. aureus* we detected in AD sample contributed to worsening the skin barrier damages, leading to the characteristic skin lesions that affected AD subject enrolled in the present study. Moreover, the pivotal role of *S. aureus* in AD was underlined by the low frequency of *S. aureus* in non-lesional skin sample of AD individual, compared to the lesional skin sample of the same subject. Interestingly, the microbiota composition of non-lesional skin belonging to AD and psoriatic individuals was very similar to the bacterial composition of sample from the healthy control. These findings suggested that the cutaneous dysbiosis we observed in psoriatic and AD subjects was directly linked to the skin damages that characterize psoriasis and AD. Moreover, bacteria belonging to *Parococcus* genera, which have been observed to be increased in psoriasis skin sample, seem to be involved in the formation of skin pustules and they may have a direct role in the maintenance and worsening of psoriatic skin lesions [30]. Cutaneous bacteria have already been observed to be directly involved in the pathogenesis of several skin diseases, in particular in psoriasis and AD, where patients show a significant difference between the microbiota composition of lesional skin and non-lesional skin [31].

S. aureus, for example, is thought to play a pivotal role in the pathogenesis of these diseases, being involved not only in the pathology onset, but also in its progression, leading to an exacerbation of inflammatory response [31]. Moreover, differences in bacterial composition often observed in different skin sites may be directly involved in the different severity of cutaneous lesions on specific skin areas.

Although, several contradictory data about the specific role of cutaneous microbiota exist due to different sampling techniques. Some studies analyze the microbiota composition using skin swabs, while others investigate the bacterial composition from the complete epidermis and dermis, leading to different results [31]. To date, there are no enough information about the specific role of the skin microbiota in cutaneous diseases, as it is not clear if the bacterial dysbiosis often associated to these dyseases is the leading cause or a consequence of the pathological status. Interestingly, several evidences underlined that also intestinal bacteria seem to be directly involved in the onset and in the maintenance of allergic diseases, suggesting the possibility of preventing or treating AD and psoriasis by influencing the intestinal microbiota. The gut dysbiosis, associated to disruption of intestinal barrier function, may lead to a significant increase in local and systemic inflammation that is often associated to allergic diseases [32, 33]. AD patients, in particular, showed several changes in the gut microbiota composition, as bifidobacteria were significantly lower in comparison to

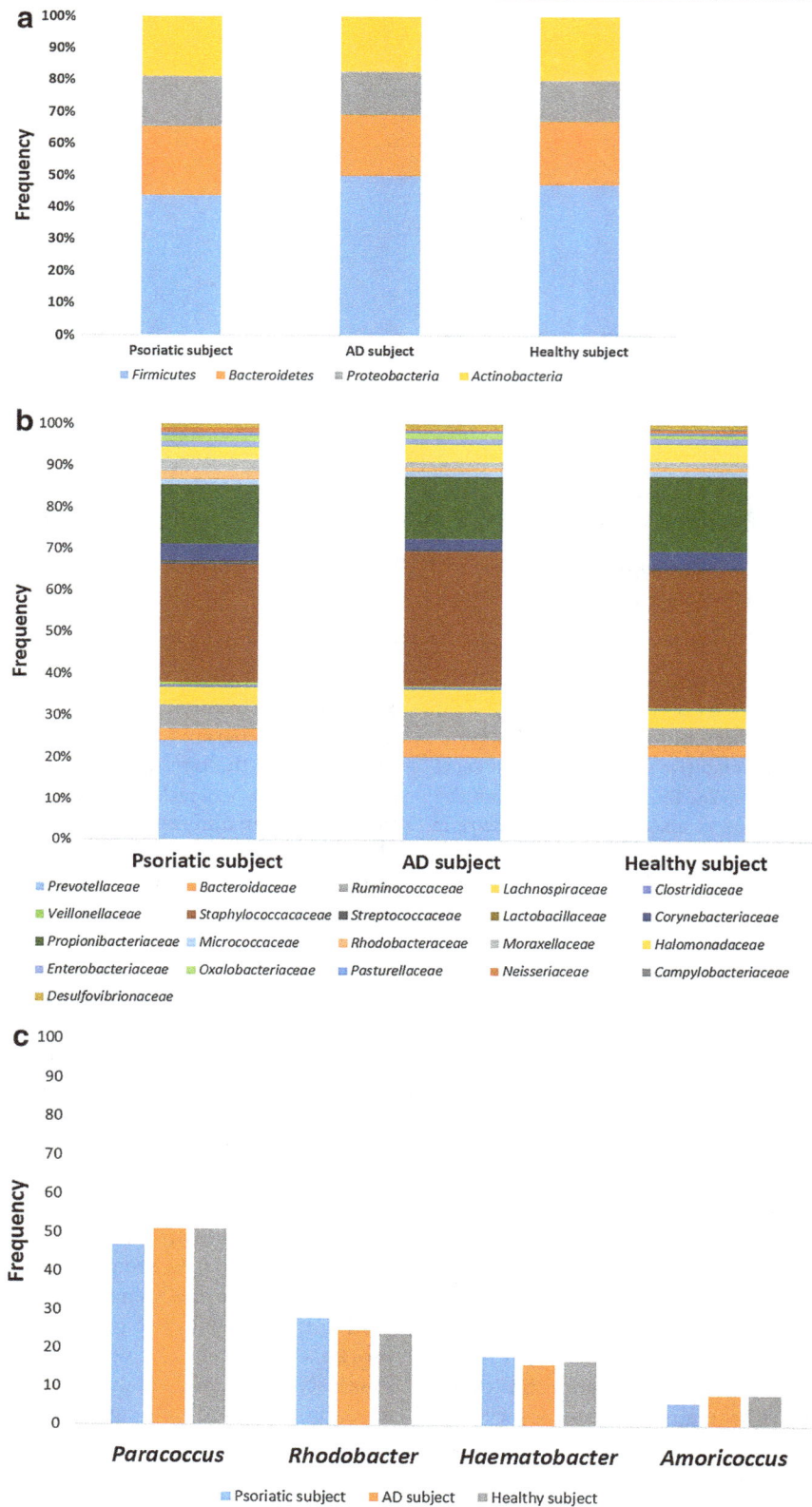

Fig. 4 Comparison between non-lesional skin samples of AD, psoriatic and healthy subjects. Comparison between bacterial phyla composition (**a**); comparison between bacterial family composition (**b**); comparison between bacterial genera composition among *Rhodobacteraceae* family (**c**)

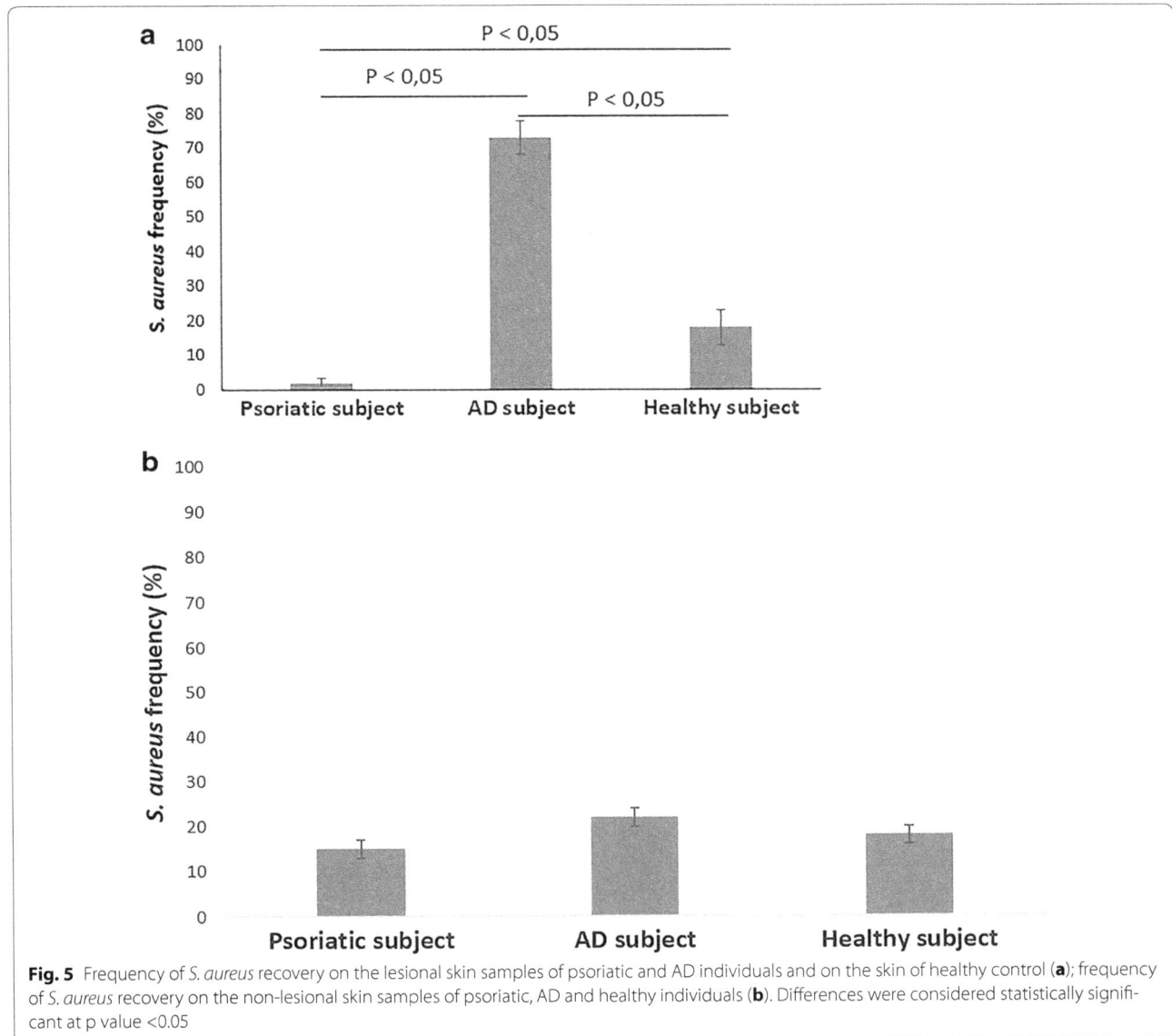

Fig. 5 Frequency of *S. aureus* recovery on the lesional skin samples of psoriatic and AD individuals and on the skin of healthy control (**a**); frequency of *S. aureus* recovery on the non-lesional skin samples of psoriatic, AD and healthy individuals (**b**). Differences were considered statistically significant at p value <0.05

healthy subjects, while the number of staphylococci was significantly higher in AD individuals compared with controls. Consequently, a decrease of anti-inflammatory molecules due to the reduction of bifidobacteria and a parallel increase in pro-inflammatory molecules due to the proliferation of staphylococci in the intestinal environment, may lead to the worsening of inflammation status and symptomatology of allergic diseases [32].

Conclusions

In conclusion, significant differences between the skin microbiota of psoriatic individual and healthy and AD subjects were observed. The majority of studies on AD- and psoriasis-associated skin microbiota focused their attention on the microbial population belonging to shoulder, finger, arm, forearm, elbow, abdomen, knee and leg, while we analyzed the area behind the left ear, highlighting how the skin area analyzed also could influence the microbiota composition in psoriasis and AD.

The forearm, for example, has been observed to be colonized mainly by microorganisms belonging to *Proteobacteria* and *Bacteroidetes* phyla, as well as the antecubital fossa that present also a high abundance of *Staphylococcaceae*. In popliteal fossa, instead, the most abundant microorganisms belong to the *Staphylococcaceae* family, while the inguinal crease is colonized mainly by *Corynebacterineae* [30]. Interestingly, the different skin sites present not only different kind of microorganisms, but they differ also for evenness and richness of bacterial communities [34]. Consequently, when a dysbiosis of the skin microbiota occurs, the kind of bacteria located on various skin sites can differently influence the onset and the progression of cutaneous diseases.

However, one limit of the present study was the low number of subjects enrolled, but our purpose was to minimize all variables that could influence the skin microbiota composition, applying stringent criteria of patient selection. Moreover, another vial of the present study was the lack of information about the family history of AD and psoriasis in the maternal or paternal line. However, the choice to enroll these three correlated-individuals with similar lifestyle have been taken to reduce the study variables, as previous studies enrolled subjects with different lifestyles and geolocation that could influence the skin microbiota composition. Further analysis will be needed to examine greater number of lesions in order to evaluate the connection of skin microbiota composition with the progression of inflammatory diseases. Furthermore, also patients with severe AD might be involved in the study to verify the correlation between the skin microbiota, and in particular the presence of *S. aureus*, and the disease severity.

Authors' contributions

LD, GA, PP and OR designed the study. GA and PP collected clinical samples. MT and RDG processed clinical samples and performed metagenomics analysis. MT and RDG performed the statistical analysis. LD, GA, PP and OR interpreted data. LD and MT wrote the paper. All authors read and approved the final manuscript.

Author details

[1] Clinical Chemistry and Microbiology Laboratory, IRCCS Galeazzi Orthopaedic Institute, Via R. Galeazzi 4, 20164 Milan, Italy. [2] Medical Technical Sciences Laboratory, Department of Biomedical Science for Health, University of Milan, Via Mangiagalli 31, 20133 Milan, Italy. [3] Clinical Dermatology, IRCCS Galeazzi Orthopaedic Institute, Via Galeazzi 4, 20164 Milan, Italy. [4] Department of Biomedical Science for Health, University of Milan, Milan, Italy. [5] SOD Immunoallergy Caraggi University-Hospital, Largo Giovanni Alessandro Brambilla, 3, 50134 Florence, Italy.

References

1. Zeeuwen PL, Kleerebezem M, Timmerman HM, Schalkwijk J. Microbiome and skin diseases. Curr Opin Allergy Clin Immunol. 2013;13:514–20.
2. Dominguez-Bello MG, Costello EK, Contreras M, Magris M, Hidalgo G, Fierer N, Knight R. Delivery mode shapes the acquisition and structure of the initial microbiota across multiple body habitats in newborns. Proc Natl Acad Sci USA. 2010;107:11971–5.
3. Capone KA, Dowd SE, Stamatas GN, Nikolovski J. Diversity of the human skin microbiome early in life. J Invest Dermatol. 2011;131:2026–32.
4. Grice EA, Kong HH, Renaud G, Young AC, Comparative Sequencing Program NISC, Bouffard GG, et al. A diversity profile of the human skin microbiota. Genome Res. 2008;18:1043–50.
5. Grice EA. The skin microbiome: potential for novel diagnostic and therapeutic approaches to cutaneous disease. Semin Cutan Med Surg. 2014;33:98–103.
6. Drago L, Iemoli E, Rodighiero V, Nicola L, De Vecchi E, Piconi S. Effects of Lactobacillus salivarius LS01 (DSM 22775) treatment on adult atopic dermatitis: a randomized placebo-controlled study. Int J Immunopathol Pharmacol. 2011;24:1037–48.
7. Iemoli E, Trabattoni D, Parisotto S, Borgonovo L, Toscano M, Rizzardini G, et al. Probiotics reduce gut microbial translocation and improve adult atopic dermatitis. J Clin Gastroenterol. 2012;46:33–40.
8. Iwase T, Uehara Y, Shinji H, Tajima A, Seo H, Takada K, et al. *Staphylococcus epidermidis* Esp inhibits *Staphylococcus aureus* biofilm formation and nasal colonization. Nature. 2010;465:346–9.
9. Drago L, Toscano M, Pigatto PD. Probiotics: immunomodulatory properties in allergy and eczema. G Ital Dermatol Venereol. 2013;148:505–14.
10. Leung DY, Travers JB, Giorno R, Norris DA, Skinner R, Aelion J, et al. Evidence for a streptococcal superantigen driven process in acute guttate psoriasis. J Clin Invest. 1995;96:2106–12.
11. Tagami H. The role of complement-derived mediators in inflammatory skin diseases. Arch Dermatol Res. 1992;284:2–9.
12. Alekseyenko AV, Perez-Perez GI, De Souza A, Strober B, Gao Z, Bihan M, et al. Community differentiation of the cutaneous microbiota in psoriasis. Microbiome. 2013;1:31.
13. Arpaia N, Campbell C, Fan X, Dikiy S, Dikiy S, van der Veeken J, deRoos P, et al. Metabolites produced by commensal bacteria promote peripheral regulatory T-cell generation. Nature. 2013;504:451–5.
14. Hanifin JM, Rajka G. Diagnostic features of atopic dermatitis. Acta Derm Venereol. 1980;1980:44–7.
15. Bager P, Wohlfahrt J, Westergaard T. Caesarean delivery and risk of atopy and allergic disease: meta-analyses. Clin Exp Allergy. 2008;38:634–42.
16. Bruggemann H, Henne A, Hoster F, Liesegang H, Wiezer A, Strittmatter A, et al. The complete genome sequence of *Propionibacterium acnes*, a commensal of human skin. Science. 2004;305:671–3.
17. Gao Z, Tseng CH, Strober BE, Pei Z, Blaser MJ. Substantial alterations of the cutaneous bacterial biota in psoriatic lesions. PLoS One. 2008;3:e2719.
18. Eady EA, Ingham E. *Propionibacterium acnes* –friend of foe? Rev Med Microbiol. 1994;5:163–73.
19. Blaser MJ, Kirschner D. The equilibria that allow bacterial persistence in human hosts. Nature. 2007;449:843–9.
20. Weisenseel P, Laumbacher B, Besgen P, Ludolph-Hauser D, Herzinger T, Roecken M, et al. Streptococcal infection distinguishes different types of psoriasis. J Med Genet. 2002;39:767–8.
21. Prinz JC. The role of streptococci in psoriasis. Hautarzt. 2009;60:109–15.
22. Yang TH, Lai YH, Lin TP, Liu WS, Kuan LC, Liu CC. Chronic exposure to *Rhodobacter sphaeroides* extract Lycogen™ prevents UVA-induced malondialdehyde accumulation and procollagen I down-regulation in human dermal fibroblasts. Int J Mol Sci. 2014;5:1686–99.
23. Liu WS, Chen MC, Chiu KH, Wen ZH, Lee CH. Amelioration of dextran sodium sulfate-induced colitis in mice by *Rhodobacter sphaeroides* extract. Molecules. 2012;17:13622–30.
24. Liu WS, Kuan YD, Chiu KH, Wang WK, Chang FH, Liu CH, et al. The extract of Rhodobacter sphaeroides inhibits melanogenesis through the MEK/ERK signaling pathway. Mar Drugs. 2013;11:1899–908.
25. Drago L, Toscano M, De Vecchi E, Piconi S, Iemoli E. Changing of fecal flora and clinical effect of *L. salivarius* LS01 in adults with atopic dermatitis. J Clin Gastroenterol. 2012;46:56–63.
26. Watanabe S, Narisawa Y, Arase S, Okamatsu H, Ikenaga T, Tajiri Y, et al. Differences in fecal microflora between patients with atopic dermatitis and healthy control subjects. J Allergy Clin Immunol. 2003;111:587–91.
27. Higaki S, Morohashi M, Yamagishi T, Hasegawa Y. Comparative study of staphylococci from the skin of atopic dermatitis patients and from healthy subjects. Int J Dermatol. 1999;38:265–9.
28. Sharp MJ, Rowe J, Kusel M, Sly PD, Holt PG. Specific patterns of responsiveness to microbial antigens staphylococcal enterotoxin B and purified protein derivative by cord blood mononuclear cells are predictive of risk for development of atopic dermatitis. Clin Exp Allergy. 2003;33:435–41.
29. Nomura I, Tanaka K, Tomita H, Katsunuma T, Ohya Y, Ikeda N, et al. Evaluation of the staphylococcal exotoxins and their specific IgE in childhood atopic dermatitis. J Allergy Clin Immunol. 1999;104:441–6.

30. van Rensburg JJ, Lin H, Gao X, Toh E, Fortney KR, Ellinger S, et al. The Human Skin Microbiome Associates with the Outcome of and Is Influenced by Bacterial Infection. MBio. 2015;6:e01315–415.

31. Zeeuwen PLJM, Kleerebezem M, Timmerman HM, Schalkwijk J. Microbiome and skin diseases. Curr Opin. 2013;13:514–20.

32. Drago L, Toscano M, De Vecchi E, Piconi S, Iemoli E. Changing of fecal flora and clinical effect of *L. salivarius* LS01 in adults with atopic dermatitis. J Clin Gastroenterol. 2013;46:S56–63.

33. Majamaa H, Isoulari E. Evaluation of the gut mucosal barrier: evidence for increased antigen transfer in children with atopic eczema. J Allergy Clin Immunol. 1996;97:985–90.

34. Grice EA, Kong HH, Conlan S, Deming CB, Davis J, Young AC, et al. NISC Comparative Sequencing Program et al. Topographical and temporal diversity of the human skin microbiome. Science. 2009;324:1190–2.

11

Hymenoptera sting reactions in southern Italy forestry workers: our experience compared to reported data

Luisa Ricciardi[1]*[ID], Francesco Papia[1], Giuseppe Cataldo[1], Mario Giorgianni[2], Giovanna Spatari[2] and Sebastiano Gangemi[1]

Abstract

Background: Hymenoptera sting reactions are among life-threatening causes of allergy. Several epidemiology studies have assessed the risk of these kind of reactions, among the general population, around 3% of adults. This incidence increases among highly at risk populations such as outdoor workers. Hymenoptera stings among forestry workers (FW) are occupational triggers but it has not yet been well defined which is the real incidence of anaphylaxis in these workers, not even in Italy. Two Italian studies reported on the risk of hymenoptera stings (HS) in northern Italy (NI) and central Italy (CI) FW while no data is available on the prevalence in southern Italy (SI) ones.

Methods: A population of 341 SI FW (301 males and 40 females, mean age 51 years, range 43–63 years), who worked in Sicily, was investigated submitting a standardized questionnaire dealing with reactions to Hymenoptera stings, such as large local reactions (LLR) and systemic reactions (SR).

Results: HS occurred in 203 FW (59%) and caused reactions in 77 (22%); LLR occurred in 46 (13%) and SR in 31 (9%); SR were life threatening in 9/341 (3%) FW and were treated with epinephrine at the emergency unit as workers did not carry an epinephrine auto-injector. A SR at a subsequent HS followed a LLR in 21/46 FW (46%).

Conclusions: FW in SI have a generic risk of HS anaphylaxis as in the general population but a higher risk of SR and LLR respect to forestry populations from different Italian geographical areas.SR among SI FW occurred in 9% of them, while published data report the incidence of SR around 2 and 4%, respectively, in the Centre and North Italy FW. The incidence of LLR in SI FW was also higher (13%) than in CI (2%) and NI (10%) ones. Previous LLR in our SI population represented a high risk factor for developing a SR and therefore a red flag for future anaphylaxis and prescription of an epinephrine auto-injector.

Background

Hymenoptera stings (HS), even if in the vast majority cause only minor problems, account, even nowadays in the third millennium, for deaths usually resulting from immunologic mechanisms.

Self-reported systemic HS reactions among adults range from 0.5 to 3.3% in the US [1] while in Europe studies report the prevalence of systemic reactions (SR) between 0.3 and 7.5% [2]; mortality due to HS has been reported ranging from 0.03 to 0.48 fatalities per 1,000,000 population per year [3].

Quality of life of subjects who have experienced a SR after a HS is impaired as these subjects usually develop emotional distress during day life [4]. Furthermore, HS are among the commonest triggers of occupational anaphylaxis especially in outdoor workers such as beekeepers [5], gardeners [6], farmers, truck drivers, masons [7] and forestry workers (FW) [8]. Some authors investigated the prevalence of reactions to HS among FW. Japanese FW have a percentage of SR to HS significantly higher than control subjects do [9]. Incorvaia [10] and Copertaro [11] studied northern Italy (NI) and central Italy

*Correspondence: lricciardi@unime.it
[1] Department of Clinical and Experimental Medicine, School and Division of Allergy and Clinical Immunology, University of Messina, Messina, Italy
Full list of author information is available at the end of the article

(CI) populations of FW, respectively in order to evaluate the prevalence of HS. Up to now, no data is available on southern Italy (SI) FWs' risk of HS reactions.

Methods

We carried out an observational retrospective study on a population of FW from Sicily, a SI region, submitting a standardized fully anonymous questionnaire dealing with reactions to HS.

The reactions to HS were classified into large local reactions (LLR), defined as a swelling exceeding a diameter of 10 cm that lasted longer than 24 h, or SR according to Mueller's classification [12] with skin, gastrointestinal, respiratory and cardiovascular systems' involvement. Life threatening SR, defined as anaphylaxis, were the reactions characterized by a rapid onset of airway, breathing, circulatory, or gastrointestinal problems defined according to EAACI and WAO Guidelines [13, 14].

A physician administered a questionnaire to the FW in order to collect information about age, sex, HS, stinging insect, average number of stings respect to how long they had been working, frequency of stinging, degree of reaction to a HS.

Results

The population of FW consisted of 341 workers, mean age 51 years (range 43–63 years), 301 males and 40 females; HS occurred in 203 FW (59%), all during working hours. The culprit Hymenoptera, recognized by each stung FW, was a Vespid in 108 and an Apid in nine workers. Stings received by the other FW were most likely from Vespids as they did nor remember to have removed the sting. In average FW included in the study had been working for 23 years. Since their employment, 64 workers had received from 1 to 3 stings, 86 between 3 and 5 while 53 more than 5. HS reactions occurred in 77 FW (22%). LLR occurred in 46 FW (13%) and about half of them, 21 (46%), after a second sting in a further occasion, had a SR. LLR were also more frequent in workers who medially had been working for more years. The overall number of FW who had a SR was of 31/341 (9%).

These reactions had been treated with topical or systemic corticosteroids or antihistamines. SR were life threatening in 9/341 (3%) and were treated with epinephrine at the emergency unit together with systemic antihistamines such as clorpheniramine and corticosteroids as methylprednisolone. Furthermore, all the workers who had life-threatening SR were among those who had received more than five stings. No FW carried an epinephrine auto-injector.

Discussion

FW are at high risk of HS and may develop occupation-related allergies but rarely surveys on the natural history of HS, among these or other outdoor workers, are reported [15].

In Italy (Table 1) surveys on NI [10] and CI [11] FW, investigating the incidence of HS reactions in these populations, reported SR in 4 and 2% of FW, respectively while LLR occurred in 10 and 2%, respectively. Data were lacking on the incidence of HS reactions in SI FW and therefore we carried out the present survey.

A higher incidence of SR (9%) and LLR (13%) in SI FW was shown, compared to NI and CI ones, even if a lower percentage of SI FW was stung (Fig. 1).

HS occurred in 203/341 SI FW (59%) compared to 76/112 (68%) in NI and 179/206 (87%) in CI ones. Nonetheless, among SI FW, only 64 workers received no more than three stings while 86 from 3 to 5 and 53 more than 5. The higher incidence of both systemic and LLR in SI FW could be correlated to the shortness of interval between stings [16]. Hymenoptera allergy is one of the allergic disease problems related to climate change which is involving also Sicily [17]. A warming climate can cause dramatic shifts on these insects' populations from extinction but usually to overpopulation with a significant increase in the number of people seeking care for stings [18].

The high incidence of LLR in our FW population is unusually high compared to the general population as previously reported [19] but up to now we are unable to explain this singularity. Only in highly exposed subjects, such as beekeepers [20] or subjects from a rural population in the Mediterranean area [21] a prevalence has been reported. It must be underlined that Sicilian FW, such as the population we examined, work in a similar geographical area.

Table 1 General data and kind of reaction to Hymenoptera stings in FW from SI (current report), CI and NI (as previously published 10, 11)

	FW	Mean age	Males	Females	N° HS[a]	LLR	SR
FW SI	341	51	301	40	203 (59%)	46 (13%)	31 (9%)
FW CI	206	39.6	180	26	179 (87%)	4 (2%)	4 (2%)
FW NI	112	39	112	/	77 (68%)	11 (10%)	5 (4%)

[a] Hymenoptera stings

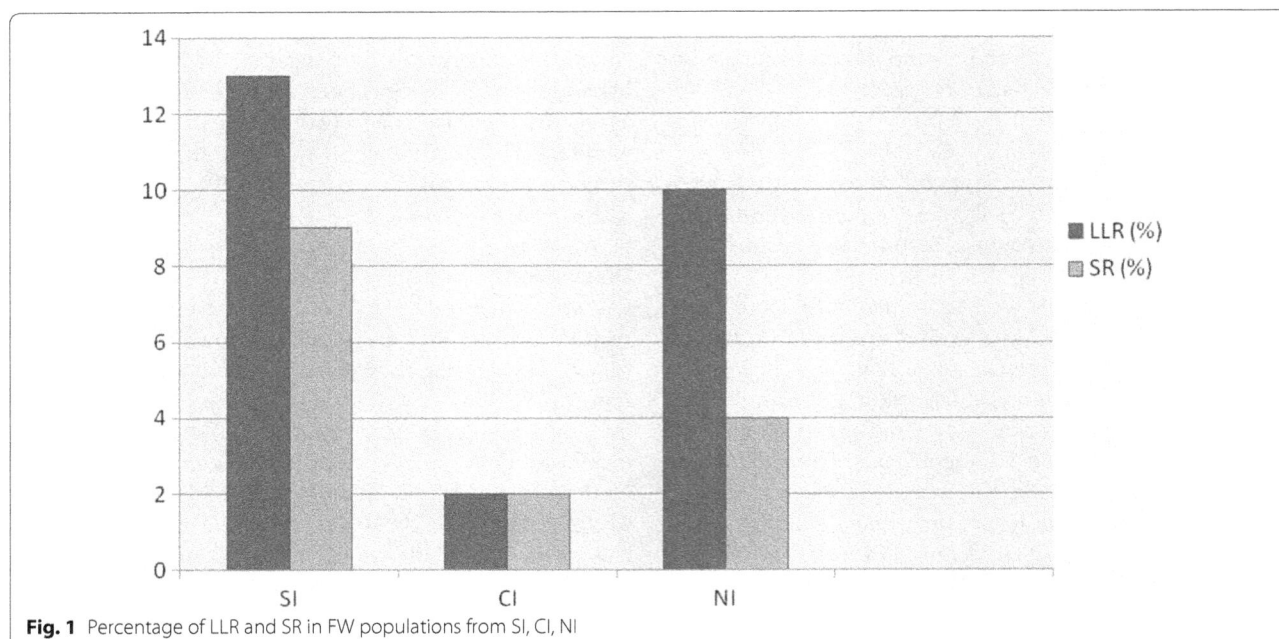

Fig. 1 Percentage of LLR and SR in FW populations from SI, CI, NI

Our data confirm what already reported in literature on how strong impact, hymenoptera venom allergy, has on work causing in some cases work disability [22].

As far as LLR in SI FW, they not also occurred with a higher incidence (13%) but a SR followed at a subsequent HS (21/46) in a high percentage of FW (46%).

LLR in SI FW represented a high risk factor for developing a SR and consequently a red flag for future anaphylaxis with the need of an epinephrine auto-injector prescription beforehand [23]. This accounts for the suggestion of a thorough allergy screening and follow-up in subjects with a high occupational risk of Hymenoptera stinging.

Authors' contributions

All the authors actively contributed in the manuscript. LR wrote the manuscript, SG, drafted the study, MG and GS submitted the questionnaire, FP and GC analyzed data from the questionnaire. All authors read and approved the final manuscript.

Author details

[1] Department of Clinical and Experimental Medicine, School and Division of Allergy and Clinical Immunology, University of Messina, Messina, Italy. [2] Department of Biomedical Sciences, Dental, Morphological and Functional Investigations, University of Messina, Messina, Italy.

References

1. Golden DB. Anaphylaxis to insect stings. Immunol allergy Clin North Am. 2015;35:287–302.
2. Bilò B, Rueff F, Mosbech H, Bonifazi F, Oude_Elmerink JN, EAACI Interest group on Insect Venom hypersensitivity. Diagnosis of hymenoptera venom allergy. Allergy. 2005;60:1339–49.
3. Pastorello EA, Rivolta F, Bianchi M, Mauro M, Pravettoni V. Incidence of anaphylaxis in the emergency department of a general hospital in Milan. J Chromatogr B Biomed Sci Appl. 2001;756:11–7.
4. Paolucci G, Folletti I, Toren K, Muzi G, Murgia N. Hymenoptera venom allergy: work disability and occupational impact of venom immunotherapy. BMJ Open. 2014;4:005593.
5. Muller UR. Bee venom allergy in beekeepers and their family members. Curr Opin Allergy Clin Immunol. 2005;5:343–7.
6. Perez-Pimiento A, Prieto-Lastra L, Rodriguez-Cabreros M, Reano-Martos M, Garcia-Cubero A, Garcia-Loria J. Work-related anaphylaxis to wasp sting. Occup Med. 2007;57:602–4.
7. Bonadonna P, Schiappoli M, Dama A, Olivieri M, Perbellini L, Senna G, Passalacqua G. Is hymenoptera venom allergy an occupational disease? Occup Environm Med. 2008;65:217–8.
8. Siracusa A, Folletti I, van Gerth Wijk R, Jeebay MF, Moscato G, Quirce S, et al. Occupational anaphylaxis—an EAACI task force consensus statement. Allergy. 2015;70:141–52.
9. Shimizu T, Hori T, Tokuyama K, Morikawa A, Kuroume T. clinical and immunologic surveys of Hymenoptera hypersensitivity in Japanese forestry workers. Ann Allergy Asthma Immunol. 1995;74:495–500.
10. Incorvaia C, Senna G, Mauro M, Bonadonna P, Marconi I, Asero E, Nitti F. Prevalence of allergic reactions to Hymenoptera stings in northern Italy. Eur Ann Allergy Clin Immunol. 2004;36:372–4.
11. Copertaro A, Pucci S, Bracci M, Barbaresi M. Hymenoptera stings in forestry department agents: evaluation of risk. Med Lav. 2006;97:676–81.
12. Mueller H. Diagnosis and treatment of insect sensitivity. J Asthma Res. 1966;3:331–3.
13. Muraro A, Roberts G, Worm M, Bilò MB, Brockow K, Fernandez Rivas M, et al. Anaphylaxis: guidelines from then european academy of allergy and clinical immunology. Allergy. 2014;69:1026–45.
14. Simons FE, Ardusso LR, Dimov V, Ebisawa M, El-Gamal YM, Lockey RF, et al. World Allergy Organization Anaphylaxis Giudelines: 2013 update of the evidence base. Int Arch Allergy Immunol. 2013;162:193–204.
15. Hayashih Y, Hirata H, Watanabe M, Yoshida N, Yojoyama T, Murayama Y, et al. Epidemiologic investigation of Hornet and Paper Wasp Stings in forest workers and electrical facility field workers in Japan. Allergol Int. 2014;63:21–6.
16. Pucci S, Antonicelli L, Bilò MB, Garritani MS, Bonifazi F. Allergy. 1994;49:894–6.
17. Viola F, Liuzzo L, Noto LV, Lo Conti F, La Loggia G. Spatial distribution of temperature trends in Sicily. Int J Climatol. 2014;34:1–17.

18. Demain JG, Gessner B, McLaughlin J, Sikes D, Foote J. Increasing insect reactions in Alaska:is this related to climate change? Allergy Asthma Proc. 2009;30:238–43.

19. Pucci S, D'Alò S, De Pasquale T, Illuminati I, Makri E, Incorvaia C. Risk of anaphylaxis in patients with large local reactions to hymenoptera stings: a retrospective and prospective study. Clin Mol Allergy. 2015;9(13):21.

20. Annila IT, Karjalainen ES, Annila PA, Kuusisto PA. Bee and wasp sting reactions in current beekeepers. Ann Allergy Asthma Immunol. 1996;77:423–7.

21. Fernandez J, Blanca M, Soriano V, Sanchez J, Juarez C. Epidemiological study of the prevalence of allergic reactions to Hymenoptera in a rural population in the Mediterranean area. Clin Exp Allergy. 1999;29:1069–74.

22. Kahan E, Ben-Moshe R, Derazne E, Tamir R. The impact of Hymenoptera venom allergy on occupational activities. Occup Med. 1997;47:273–6.

23. Ridolo E, Montagni M, Bonzano L, Savi E, Peveri S, Costantino MT, et al. How far from correct is the use of adrenaline auto-injectors? A survey in Italian patients. Intern Emerg Med. 2015;10:937–41.

12

Hypersensitivity pneumonitis: a complex lung disease

Gian Galeazzo Riario Sforza* ⓘ and Androula Marinou

Abstract

Hypersensitivity pneumonitis (HP), also called extrinsic allergic alveolitis, is a respiratory syndrome involving the lung parenchyma and specifically the alveoli, terminal bronchioli, and alveolar interstitium, due to a delayed allergic reaction. Such reaction is secondary to a repeated and prolonged inhalation of different types of organic dusts or other substances to which the patient is sensitized and hyper responsive, primarily consisting of organic dusts of animal or vegetable origin, more rarely from chemicals. The prevalence of HP is difficult to evaluate because of uncertainties in detection and misdiagnosis and lacking of widely accepted diagnostic criteria, and varies considerably depending on disease definition, diagnostic methods, exposure modalities, geographical conditions, agricultural and industrial practices, and host risk factors. HP can be caused by multiple agents that are present in work places and in the home, such as microbes, animal and plant proteins, organic and inorganic chemicals. The number of environment, settings and causative agents is increasing over time. From the clinical point of view HP can be divided in acute/subacute and chronic, depending on the intensity and frequency of exposure to causative antigens. The mainstay in managing HP is the avoidance of the causative antigen, though the complete removal is not always possible due to the difficulties to identify the agent or because its avoidance may lead to major changes in life style or occupational settings. HP is a complex syndrome that needs urgently for more stringent and selective diagnostic criteria and validation, including wider panels of IgG, and a closer collaboration with occupational physicians, as part of a multidisciplinary expertise.

Background

Hypersensitivity pneumonitis (HP), also called extrinsic allergic alveolitis, is a respiratory syndrome involving the lung parenchyma and specifically the alveoli, terminal bronchioli, and alveolar interstitium, due to a delayed allergic reaction. Such reaction is secondary to a repeated and prolonged inhalation of different types of organic dusts or other substances to which the patient is sensitized and hyper responsive, primarily consisting of organic dusts of animal or vegetable origin, more rarely from chemicals [1]. In this condition, that was first described in 1713 by the Italian researcher Bernardino Ramazzini in subjects belonging to 52 different professions, a repeated exposure to particles sufficiently small (diameter < 5 μm) to reach the alveoli and to trigger an immune response is necessary. The most at risk professional categories are workers in environments or settings contaminated by organic dust of various origin, mostly farmers or breeders. A lot of substances may be linked to this condition such as avian dust, mold, paint catalyst, sugar cane dust, hay dust, mushrooms, rat or gerbil urine, tobacco, heating and cooling systems water, maple bark dust, redwood bark dust, beer brewing, cork dust, plastic residue, epoxy resin, enzyme detergents, wheat mold or dust. The syndrome is greatly variable in symptoms severity, clinical presentation and prognosis, depending on the nature of causative agent, the duration of exposure, the host factors and the characteristics of the antigen [2]. In most cases, HP can be reversed promptly identifying and removing the causative agent(s), which can be found in a lot of settings, including home, workplace, and recreational environments [3].

*Correspondence: griariosforza@asst-nordmilano.it
Division of Sub Acute Care, Sesto San Giovanni Hospital, ASST Nord Milano, Sesto San Giovanni, Italy

Prevalence

The prevalence of HP is difficult to evaluate because of uncertainties in detection and misdiagnosis and lacking of widely accepted diagnostic criteria, and varies considerably depending on disease definition, diagnostic methods, exposure modalities, geographical conditions, agricultural and industrial practices, and host risk factors [2]. Moreover, HP develops only in a small part of individuals exposed to causing agents, while the majority of individuals exposed to the same agent are sensitized but asymptomatic or do not even become sensitized, suggesting the existence of a genetic predisposition [4]. To further complicate the issue, in some patients HP might be a reaction to a single environmental agent, whereas in other patients the lung disease might represent a reaction to a number of inhaled antigens, none of which appears to be exclusively responsible for the disease. Anyway, estimated prevalence varies by region, climate, and farming practices. In the US HP accounted for less than 2% of the patients with interstitial lung disease (ILD), whose yearly incidence was calculated to be about 30 per 100,000 [5]. A study carried out in Wisconsin on 1400 individuals estimated HP prevalence at 4.2% [6], while other data estimates HP affecting from 0.5 to 19.0% of exposed farmers [7]. In Europe, according to ILD registries, HP affects from 4 to 15% of all ILD cases [8], even if disease prevalence widely varies in different countries and within the same country due to geographic, seasonal, and climatic factors [9]. In a study of 431 incident cases in central Denmark, HP was the third most common ILD (7%), after idiopathic pulmonary fibrosis (28%) and connective tissue diseases (14%) [10]. In a Brazilian database including 3168 cases of ILD, prevalence of HP was 15%, the second place after connective tissue diseases 17% [11].

Causative agents

Hypersensitivity pneumonitis can be caused by multiple agents that are present in work places and in the home, such as microbes, animal and plant proteins, organic and inorganic chemicals (Table 1). The number of environment, settings and causative agents is increasing over time. A relatively recent example are metal workers exposed to aerosolized metal working liquid often containing mycobacteria [12]. Studying an outbreak of metal fluid HP in an automobile manufacturing plant in Ontario, Canadian researchers found that when mycobacteria are established in the biofilms of the fluid system it is very difficult, if not impossible, to eradicate them [13]. HP has been observed also in wood transformation plants [14], peat moss packaging units [15] and in saxophone player, in this case caused by molds that grow inside the instrument [16]. These isolated cases underline the importance of a carefully taken environmental history in presence of symptoms suggesting the presence of an HP. On the other side, even in the context of a single specific exposure, there can be several potential antigens that might trigger the inflammatory pulmonary response [17]. One example of this complexity is the bird-fancier's disease, in which the causative bird-related antigens include immunoglobulins, intestinal mucin present in bird droppings or blooms, a waxy substance coating the feathers of birds [18]. Another example is the complex ecosystem that could be observed in a contaminated humidifier system, such as *Klebsiella* species bacteria and Pullularia, Aureobasidium, Curvularia, Chaetomium, Penicillium, and Cephalosporium molds. Small amounts of these antigens also can be present in lake water, soil, and outdoor air in summertime [19]. The continuous research of etiologic agents in occupational and non occupational exposures is of outstanding importance because an extensive knowledge of these causative substances not only allows a better diagnosis and treatment but also leads to a reduction of the exposure.

Pathogenesis

Inhaled antigens less than 5 μm in diameter may reach the lung parenchyma, moving to the lymphatic vessels and depositing at the level of respiratory bronchioles. Pathogens involved in HP cause similar clinical features, with an almost exclusive involvement of distal airways, alveolar and interstitial infiltration by inflammatory cells, and high titers of serum precipitating antibodies against the antigens responsible of the alveolar inflammation (precipitins), with normal levels of IgE and eosinophils. The pathogenesis of HP is quite similar regardless of the causative agent: the inflammatory response of the alveolar mucosa is a hypersensitivity reaction of type 3 (immune-complex-mediated) or type 4 (T lymphocytes mediated) [21]. The pathology is characterized by a bronchiolocentric interstitial mononuclear cell infiltration, small non-necrotizing epithelioid cell granulomas poorly formed, diffuse cellular pneumonitis and variable degrees of pulmonary fibrosis. Granulomas were commonly observed in the bronchiolar wall and alveolar ducts in subacute hypersensitivity pneumonitis; they are less than 150 μm in diameter, smaller than those observed in sarcoidosis [22]. Precipitins against causative antigen and immunoglobulin and complement were demonstrated in vessel walls [23]. T-lymphocytes mediated hypersensitivity response is the most important type 4 immune reaction in the pathogenesis of HP. Th1-cytokine network plays a key role in the development of HP [24], and later in the chronic form develops a Th2-like immune response. In fact, the features associated with chronic HP include a gradual increase in CD4+ T cells and in the CD4+/CD8+ ratio, a modification toward

Table 1 Hypersensitivity pneumonitis causative antigens

Antigen	Source	Disease
Microbes		
Alternaria species	Wood or wood pulp	Woodworker's lung
Aspergillus clavatus	Moldy grains	Malt-worker's lung
Aspergillus species	Tobacco mold	Tobacco-worker's lung
Aspergillus species	Moldy malt	Malt-worker's lung
Aspergillus versicolor	Animal bedding	Dog house disease
Aureobasidium pullulans	Moldy sequoia dust	Sequoiosis
Aureobasidium species	Contaminated water	Sauna-taker's disease
Bacillus subtilis	Detergent enzymes	Detergent-worker's lung
Botrytis cinerea	Grape mold	Winegrower's lung or Späetlase lung
Candida albicans	Saxophone mouthpiece	Sax lung
Cephalosporium	Sewage	Sewage-worker's lung
Cryptostroma corticale	Moldy maple bark	Maple bark–stripper's lung
Merulius lacrymans	–	Dry rot lung
Mixed amoeba, fungi, and bacteria	Cold mist and other humidifiers, air conditioners	Nylon plant or office worker's or air conditioner's lung, ventilation pneumonitis
Mycobacterium avium	Contaminated water	Hot tub lung
Mycobacterium species, Gram negative bacilli	Metal-cutting fluid	Machine-worker's lung
Mucor stolonifer	Paprika	Paprika-splitter's lung
Penicillium casei	Cheese mold	Cheese-washer's lung
Penicillium chrysogenum	Moldy wood dust	Woodworker's lung
Penicillium frequentans	Moldy cork	Suberosis
Saccharopolyspora rectivirgula (micropolyspora faeni)	Moldy hay	Farmer's lung
Thermoactinomyces vulgaris	Moldy hay, compost	Farmer's lung, mushroom-worker's lung, composter's lung
Thermoactinomyces sacchari	Sugar cane residue	Bagassosis
Thermophilic actinomycetes	Moldy plant materials	Farmer's lung
Trichosporon cutaneum	Mold in Japanese homes	Summer-type HP
Animals		
Animal fur protein	Animal fur	Furrier's lung
Avian proteins	Bird excreta, blood, or feather	Bird-breeder's lung, bird-fancier's lung, pigeon-breeder's lung
Gerbil proteins	Gerbil	Gerbil-keeper's lung
Fish	Fish meal dust	Fishmeal-worker's lung
Mollusk shell protein	Mollusk shell dust	Oyster shell lung
Ox and pork protein	Pituitary snuff	Pituitary snuff–taker's lung
Rat proteins	Rat urine or serum	Rodent-handler's lung
Silk worm larvae proteins	Silk worm larvae	Sericulturist's lung
Wheat weevil	Flour	Miller's lung
Plants		
Coffee	Coffee bean dust	Coffee-worker's lung
Lycoperdon species	Puffballs	Lycoperdonosis
Soybean	Soybean hulls	Soybean-worker's lung
Chemicals		
Anhydrides	Plastics	Chemical-worker's lung, plasticworker's lung, epoxy-worker's lung
Bordeaux mixture	Vineyard fungicide	Vineyard-sprayer's lung
Isocyanates	Paints, plastics	Paint-refinisher's lung
Pauli's reagent	–	Pauli's reagent lung
Pyrethrum	Insecticides	Insecticide lung

Table 1 continued

Antigen	Source	Disease
Metals		
Cobalt	–	Hard metal lung disease
Beryllium	–	Berylliosis

Derived and adapted from Costabel et al [20]

TH2 T cell differentiation and cytokine profile as well as a decline of CD8+ T cells [25]. In acute HP, pulmonary parenchyma inflammation appears to be mainly mediated by a type 3 response, as suggested by the presence of high titers of antigen-specific precipitating IgG in the serum, and an increase in lung neutrophils. Subacute and chronic forms of HP are characterized by a T cell-mediated immune response with increased T-cell migration and developing of a characteristic T-lymphocytic alveolitis [25]. The genetic factors determining individual predisposition to HP are still unclear, but in pigeon breeders disease (PBD) patients Camarena et al. [26] showed a significant increase of the alleles HLA-DRB1*1305 and HLA-DQB1*0501, while a decrease of HLA-DRB1*0802 was noticed in patients versus both control groups. Moreover, PBD patients had an increased frequency of TNF-2(-)(308) compared with both control groups. This subpopulation of patients exhibiting the TNF-2(-)(308) allele were younger, and displayed more lymphocytes in their bronchoalveolar lavages. These results suggest that genetic factors located within the MHC region contribute to the development of PBD.

Clinical presentation

From the clinical point of view HP can be can be divided in acute/subacute, and chronic phenotypes, depending on the intensity and frequency of exposure to causative antigens. See Table 2 for classification and diagnostic criteria.

The acute form occurs after hours or days of antigen exposure, that generally is a short-term and intermittent exposure. The patient's symptoms begin with fever, cough, dyspnea, asthenia and malaise that may persist for about a week after the causative agent exposure ends. The exacerbations might coincide with returning to work and subside when the subject is away from the working environment or from the allergenic setting for a sufficient period. On the chest auscultation could be noted widespread crackles in both chest walls, but sometimes auscultation is negative. The radiologic manifestations of acute HP are those of acute pulmonary edema, a high-resolution CT could be performed to better evaluate these patients [27]. The high-resolution CT scans could show patchy or diffuse bilateral ground-glass opacities and, especially in subacute forms, poorly defined small centrilobular nodules and lobular areas of decreased attenuation. The ground-glass opacities primarily reflect a diffuse lymphocytic interstitial pneumonitis, while the poorly defined centrilobular nodules may be caused by cellular bronchiolitis or focal areas of organizing pneumonia. The lobular areas of decreased attenuation and air trapping are presumably caused by small-airway obstruction by cellular bronchiolitis or, less commonly, by constrictive bronchiolitis [28]. During the acute episode respiratory function is reduced, also with DLCO alteration. Blood tests may show a slight eosinophilia with normal levels of IgE.

Subacute HP, a phenotype particularly difficult to identify, as demonstrated by the cluster analysis of 168 patients with HP performed by the international HP Study Group [3], is caused by a more prolonged exposure to the agent compared with the acute form. The onset is clinically sneaky, with productive cough, dyspnea, asthenia. For the rest, the subacute form is not particularly different than the acute form and the classification of HP should be restricted to two phenotypes, as suggested by the recent EAACI Position Paper on Occupational HP [29]. Chronic HP occurs as consequence of a continuous exposure to the pathogen, which causes a constant inflammation eliciting over time an irreversible pulmonary fibrosis. The chronic form has a more insidious onset than the subacute one, developing over a period of months or years, with progressive dyspnea with episodes of wheezing and recurrent low-grade fever. Symptoms, followed over time by a respiratory failure often evolve to pulmonary fibrosis [11]. Chest X-ray shows a diffuse interstitial fibrosis; spirometry demonstrates a restrictive syndrome, sometimes with obstructive patterns. DLCO is very low. In the chronic form, several months of low-level exposure to the offending allergen can result in very insidious respiratory symptoms with dyspnea, cough, sometimes mucopurulent sputum, anorexia and weight loss. The pattern of the chronic form can be similar to other forms of fibrotic pulmonary disease, evolving in most cases towards a progressive and irreversible disease despite avoidance of exposure to the causative agent and steroid treatment.

Diagnosis

HP is often unrecognized and frequently misdiagnosed as respiratory infection or idiopathic interstitial lung disease because of its relatively low incidence in the general

Table 2 Classification and diagnostic criteria of hypersensitivity pneumonitis

Characteristics	Acute/subacute HP	Chronic HP
Exposure to causal antigen	Intermittent high-level exposure	Continuous low-level exposure
Onset of symptoms	2–9 h after exposure; may evolve to gradually increasing symptoms over days to weeks	Insidious, over weeks to months
Nature of symptoms	Cough and dyspnea, but predominantly influenza-like symptoms	Progressive symptoms (dyspnea, cough, and weight loss), sometimes punctuated by intermittent attacks of symptoms or slowly increasing
Physical signs	Fever	Inspiratory crackles; cyanosis; digital clubbing; cor pulmonale
Outcome	Symptoms peak within 6–24 h after exposure, lasting hours to days. Symptoms recur on re-exposure and may progress to severe dyspnea	End-stage fibrotic disease and/or emphysema. Exacerbations may occur despite avoidance of exposure

Derived and adapted from the cluster analysis of the HP Study Group [3]

population. Moreover, the wide variability in clinical presentation of the disease HP often leads to the risk of underdiagnosis, unless the condition is specifically considered as a diagnostic possibility. In some patients, respiratory symptoms are the main feature of the clinical presentation, whereas in others people, systemic manifestations such as anorexia and weight loss overshadow other symptoms that, when present, might be intermittent, corresponding to episodic exposures to the causative agent, or might be always present, as in chronic form of the disease.

A high index of suspicion and a careful history, conducted in a systematic manner to insure that all relevant environmental and occupational information are obtained, are the main keys to make a correct diagnosis of HP. Once the suspicion of HP arises on the basis of initial history-taking, the diagnostic procedure could aim not only to identify the causative agent, but also to establish a temporal relationship between environmental exposures and initial onset of symptoms as well as temporary clinical manifestations. The diagnosis is often suspected when there is evidence of a respiratory disease with a history of relevant environmental or occupational setting and a clear relationship between symptoms and exposure. Physical examination and routine laboratory tests are generally not helpful, with total IgG often elevated, rheumatoid factor often positive, and peripheral eosinophil count generally normal as well as serum IgE levels. The suspected causative agent could be identified with the identification of specific precipitating antibodies in the patient's serum, although specific precipitins can be found in many, but not all, patients with HP because of the low sensitivity due to poorly purified antigens, because of failure to adequately concentrate the patient's serum prior to testing or, finally, because of the lack of the causative agent in the test panel [3, 30]. Moreover, it should be underlined that from 40 to 50% of asymptomatic individuals exposed to the same causative antigen have specific serum IgG antibodies [31]. In

patients with a suspect of HP, a careful environmental and occupational history should guide the use of specific panels of precipitating antibodies, but the lack of consensus on disease definition limits the possibility to reach a certain diagnosis, although many diagnostic criteria for HP have been proposed [3]. Aiming at validating clinical diagnostic criteria for HP, in 2003 the HP study group analyzed a prospective cohort of consecutive patients with HP, identifying six significant predicting factors: (1) exposure to a known causative antigen, (2) presence of precipitins to the suspected causative antigen, (3) recurrent respiratory and systemic symptoms, (4) inspiratory crackles detected by physical examination, (5) symptoms occurring 4–8 h after exposure, (6) weight loss [27]. Pulmonary function tests can be normal in acute HP, while in chronic forms they typically demonstrate a restrictive pattern with small lung volumes and decreased (DLCO), although none of these features are specific to HP. Chest X-ray may provide some information regarding the extent of lung involvement: patients with acute or subacute HP may show bilateral interstitial and alveolar nodular infiltrates that could be patchy or homogeneous, while in chronic disease are present diffuse reticulonodular infiltrates and fibrosis, and honeycombing may occur. However, chest X-ray alone is not diagnostic, and a normal chest X-ray does not exclude the presence of HP. Instead of chest X-ray, high resolution CT (HRCT) scan has become important in the diagnosis of HP. In subacute form HRCT shows lobular areas of decreased attenuation or air-trapping, patchy or diffuse ground-glass opacities, and small centrilobular nodules [32]. In chronic HP the most common findings are traction bronchiectasis, interlobular septal thickening, and intralobular reticulation, with a distribution mainly peribronchovascular with no areas of predominance [33]. Other diagnostic procedures can be helpful in the diagnosis of HP, such as bronchoalveolar lavage (BAL) fluid analysis and lung biopsies. The presence of a lymphocyte count greater than or equal to 25% in BAL suggests a granulomatous disease such as sarcoidosis or HP, while a lymphocyte count greater than 50% is suggestive of HP, especially when associated with a neutrophils count greater than 3% and a mast cell count greater than 1% [34]. The utility of transbronchial biopsies (TBB) is limited by non specific results obtained in up to 48% of samples, however the presence of some findings such as diffuse lymphocytic infiltrates can be strongly suggestive for HP [35]. Surgical lung biopsies are more sensitive than TBB, and in subacute stages of disease the histologic findings can show the presence of interstitial lymphoplasmocytic pneumonitis, giant cells or non-necrotizing granulomas and cellular bronchiolitis. In the chronic stages of HP a predominantly fibrotic pattern mimics other types of interstitial lung disease particularly usual interstitial pneumonia (UIP), and a certain diagnosis can be always supported by clinical and radiological findings [36]. In conclusion, no gold standard for diagnosis of HP is currently available. Occupational or environmental exposure to a known causative agent, recurrent symptoms after exposure, inspiratory crackles, positivity of precipitating antibodies, and eventually weight loss were indicative findings of HP, together with BAL, HRCT, and, if needed, other diagnostic procedures such as lung biopsy.

Treatment

The mainstay in managing HP is the avoidance of the causative antigen, though the complete removal is not always possible due to the difficulties to identify the agent or because its avoidance may lead to major changes in life style or occupational settings [37]. Some studies have suggested that HP could be not always a progressive disease, even if the job was not changed [38], suggesting a complex interaction between environmental and genetic factors [39]. If the allergen avoidance is not feasible or does not result in a complete symptoms relief, corticosteroid therapy is indicated. Corticosteroids may be useful either in relieving acute symptoms, or in subacute and chronic forms of HP, but they do not appear to have any effect on the long-term outcome of disease [40]. Anyway, a reasonable scheme therapy is oral prednisone between 40 and 60 mg, or equivalent doses for other corticosteroids, administered for a few days to 2 weeks in acute HP or for 4–8 weeks in subacute/chronic forms, followed by a gradual tapering to a maintenance dose of approximately 10 mg/day, or, if the patient clinical response is particularly good, to the discontinuation of the corticosteroid treatment. However, it should be emphasized that the efficacy of corticosteroid treatment lasting 12 weeks is not significantly superior to that of 4 weeks' duration [41]. Interestingly, recurrence of acute farmer's lung was more frequent among patients treated with corticosteroids who had also a prolonged antigen exposure, raising

the hypothesis that steroid therapy was also suppressing the counter regulatory immune response. Depending on the patient clinical features, some supportive therapies may be prescribed, such as oxygen therapy if blood oxygen saturation is permanently under 90%, bronchodilators to open the airways, and opioids to control shortness of breath or chronic cough that is resistant to other treatments. If opioids are used several times a day, for several weeks or longer, it can lead to physical dependence and possibly addiction. In some cases the chronic form could not respond to corticosteroid treatment, evolving toward a progressive pulmonary fibrosis; in this eventuality lung transplantation should be considered, but it is important to remember that the procedure is not a cure: if after transplantation the patient will be exposed again to the causative antigen, a new allergic inflammation may severely damage again also the transplanted lung. Treatment is more successful when HP is diagnosed in the early stages of the disease, before permanent irreversible lung damage has occurred.

Prognosis

Even though mortality trends are poor in the literature, in England and Wales from 1968 to 2008 878 deaths due to HP were described, with a mortality rate higher in men than women and with increasing age [42]. In a Danish cohort selected from high-quality registry, which provides real-life data with a diagnosis based on the current diagnostic criteria, the 5-year survival in the HP group was 93% [43]. Depending on the causative antigen, some studies suggested that bird-fancier's hypersensitivity pneumonitis might have a worse prognosis than farmer's lung, probably because patients with fibrosis on HRCT and/or lung biopsy have a poorer prognosis [44]. Factors associated with worse prognosis include an exposure for a longer period [45], older age, a histologic pattern of either fibrotic NSIP or UIP [46], digital clubbing [47], and a greater intensity of exposure [3].

Conclusions

HP is a complex syndrome that needs urgently for more stringent and selective diagnostic criteria and validation, including wider panels of IgG, and a closer collaboration with occupational physicians, as part of a multidisciplinary expertise. The occupational HP was recently defined by the EAACI Position Paper on Occupational HP [29], and the definition proposed may partly be applied to the proportion of cases of non-occupational HP. The disease has not only protean clinical manifestations, but also a substantial overlap with other ILDs, and its pathogenesis is not fully understood. Further research is warranted to develop prognostic markers that can drive clinical decision making, even to establish worldwide registers and multicenter networks including tissue and imaging repository, to increase our knowledge on evolution of the different disease forms. Corticosteroids may improve symptoms in the short term, but additional studies are needed to test their long term effects and other immunosuppressive drugs in HP patients. Finally, there is no evidence on the efficacy of anti-fibrotic agents such as nintedanib and pirfenidone in the treatment of chronic HP [48], making it necessary further research.

Authors' contributions

GGRS designed the study, made data analysis and interpretation, and revised the manuscript. AM made data collection and drafting the manuscript. Both authors read and approved the final manuscript.

References

1. Fink JN, Ortega HG, Reynolds HY, et al. Needs and opportunities for research in hypersensitivity pneumonitis. Am J Respir Crit Care Med. 2005;171(7):792–8.
2. Selman M, Pardo A, King TE Jr. Hypersensitivity pneumonitis: insights in diagnosis and pathobiology. Am J Respir Crit Care Med. 2012;186(4):314–24.
3. Lacasse Y, Girard M, Cormier Y. Recent advances in hypersensitivity pneumonitis. Chest. 2012;142:208–17.
4. Spagnolo P, Richeldi L, du Bois RM. Environmental triggers and susceptibility factors in idiopathic granulomatous diseases. Semin Respir Crit Care Med. 2008;29:610–9.
5. Lacasse Y, Cormier Y. Hypersensitivity pneumonitis. Orphanet J Rare Dis. 2006;1:25.
6. Gruchow HW, Hoffmann RG, Marx JJ Jr, Emanuel DA, Rimm AA. Precipitating antibodies to farmer's lung antigens in a Wisconsin farming population. Am Rev Respir Dis. 1981;124(4):411–5.
7. Ohshimo S, Bonella F, Guzman J, Costabel U. Hypersensitivity pneumonitis. Immunol Allergy Clin N Am. 2012;32:537–56.
8. Thomeer MJ, Costabel U, Rizzato G, Poletti V, Demedts M. Comparison of registries of interstitial lung diseases in three European countries. Eur Respir J Suppl. 2001;32:114s–8s.
9. Grant IW, Blyth W, Wardrop VE, Gordon RM, Pearson JC, Mair A. Prevalence of farmer's lung in Scotland: a pilot survey. Br Med J. 1972;1:530–4.
10. Hyldgaard C, Hilberg O, Muller A, Bendstrup E. A cohort study of interstitial lung diseases in central Denmark. Respir Med. 2014;108(5):793–9.
11. Pereira CAC, Gimenez A, Kuranishi L, Storrer K. Chronic hypersensitivity pneumonitis. J Asthma Allergy. 2016;9:171–81.
12. Bracker A, Storey E, Yang C, Hodgson MJ. An outbreak of hypersensitivity pneumonitis at a metalworking plant: a longitudinal assessment of intervention effectiveness. Appl Occup Environ Hyg. 2003;18:96–108.
13. Trafny EA. Microorganisms in metalworking fluids: current issues in research and management. Int J Occup Med Environ Health. 2013;26(1):4–15.
14. Veillette M, Cormier Y, Israël-Assayag E, Mériaux A, Duchaine C. Hypersensitivity pneumonitis in a hard wood processing plant: impact and etiology. J Occup Environ Hyg. 2006;3:301–7.
15. Cormier Y, Israel-Assayag E, Bedard G, Duchaine C. Hypersensitivity pneumonitis in peat moss processing plant workers. Am J Respir Crit Care Med. 1998;158(2):412–7.
16. Metzger F, Haccuria A, Redoux G, Nolard N, Dalphin J-C, DeVuyst P. Hypersensitivity pneumonitis due to molds in a saxophone player. Chest. 2010;138:724–6.
17. McSharry C, Anderson K, Boyd G. A review of antigen diversity causing lung disease among pigeon breeders. Clin Exp Allergy. 2000;30:1221–9.
18. Hisauchi-Kojima K, Sumi Y, Miyashita Y, Miyake S, Toyoda H, Kurup VP, et al. Purification of the antigenic components of pigeon dropping extract, the responsible agent for cellular immunity in pigeon breeder's disease. J Allergy Clin Immunol. 1999;103:1158–65.
19. Patterson R, Mazur N, Roberts M, Scarpelli D, Semerdjian R, Harris KE. Hypersensitivity pneumonitis due to humidifier disease: seek and ye shall find. Chest. 1998;114:931–3.
20. Costabel U, Bonella F, Guzman J. Chronic hypersensitivity pneumonitis. Clin Chest Med. 2012;33(1):151–63.
21. Selman M, Buendía-Roldán I. Immunopathology, diagnosis and management of hypersensitivity pneumonitis. Semin Respir Crit Care Med. 2012;33:543–54.
22. Katzenstein AL. Surgical pathology of the non-neoplastic lung disease. 4th ed. Philadelphia: Saunders Elsevier; 2006. p. 151–8.
23. Ghose T, Landrigan P, Killeen R, et al. Immunopathological studies in patients with farmer's lung. Clin Allergy. 1974;4:119–29.
24. Ando M, Suga M, Kohrogi H. A new look at hypersensitivity pneumonitis. Curr Opin Pulm Med. 1999;5:299–304.
25. Barrera L, Mendoza F, Zuñiga J, Estrada A, Zamora AC, Melendro EI, Ramírez R, Pardo A, Selman M. Functional diversity of T-cell subpopulations in subacute and chronic hypersensitivity pneumonitis. Am J Respir Crit Care Med. 2008;177:44–55.
26. Camarena A, Juárez A, Mejía M, Estrada A, Carrillo G, Falfán R, Zuñiga J, Navarro C, Granados J, Selman M. Major histocompatibility complex and tumor necrosis factor-alpha polymorphisms in pigeon breeder's disease. Am J Respir Crit Care Med. 2001;163(7):1528–33.
27. Lacasse Y, Selman M, Costabel U, et al. Clinical diagnosis of hypersensitivity pneumonitis. Am J Respir Crit Care Med. 2003;168:952–8.
28. Hansell DM, Wells AU, Padley SP, Müller NL. Hypersensitivity pneumonitis: correlation of individual CT patterns with functional abnormalities. Radiology. 1996;199:123–8.
29. Quirce S, Vandenplas O, Campo P, Cruz MJ, de Blay F, Koschel D, Moscato G, Pala G, Raulf M, Sastre J, Siracusa A, Tarlo SM, Walusiak-Skorupa J, Cormier Y. Occupational hypersensitivity pneumonitis: an EAACI Position Paper. Allergy. 2016;71:765–79.
30. Krasnick J, Meuwissen HJ, Nakao MA, et al. Hypersensitivity pneumonitis: problems in diagnosis. J Allergy Clin Immunol. 1996;97:1027–30.
31. Rodrigo MJ, Benavent MI, Cruz MJ, Rosell M, Murio C, Pascual C, et al. Detection of specific antibodies to pigeon serum and bloom antigens by enzyme linked immunosorbent assay in pigeon breeder's disease. Occup Environ Med. 2000;57:159–64.
32. Silva CIS, Churg A, Müller NL. Hypersensitivity pneumonitis: spectrum of high-resolution CT and pathologic findings. AJR Am J Roentgenol. 2007;188:334–44.
33. Tateishi T, Ohtani Y, Takemura T, et al. Serial high-resolution computed tomography findings of acute and chronic hypersensitivity pneumonitis induced by avian antigen. J Comput Assist Tomogr. 2011;35:272–9.
34. Meyer KC, Raghu G, Baughman RP, on behalf of the American Thoracic Society Committee on BAL in interstitial lung disease, et al. An official American Thoracic Society clinical practice guideline: the clinical utility of bronchoalveolar lavage cellular analysis in interstitial lung disease. Am J Respir Crit Care Med. 2012;185(9):1004–14.
35. Lacasse Y, Fraser RS, Fournier M, Cormier Y. Diagnostic accuracy of transbronchial biopsy in acute farmer's lung disease. Chest. 1997;112:1459–65.
36. Barrios RJ. Hypersensitivity pneumonitis: histopathology. Arch Pathol Lab Med. 2008;132:199–203.
37. Fernández Pérez ER, Swigris JJ, Forssén AV, et al. Identifying an inciting antigen is associated with improved survival in patients with chronic hypersensitivity pneumonitis. Chest. 2013;144(5):1644–51.
38. Cormier Y, Bélanger J. Long-term physiologic outcome after acute farmer's lung. Chest. 1985;87:796–800.
39. Spagnolo P, Grunewald J, du Bois RM. Genetic determinants of pulmonary fibrosis: evolving concepts. Lancet Respir Med. 2014;2:416–28.
40. Kokkarinen JI, Tukiainen HO, Terho EO. Effect of corticosteroid treatment on the recovery of pulmonary function in farmer's lung. Am Rev Respir Dis. 1992;145:3–5.
41. Monkare S, Haahtela T. Farmer's lung—a 5-year follow-up of eighty-six patients. Clin Allergy. 1987;17(2):143–51.

42. Hanley A, Hubbard RB, Navaratnam V. Mortality trends in asbestosis, extrinsic allergic alveolitis and sarcoidosis in England and Wales. Respir Med. 2011;105:1373–9.

43. Hyldgaard C, Hilberg O, Muller A, Bendstrup E. A cohort study of interstitial lung diseases in central Denmark. Respir Med. 2014;108:793–9.

44. Vourlekis JS, Schwarz MI, Cherniack RM, et al. The effect of pulmonary fibrosis on survival in patients with hypersensitivity pneumonitis. Am J Med. 2004;116:662–8.

45. de Gracia J, Morell F, Bofill JM, Curull V, Orriols R. Time of exposure as a prognostic factor in avian hypersensitivity pneumonitis. Respir Med. 1989;83:139–43.

46. Miyazaki Y, Tateishi T, Akashi T, Ohtani Y, Inase N, Yoshizawa Y. Clinical predictors and histologic appearance of acute exacerbation in chronic hypersensitivity pneumonitis. Chest. 2008;134:1265–70.

47. Sansores R, Salas J, Chapela R, Barquin N, Selman M. Clubbing in hypersensitivity pneumonitis. Its prevalence and possible prognostic role. Arch Intern Med. 1990;150:1849–51.

48. Adegunsoye A, Strek ME. Therapeutic approach to adult fibrotic lung diseases. Chest. 2016;150(6):1371–86.

Interleukin-17-producing decidual CD4+ T cells are not deleterious for human pregnancy when they also produce interleukin-4

Letizia Lombardelli[1], Federica Logiodice[1], Maryse Aguerre-Girr[2], Ornela Kullolli[1], Herman Haller[5], Ysabel Casart[2], Alain Berrebi[3], Fatima-Ezzahra L'Faqihi-Olive[2], Valérie Duplan[2], Sergio Romagnani[1], Enrico Maggi[1], Daniel Rukavina[4], Philippe Le Bouteiller[2] and Marie-Pierre Piccinni[1]*

Abstract

Background: Trophoblast expressing paternal HLA-C antigens resemble a semiallograft, and could be rejected by maternal CD4+ T lymphocytes. We examined the possible role in human pregnancy of Th17 cells, known to be involved in allograft rejection and reported for this reason to be responsible for miscarriages. We also studied Th17/Th1 and Th17/Th2 cells never investigated before. We defined for the first time the role of different Th17 subpopulations at the embryo implantation site and the role of HLA-G5, produced by the trophoblast/embryo, on Th17 cell differentiation.

Methods: Cytokine production by CD4+ purified T cell and T clones from decidua of normal pregnancy, unexplained recurrent abortion, and ectopic pregnancy at both embryo implantation site and distant from that site were analyzed for protein and mRNA production. Antigen-specific T cell lines were derived in the presence and in the absence of HLA-G5.

Results: We found an associated spontaneous production of IL-17A, IL-17F and IL-4 along with expression of CD161, CCR8 and CCR4 (Th2- and Th17-type markers) in fresh decidua CD4+ T cells during successful pregnancy. There was a prevalence of Th17/Th2 cells (producing IL-17A, IL-17F, IL-22 and IL-4) in the decidua of successful pregnancy, but the exclusive presence of Th17 (producing IL-17A, IL-17F, IL-22) and Th17/Th1 (producing IL-17A, IL-17F, IL-22 and IFN-γ) cells was found in the decidua of unexplained recurrent abortion. More importantly, we observed that Th17/Th2 cells were exclusively present at the embryo implantation site during tubal ectopic pregnancy, and that IL-4, GATA-3, IL-17A, ROR-C mRNA levels increased in tubal biopsies taken from embryo implantation sites, whereas Th17, Th17/Th1 and Th1 cells are exclusively present apart from implantation sites. Moreover, soluble HLA-G5 mediates the development of Th17/Th2 cells by increasing IL-4, IL-17A and IL-17F protein and mRNA production of CD4+ T helper cells.

Conclusion: No pathogenic role of decidual Th17 cells during pregnancy was observed. Indeed, a beneficial role for these cells was observed when they also produced IL-4. HLA-G5 could be the key feature of the uterine microenvironment responsible for the development of Th17/Th2 cells, which seem to be crucial for successful embryo implantation.

Keywords: Th17, Pregnancy, IL-17, IL-4, Spontaneous abortion, Ectopic pregnancy

*Correspondence: mppiccinni@hotmail.com
[1] Department of Experimental and Clinical Medicine and DENOTHE Excellence Center, University of Florence, Largo Brambilla 3, 50134 Florence, Italy
Full list of author information is available at the end of the article

Background

The conceptus, because of the presence of paternal classical MHC class I antigens (HLA-C) [1], is thought to resemble a semiallograft [2]. Paternal antigens expressed by trophoblast could be processed and presented, together with self MHC class II, to the specific maternal CD4+ T helper cells by maternal antigen presenting cells (APCs). Consequently, the activated maternal effector CD4+ T helper cells could release various cytokines.

On the basis of the cytokines produced, the human effector CD4+ T helper cells have been classified as T helper (Th)1, (Th)2 and, more recently, as (Th17) cells [3, 4]. Indeed, CD4+ Th1 cells, which produce interleukin (IL)-2, tumor necrosis factor (TNF)-α and interferon (IFN)-γ are the main effectors of phagocyte-mediated host defense, which is highly protective against infections sustained by intracellular parasites. On the other hand, CD4+ Th2 cells, which are mainly responsible for phagocyte-independent host defense against extracellular parasites, including nematodes, produce IL-5 (promoting the growth and the differentiation of eosinophils) and IL-4 (which together with IL-13 stimulates IgE and IgG1 antibody production and inhibits several macrophage functions) [3]. An additional subset of CD4+ T helper cells identified as Th17 produces IL-17A, IL17F, IL-21, IL-26 and IL-22 [4–6]. There is an increasing body of evidence showing that Th17 cells constitute a novel Th cell lineage distinct from Th1 and Th2 cells [4]. It has been reported that the transcription factor retinoic-acid-related orphan receptor (ROR)-C is important for the generation of Th17 cells in vitro and in vivo [7]. Human Th17 cells appear to be quite different from mouse Th17 cells in that TGF-β1 and IL-6 are not required for generation of Th17 cells. To date, the most effective cytokines to enhance the generation or expansion of human Th17 cells are IL-1β and IL-23 [8, 9]. In addition, cytokines such as IL-23 and IL-21 promote the generation or proliferation of Th17 cells, whereas others such as IFN-γ, IL-4, and IL-27, seem to suppress their generation [5, 6, 8, 10, 11]. The major role of Th17 is the protection against extracellular bacteria by activating epithelial cells, macrophages, fibroblasts and endothelial cells, which produce chemokines and cytokines responsible for granulocyte recruitment, which contributes to chronic tissue inflammation. The pathogenic role of Th17 cells has been suggested in several murine models of chronic inflammatory disorders, such as experimental autoimmune encephalomyelitis (EAE) [11], collagen-induced arthritis [9], and bowel inflammatory disorders [12].

Importantly for pregnancy, Th1-type and Th17-type T helper cells seem to play a role in acute allograft rejection [13–18], whereas Th2 T helper cells [15] and CD4+CD25+Foxp3+ T reg cells act to enhance allograft tolerance [19]. Although the mechanisms of action of Th1- and Th2-type cytokines produced by maternal CD4+ T helper lymphocytes present at the fetomaternal interface are defined with respect to conceptus tolerance/pregnancy maintenance or are conceptus rejection/failure of pregnancy [20–24], the mechanisms of action of CD4+CD25+Foxp3+ T reg cells present during human pregnancy are not so clear [25]. It was suggested in human pregnancy that T reg cells could inhibit the majority of human T cells that spontaneously proliferate and produce IFN-γ [26]. Kallikourdis et al. [27] reported that paternal alloantigen enhanced the accumulation of CCR5+ effector Treg cells in the murine pregnant uterus. Shima et al. [28] also reported that paternal antigen-specific Ki67+ proliferating Treg cells expressed CCR5 on their surface. These findings suggest that CCR5+ proliferating T cells might induce paternal antigen-specific tolerance in humans. However, recently Inada et al. [29] reported that the frequencies of CCR5^{+} Treg cells did not change in miscarriage. Unexpectedly, this study showed that the frequencies of CCR5^{+} Treg cells and Ki67+ Treg cells are similar in cases of normal pregnancy, miscarriage with a normal embryo, and miscarriage with an abnormal embryo, suggesting that decidual T reg specific for paternal antigens could be not responsible for the success of pregnancy by inducing fetal allograft tolerance. Accordingly, in mice it seems that T reg cells are activated in the uterine lymph nodes in response to semen and seminal antigens, not spermatozoa antigens and they home back to the uterus where they prepare the endometrium for implantation [30]. Presumably, the T reg cells in part act to dampen uterine inflammation, which is induced by semen and is independent of placental antigen exposure.

In the transplant setting, it was widely believed that allograft rejection is predominantly a Th1-mediated immune response, and that Th2-type cytokines inhibiting the Th1 responses improve allograft tolerance. It has been shown that a new T helper cell subpopulation, known as Th17 has a role in early stage allograft acute rejection [13, 14]. Therefore, the role of Th17 cells in conceptus rejection pregnancy failure has been investigated. Early evidence suggests that excessive Th17 activity may promote miscarriage. The number of Th17 CCR6+ cells is increased in the peripheral blood and decidua of patients with unexplained recurrent miscarriage compared to healthy control subjects, whereas T reg cells are decreased [31]. Accordingly, it has been shown that IL-27, a key regulator of T cell responses suppressing in particular Th17 cells, is lower in deciduas of patients with unexplained recurrent abortion compared to spontaneous abortion and controls subjects [32]. An accumulation of Th17 cells has also been found in the decidua of spontaneous abortion cases [33], and the number of decidual IL-17+ cells in inevitable abortion cases involving active genital bleeding was significantly higher than that in normal pregnancy. However, it seemed that there were no significant differences in the number of decidual IL-17+ cells between missed abortion cases without genital bleeding and normal pregnancy subjects. These last results suggest that IL-17+ cells might be involved in the induction of inflammation in the late but not the early stages of abortion [33]. Thus, the role of Th17 cells in the induction of spontaneous abortion remains unclear.

It has been reported that virtually all human memory Th17 cells are contained within the CD161+ fraction of circulating and tissue-infiltrating CD4+ T cells [10, 12]. Interestingly, human Th17 cells express molecules distinct from Th1 cells, such as IL-23R and RORC, but other molecules are shared with Th1 cells, such as the T-box 21 (TBX21) and IL-12Rβ2. Furthermore, a portion of human IL-17A-producing cells were found to also produce IFN-γ (they are named Th17/Th1) and both Th17 and Th17/Th1 exhibit plasticity towards Th1 cells in response to IL-12 produced in by APCs [11]. This plasticity of Th17 cells to Th1 cells has recently been observed even in mice, where it was found to be related to the activity of IL-12, or the prolonged exposure to IL-23 of Th17 cells [34]. Thus, naive CD4+ CD161+ T cells that behave as precursors of Th17 cells [10] could differentiate into Th17, Th17/Th1 and finally into Th1 cells, in response to cytokines present in the microenvironment of CD4+ T cells. The association of IL-17 and IL-4 production by CD4+ T helper cells has also been observed recently in allergic disorders [35]. A small proportion of CCR6(+)CD161(+) CD4(+) T cell clones showed the ability to produce both IL-17A and IL-4 (Th17/Th2). Th17/Th2 clones also produced IL-5, IL-13, IL-21, and IL-22 and displayed the ability to induce the in vitro secretion of IgE. Very few Th17/Th2 cells were found among circulating CD4(+) T cells from normal subjects (0.04 %), but their proportions were significantly increased in the circulation of patients with chronic asthma (1.3 %). Th17/Th2 cells could not be derived from naive umbilical cord blood CD4(+) T cells under any experimental condition. However, when circulating memory CCR6(+)CD161(+)CD4(+) T cells were cloned under appropriate polarizing conditions, Th17/Th2 clones originated in the presence of IL-4, suggesting that an IL-4-rich microenvironment may induce the shifting of memory Th17 cells into Th17/Th2 cells.

The aims of our study were (1) to define the role of Th17 cells in pregnancy, in particular to investigate if, as was reported by Wang et al. [31], these cells are responsible for miscarriages; (2) to define to which Th17-type subpopulation (Th17/Th1 or Th17/Th2 cells) the decidual Th17 cells belong and to ascertain whether one of these two Th17-type profiles is preferentially associated with pregnancy failure or successful pregnancy; (3) to find a putative soluble factor present at the fetomaternal interface responsible, at least in part, for the differentiation of decidual CD4+ T cells into Th17/Th2 cells.

Methods
Subjects

Among the 36 pregnant women studied (Table 1), 30 pregnant women, agreed to participate to the study at Hôpital Paule de Viguier, Toulouse, France. An additional six pregnant women suffering from ectopic pregnancy agreed to participate in the study at Hospital of Rijeka, Croatia. All subjects received verbal and written information about the aim and the design of the research, and all pregnant women signed the informed consent. The study was approved by local ethics committees of Hôpital Paule de Viguier, Toulouse, and by the Medical Faculty, Rijeka. Twenty-six pregnant women with normal gestation and no spontaneous abortion in their past history (Table 1), had requested elective termination. Four women had histories of at least 7 ± 3 (range 4–10) prior first-trimester spontaneous abortions, which could not been explained on the basis of conventional criteria (normal parental chromosomes, hysterosalpengography and hysteroscopy, endometrial biopsy, hormonal analysis including FSH, LH, estradiol, testosterone, cervical cultures for the presence of ureaplasma, mycoplasma and chlamydia, lupus anticoagulant, anti-phospholipid antibodies, thyroid function tests). Specimens of deciduae and peripheral blood were obtained at the time of spontaneous abortion

Table 1 Clinical data from patients (unexplained recurrent abortion, ectopic, pregnancy and controls)

	Normal pregnancy	Unexplained recurrent abortion	Ectopic pregnancy
n	26	4	6
Age (years)	28 ± 2 (25–35)	29 ± 0.9 (28–30)	32 ± 3 (29–36)
No. of Sp-ab[a]	0	7 ± 3 (4–10)	0
Gestational age (weeks)	9 ± 1 (8–12)	9 ± 1 (8–11)	8 ± 1 (6–9)

Data are expressed as mean ± SD (range)

[a] Number of patients with spontaneous abortion in past history, excluding the abortion cases discussed in this study

(at 8–11 weeks of pregnancy with normal karyotype of trophoblast). All the women were in excellent health at that time, had no history of atopy or allergy and were taking no medication. Trophoblast-invaded tubal mucosa at the implantation site and tubal mucosa distant from the implantation site was obtained from 6 women (with no spontaneous abortion in past history) whose ectopic pregnancies were terminated by surgical removal as a result of threatened tubal rupture. The mean age and the gestational age values of the three groups of patients (normal pregnancy, unexplained recurrent abortion and ectopic pregnancy) were not statistically different (Table 1).

Isolation of purified CD4+ T cells from peripheral blood and *decidua basalis* of early pregnant women

Samples of *decidua basalis* were obtained from healthy pregnant women undergoing vaginal elective termination of pregnancy (8–12 weeks of gestation with normal karyotype of trophoblast). Decidual mononuclear cells were isolated from the *decidua basalis* by collagenase digestion and gradient centrifugation as previously described [36]. Decidual CD4+ T cells were purified from non adherent cells using MACS CD4 isolation kit (positive selection, Miltenyi Biotec, Bergisch Gladbach, Germany). Purity was routinely >98 %. Peripheral blood (PB) cells from the same pregnant women were obtained as described [37]. Peripheral blood-CD4+ T cells were purified by using MACS CD4 isolation kit (positive selection, Miltenyi Biotec, Bergisch Gladbach, Germany). Purity was >99 %.

Flow cytometry

Freshly isolated decidual CD4+ T and Peripheral blood-CD4+ T cells were stained simultaneously with CD3-PE-Cy7, CD4-pacific blue, CD161-APC (BD Biosciences, Franklin Lakes, New Jersey) and either CCR3-FITC (Miltenyi Biotec, Bergisch Gladbach, Germany), IL-23R-PerCP, CCR4-mouse PE, CCR8-rat PE, CCR6-PE, CCR8-rat-PE, CXCR3 mouse-PE (R&D systems, Minneapolis, MN), or CRTH2 rat-PE (Myltenyi Biotech, Bergisch Gladbach, Germany) mAbs or their respective isotype controls: IgG1 mouse PE-Cy7, IgG1 mouse-pacific blue, IgG1 mouse APC, IgG2a rat-FITC, IgG2b mouse-PerCP, IgG1 mouse-PE, IgG2a rat-PE (BD Biosciences, Franklin Lakes, New Jersey), IgG2b-mouse PE, IgG2b-rat PE (R&D systems, Minneapolis, MN). Stained cells were acquired on a BD Biosciences LSR II flow cytometer (BD Biosciences, Franklin Lakes, New Jersey) (Data were analyzed with BD Biosciences FACSDiva software version 6.2.

Generation of CD4+ T-cell clones from peripheral blood, decidual biopsies of normal pregnancy unexplained recurrent abortion, and from Fallopian tube biopsies of ectopic pregnancy

Specimen of deciduae (separated from villus with normal karyotype) and of Fallopian tubes, were washed twice in PBS (pH 7.2) and then disrupted in small fragments (2–3 mm in diameter). Short-term T-cell lines were generated by culturing single fragments for one week in 24-well plates (Costar, Cambridge, Massachusetts) in 2 ml RPMI 1640 supplemented with 2 mM L-glutamine, 20 mM L-mercaptoethanol, 10 % FCS (complete medium) (Hyclone Laboratories, Logan, Utah) and IL-2 (Eurocitus, Milan, Italy) (20 U/ml). T-cell clones were then generated from short-term cultures of decidual and tubal T cells derived in the presence of IL-2, as well as from PBMC obtained from the same donors, using to a method described elsewhere [22].

Induction of cytokine production by T-cell clones

To induce cytokine production, 10^6 T-cell blasts from each T-cell clone were cultured in the presence of PMA (20 ng/ml; Sigma, St. Louis, MO) plus monoclonal antibody against CD3 (100 ng/ml; Ortho Pharmaceuticals, Raritan, New Jersey). After 36 h, culture supernatants were collected, filtered, and stored in aliquots at $-70°$.

Determination of cytokine concentrations in supernatants with bead-based multiplex immunoassays

The quantitative determination of the following cytokines: IL-4, IL-5, IL-13, IL-17A, I and FN-γ was performed by a bead-based multiplex immunoassay (Biorad Laboratories, Hercules, CA, USA) and IL-17F and IL-22 (Millipore, Billerica, Massachusetts) a Bioplex 200 system (Biorad Laboratories, Hercules, CA, USA), as previously described [38]. In brief, supernatant was added to antibody-conjugated beads directed against the cytokines listed above in a 96-well filter plate. After a 30-min incubation, the plate was washed and biotinylated anti-cytokine antibody solution was added before another 30-min incubation. The plate was then washed and streptavidin-conjugated PE was added. After a final wash, each well was suspended with assay buffer and analyzed with the Bioplex 200 system. Standard curves were derived from various concentrations of the different cytokine standards following the same protocol as the supernatant samples. The concentration of each cytokine (pg/ml) in each T cell clone supernatant was calculated thanks to the Bioplex200 software.

Cytokine production and mRNA expression of antigen-specific T cell lines in the absence or presence of HLA-G5

Recombinant HLA-G5 protein was purified from specific transfectant cell culture supernatants as previously described [39]. Streptokinase (SK)-specific T cell lines were generated from 5 donors as described elsewhere [40]. Briefly, 10^6 PBMC in 2 ml of complete medium were stimulated for 5 days with the SK antigen (1000 U/ml) in the absence or presence of either HLA-G5 (1 µg/ml) or recombinant human IL-4 (RD System, 200 pg/ml, Minneapolis) and IL-12 (RD System, 5000 pg/ml) as controls of cytokine modulation. Human IL-2 (Eurocetus, Milan) at 20 U/ml was then added and cultures continued for an additional 9 days. Viable T blasts were tested for their antigen specificity as follows: T cell lines, 2×10^4 T blasts were seeded in microplates and co-cultured for 48 h with irradiated (9000 rad) autologous PBMC (5×10^4) in the presence of medium alone or SK (1000 U/ml). After a 16-h pulse with 0.5 µCi ^{3}H-TdR (Amersham), cultures were harvested and radioactivity measured by liquid scintillation. The phenotype distribution of SK-specific T cells was assessed by flow cytometry analysis: the T cell lines were CD4+ cells. To induce the cytokine production by T cell lines, 10^6 T blasts from each were cultured in the presence of PMA (Sigma, 20 ng/ml, St. Louis, MO) plus anti-CD3 mAb (BD Bioscience, 100 ng/ml, Franklin Lakes, New Jersey). After 36 h, culture supernatants were collected and stored at −80 °C. IL-4, IL-17A, IFN-γ and IL-17F were quantified by bead-based multiplex assay. Values of the cytokine content 5 SD over those of control supernatants obtained by stimulation of irradiated feeder cells alone were considered as an effective secretion.

Quantification by real-time quantitative RT-PCR of IL-4, IL-17A, IL-17F, IL-23R, IFN-γ RORC, and GATA3 mRNA

Total RNA was extracted from freshly isolated PB and decidual CD4+ T cells, Fallopian tube biopsies and streptokinase (SK)-specific T cell lines by using Trizol (Invitrogen, Carlsbad, CA) and treated with DNase I (Qiagen, Venlo, NL). First strand cDNA was prepared from 1–5 µg of each RNA sample using Superscript II Reverse transcriptase according to the manufacturer's instructions (Invitrogen). Total RNA was extracted with RNAsy Kit and treated with DNase I (Qiagen, Venlo, NL), and cDNA was synthetized by using TaqMan Reverse Transcription Reagents (Applied Biosystem, Warrington, UK). RT-PCR was then performed by using TaqMan methodology, as described [40]. Quantitative analysis of IL-4, IL-17A, IL-17F, IL-23R, IFN-γ, RORC, GATA 3 and β-actin was performed by using assay on Demand (Applied Biosystem, Warrington, UK). β-actin was used for normalization.

Statistics

Statistical analyses were performed using SSPS software (SPSS, Inc, Evanston, IL). Due to non parametric distribution, all comparisons between cytokine concentrations in basal and stimulated conditions were performed by Wilcoxon test. Th subpopulations percentages were analyzed by Chi-square test. A p value of <0.05 was considered statistically significant.

Results

Associated production of IL-17 and IL-4 and expression of Th17 and Th2-type molecules by decidual CD3+CD4+ T cells in successful pregnancy

Unstimulated decidual and peripheral blood CD4+CD3+ T cells purified from the same 9 pregnant women were cultured for 24 h and IL-4, IL-17A, IL-17F and IL-22 production was measured in the corresponding cell culture supernatants (Fig. 1a). A significant increase of IL-4 and IL-17A release (p = 0.028 and p = 0.027, respectively) was observed in the culture supernatants of freshly isolated, unstimulated in vitro decidual CD4+ T cells compared to those of peripheral blood CD4+ cells from the same pregnant women (Fig. 1a). By contrast, no significant increase of IL-17F and IL-22 production was detected in the same culture supernatants of decidual CD4+ T cells compared to those of peripheral blood CD4+ cells from the same pregnant women. These data were confirmed by the increased levels of mRNA for IL-4, IL-17A and RORC (transcriptional factor of Th17 cells) expressed by freshly isolated, unstimulated decidual CD4+ T cells compared to those of peripheral blood CD4+ cells from the same 3 pregnant women (Fig. 1b). These results show a spontaneous, associated production of both IL-17A and IL-4 by fresh decidual CD3+CD4+ T cells during normal pregnancy.

Th1 cells express CXCR3, whereas Th2 cells express CCR4, CCR8 and CRTH2 [41–43]. Recent reports [10, 12] suggest that Th17 cells express CD161, IL-23 receptor (IL-23R) CCR6 and CCR4, as Th2 cells, but not CXCR3 in human adult peripheral blood or CCR6 in human decidua. We compared the associated expression of molecules expressed by Th17 cells and molecules expressed by Th1 and Th2 cells by fresh unstimulated CD3+CD4+ T cells purified from decidua and peripheral blood of the same pregnant women (Fig. 1c, d). Using multicolor flow cytometry analysis, we found that the percentage of CD3+CD4+ cells expressing CD161 (p = 0.027) and the mean fluorescence intensity (MFI) of CD161 were increased in the decidua compared to peripheral blood of the same 8 pregnant women (Fig. 1c). More importantly, this increased expression of CD161 by decidua CD3+CD4+ cells is associated with the increased expression of CCR4 and CCR8 by decidual CD3 + CD4+

Interleukin-17-producing decidual CD4 T cells are not deleterious for human + pregnancy...

107

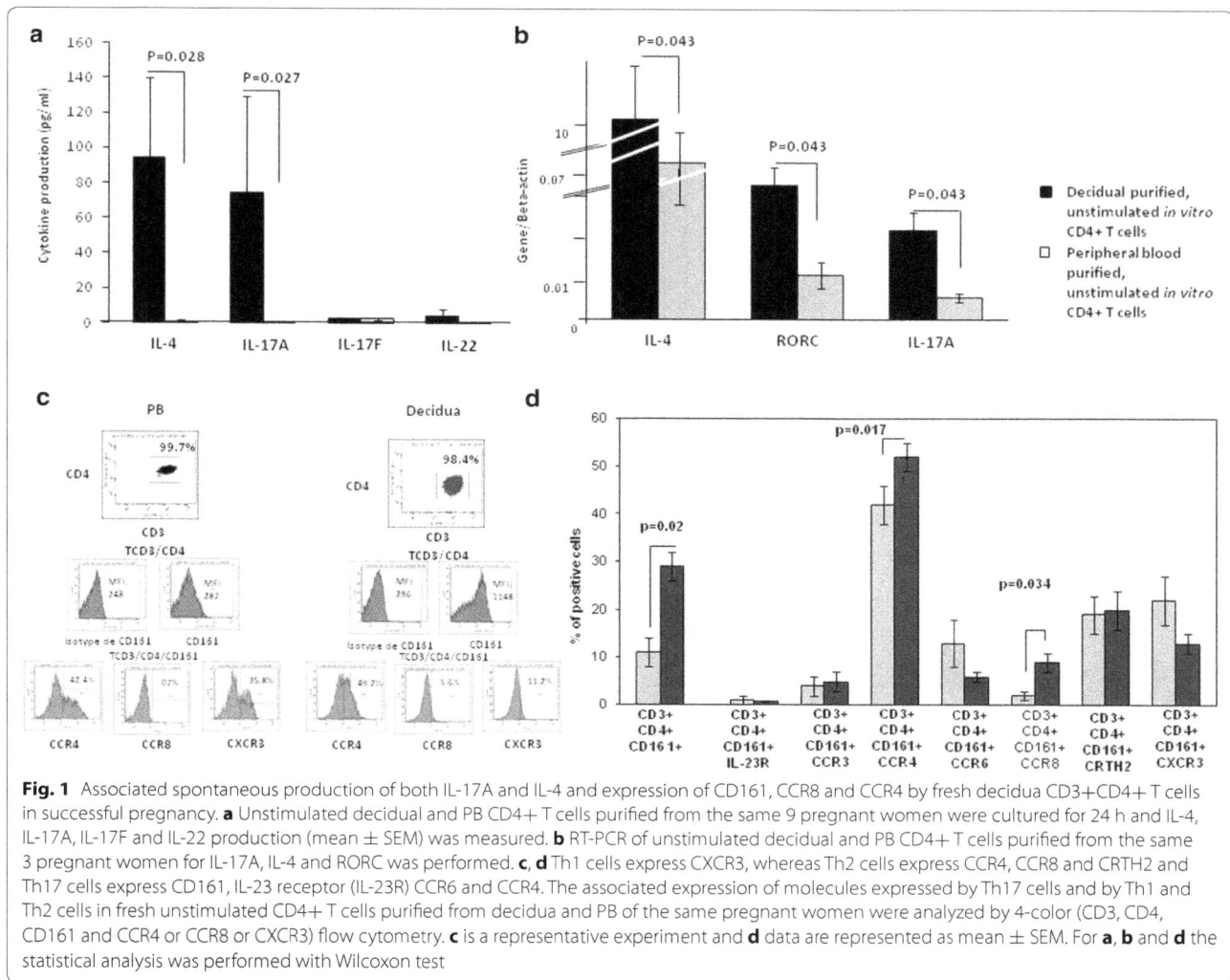

Fig. 1 Associated spontaneous production of both IL-17A and IL-4 and expression of CD161, CCR8 and CCR4 by fresh decidua CD3+CD4+ T cells in successful pregnancy. **a** Unstimulated decidual and PB CD4+ T cells purified from the same 9 pregnant women were cultured for 24 h and IL-4, IL-17A, IL-17F and IL-22 production (mean ± SEM) was measured. **b** RT-PCR of unstimulated decidual and PB CD4+ T cells purified from the same 3 pregnant women for IL-17A, IL-4 and RORC was performed. **c, d** Th1 cells express CXCR3, whereas Th2 cells express CCR4, CCR8 and CRTH2 and Th17 cells express CD161, IL-23 receptor (IL-23R) CCR6 and CCR4. The associated expression of molecules expressed by Th17 cells and by Th1 and Th2 cells in fresh unstimulated CD4+ T cells purified from decidua and PB of the same pregnant women were analyzed by 4-color (CD3, CD4, CD161 and CCR4 or CCR8 or CXCR3) flow cytometry. **c** is a representative experiment and **d** data are represented as mean ± SEM. For **a**, **b** and **d** the statistical analysis was performed with Wilcoxon test

cells compared to the peripheral blood CD3+CD4+ cells (Fig. 1d). These results indicate that decidual CD4+ T cells spontaneously expressed on their cell membrane molecules that characterize Th17 and Th2 cells.

Increased IL-4, IL-17A, IL-17F and IL-22 production by decidual CD4+ T cell clones in successful pregnancy

172 and 55 CD4+ T cell clones were respectively generated from decidual biopsies and peripheral blood obtained from 4 pregnant women (with normal pregnancy) who voluntarily underwent an elective termination of pregnancy. IL-4, IL-17A, IL-17F, IL-22 and IFN-γ were measured in the supernatant of the CD4+ T cell clones by multiplex bead-based assay.

In normal pregnancy, decidua CD4+ T cell clones produce higher levels of IL-4 (p = 0.0000004), a Th2-type cytokine, IL-17A (p = 0.015), IL-17F (p = 0.023)

and IL-22 (p = 0.006), three Th17-type cytokines, compared to peripheral blood T cell clones (Fig. 2). By contrast, IFN-γ production by T cell clones was decreased (p = 0.0001) in the decidua compared to peripheral blood (Fig. 2).

These data confirm the associated production of IL-4, IL-17A, IL-17F and IL-22 by decidual CD4+ T cells in normal pregnancy, thus showing an association between Th2-and Th17-type cytokines by decidual CD4+ T cells in normal pregnancy.

Prevalence of Th17/Th2 CD4+ cells in the decidua of successful pregnancy whereas of Th17 and Th17/Th1 cells in the decidua of unexplained recurrent abortion

It has been reported that in "inevitable" spontaneous abortion with genital bleeding and in unexplained spontaneous abortion, the number of decidual Th17

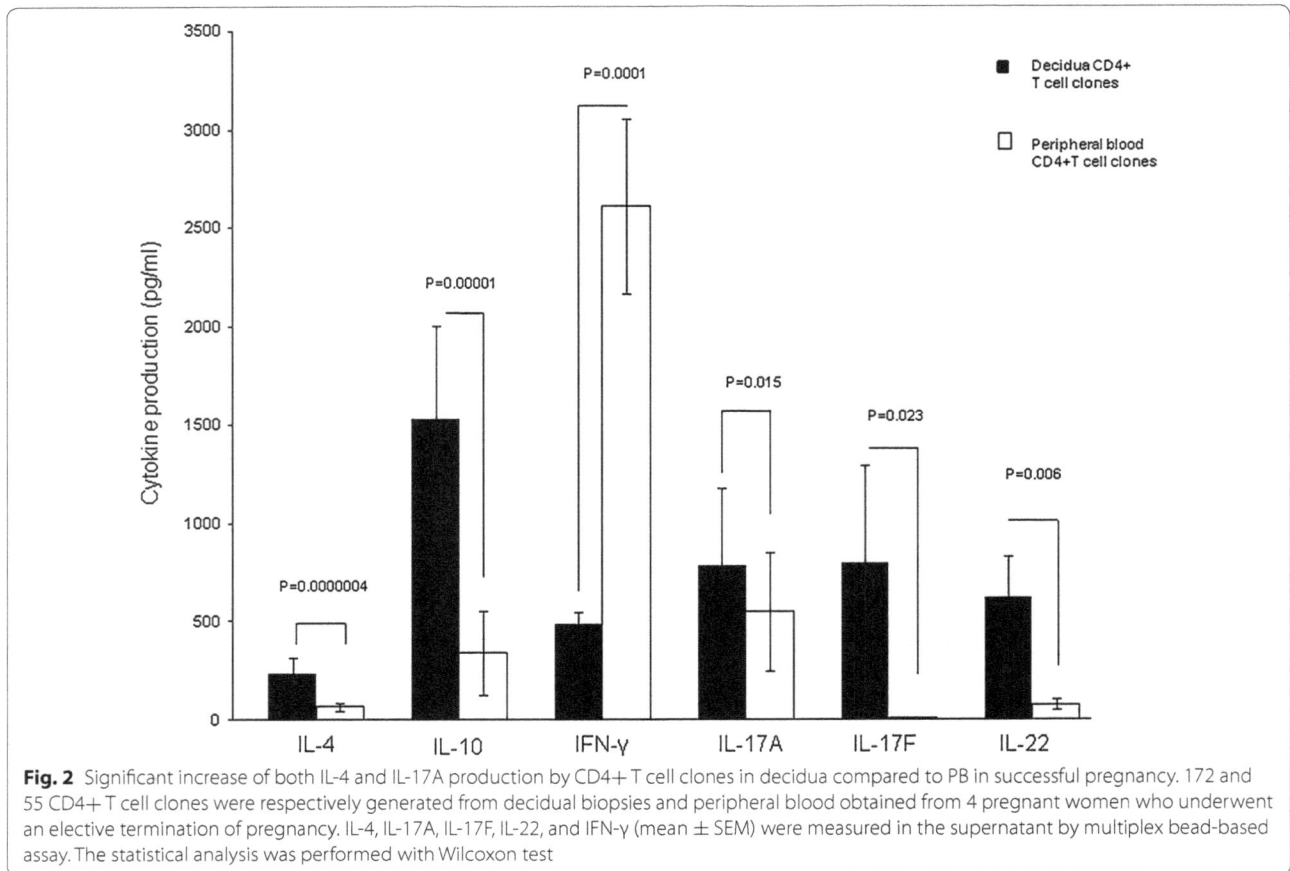

Fig. 2 Significant increase of both IL-4 and IL-17A production by CD4+ T cell clones in decidua compared to PB in successful pregnancy. 172 and 55 CD4+ T cell clones were respectively generated from decidual biopsies and peripheral blood obtained from 4 pregnant women who underwent an elective termination of pregnancy. IL-4, IL-17A, IL-17F, IL-22, and IFN-γ (mean ± SEM) were measured in the supernatant by multiplex bead-based assay. The statistical analysis was performed with Wilcoxon test

cells increased compared to normal pregnancy [31, 33]. Previously, we showed that in normal pregnancy both IL-17A, IL-17F and IL-22 are produced by decidua CD4+ T helper cells in association with IL-4. However, these previous experiments did not show whether the Th17-type cytokines (IL-17A, IL-17F and IL-22) and the Th2-type cytokine, IL-4, are produced by two different decidual CD4+ T cell subsets or if the same CD4+ T cell simultaneously produces the Th17-type and the Th2-type cytokines. In fact, part of human IL-17A-producing cells were found to also produce IL-4 (these cells were named Th17/Th2 [35] and other cells together with IL-17 can produce interferon (IFN)-γ (these cells were named Th17/Th1 [6]. To investigate the possibility that in normal pregnancy the same CD4+ cell subset can produce IL-17 and IL-4, we analyzed not only the percentages of Th1-, Th2-, Th0- and Th17-cells, but also the percentages of Th17/Th1 (producing IL-17A, IL-17F, IL-22 and IFN-γ), Th17/Th2 (producing IL-17A, IL-17F, IL-22 and IL-4) and Th17/Th0 (producing IL-17A, IL-17F, IL-22, IL-4 and IFN-γ). CD4+ T cell clones were derived from the decidua of 4 women with normal pregnancies, who

underwent an elective termination of pregnancy, and from the decidua obtained from 4 women suffering from unexplained recurrent abortion (Fig. 3). We found that 26 % of the whole CD4+ T cell clones generated from normal pregnancy produce IL-17 (54/208 T cell clones), whereas 59 % of the whole CD4+ T cell clones generated from unexplained recurrent abortion produce IL-17 (103/174 T cell clones). Thus, according to what was reported by Wang [31] and Nakashima [33], it seems that the percentage of the whole IL-17-producing T cells, without any Th17-type subpopulations analysis, is higher in unexplained recurrent abortion compared to normal pregnancy (p = 0.000001). We found that all the Th17, Th17/Th2 and Th17/Th1 T cell clones produced IL-22. There is no significant difference between the percentage of Th1, Th0 and Th17/Th0 CD4+ T cell clones generated from the decidua of normal pregnancy and those generated from spontaneous abortion (Fig. 3a). In contrast, the percentage of "proper" decidual Th17 (producing only IL-17A, IL-17F and IL-22) (p = 0.000001) and decidual Th17/Th1 (producing IFN-γ plus IL-17A, IL-17F and IL-22) T cell clones (p = 0.00001) were significantly higher in

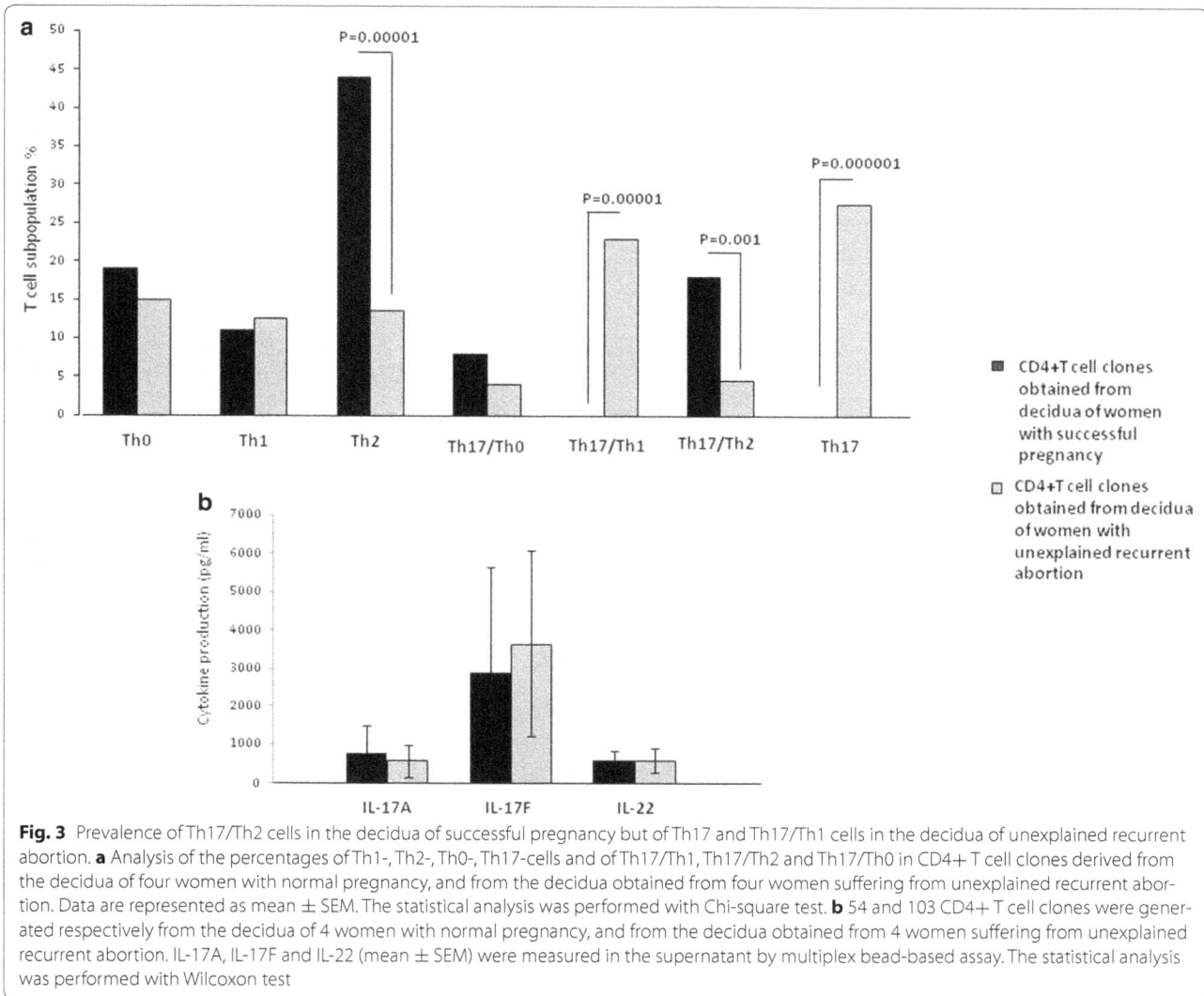

Fig. 3 Prevalence of Th17/Th2 cells in the decidua of successful pregnancy but of Th17 and Th17/Th1 cells in the decidua of unexplained recurrent abortion. **a** Analysis of the percentages of Th1-, Th2-, Th0-, Th17-cells and of Th17/Th1, Th17/Th2 and Th17/Th0 in CD4+ T cell clones derived from the decidua of four women with normal pregnancy, and from the decidua obtained from four women suffering from unexplained recurrent abortion. Data are represented as mean ± SEM. The statistical analysis was performed with Chi-square test. **b** 54 and 103 CD4+ T cell clones were generated respectively from the decidua of 4 women with normal pregnancy, and from the decidua obtained from 4 women suffering from unexplained recurrent abortion. IL-17A, IL-17F and IL-22 (mean ± SEM) were measured in the supernatant by multiplex bead-based assay. The statistical analysis was performed with Wilcoxon test

unexplained recurrent abortion compared to normal pregnancy (Fig. 3a). Noteworthy is the observation that no "proper" Th17 and Th17/Th1 T cell clones were ever detected in normal pregnancy decidua. However, the percentages of Th2 (p = 0.00001) and Th17/Th2 (producing IL-4 plus IL-17A, IL-17F and IL-22) (p = 0.001) T cell clones were significantly higher in the decidua of normal pregnancy compared to decidua of women suffering from unexplained recurrent abortion (Fig. 3a).

Measuring the levels of IL-17A and IL-17F produced by the whole IL-17-producing CD4+ T cell clones obtained from normal pregnancy (54 T cell clones) and by the whole IL-17-producing CD4+ T cell clones obtained from unexplained recurrent abortion (103 T cell clones), we did not find a significant increase in IL-17A and IL-17F production by CD4+ T cell clones generated from the decidua from unexplained recurrent abortion

compared to the IL-17A and IL-17F production by CD4+ T cell clones generated from the decidua of successful pregnancy (Fig. 3b). Similarly we did not find a significant increase in IL-17A and IL-17F production by CD4+ T cell clones generated from peripheral blood of successful pregnancy and recurrent spontaneous abortions (Additional file 1). These results also indicate that spontaneous recurrent abortions are not necessarily associated with increased levels of IL-17A and IL-17F produced by CD4+ T cells. Moreover, we measured the levels of IL-17 produced by Th17/Th2 T cell clones in normal pregnancy (18 % of T cell clones) and unexplained recurrent abortion (4.5 % of T cell clones), and we found that the levels of IL-17A produced by Th17/Th2 cells in successful pregnancy is higher (9507 ± 7000 pg/ml) compared to the levels of IL-17A produced by Th17/Th2 cells in unexplained recurrent abortion (137 ± 80 pg/ml) (p = 0.0001). These results confirmed that high IL-17 production is not associated with spontaneous recurrent abortion.

We demonstrated that IL-17A, IL-17F, IL-22, together with IL-4, were produced by the same decidual CD4+ T cell subpopulation (the Th17/Th2 cells) in normal pregnancy and not by two different CD4+ T cell subsets. Thus, IL-17 production by decidual CD4+ T cells does not seem to be associated with spontaneous abortion or unexplained spontaneous abortion, as was reported [31, 33]. IL-17 produced by decidual CD4+ T cells, if associated with IL-4 production, is not deleterious for pregnancy outcome.

Th17/Th2 CD4+ T cells are exclusively present at the implantation site of ectopic pregnancy

Decidual Th17/Th2 cells seem to be important for normal pregnancy development. We wondered whether these cells were present at the implantation site of the embryo and thus could have an important role for embryo implantation. To answer this question, we performed the same kind of cytokine analysis in ectopic tubal pregnancies.

We evaluated not only the percentage of Th1-, Th2-, Th0- and Th17-cells, but also the percentages of Th17/Th1 (producing IL-17A, IL-17F, IL-22 and IFN-γ), Th17/Th2 (producing IL-17A,IL-17F, IL-22 and IL-4) and Th17/Th0 (producing IL-17A, IL-17F, IL-22, IL-4 and IFN-γ) among the CD4+ T cell clones derived from the implantation site of the embryo (N = 133) and those distant from the implantation site in the same fallopian tube (N = 62) of 3 women suffering from ectopic pregnancy.

There is no significant difference in the percentage of pure Th2 and pure Th0 CD4+ T cell clones generated from the implantation site and distant from the implantation site (Fig. 4a). At the implantation site the percentage of Th17/Th2 (p = 0.000001) and of Th17/Th0 (p = 0.000001) CD4+ T cell clones is higher than those clones distant from the implantation site. Conversely, the percentage of Th1(p = 0.00001), pure Th17 (p = 0.00001) and Th17/Th1 (p = 0.000001) is higher apart from the implantation site compared to the embryo implantation site where these 3 types of CD4+ T cells are not present (Fig. 4a). Thus, Th17/Th1 cells are present only outside the implantation site or, as seen above, in decidua of recurrent spontaneous abortions. In other words, it seems that Th17/Th1 and pure Th17 cells, together with Th1 cells, are observed at locations where no implantation of the embryo occurs or when the implantation failed or is not maintained. By contrast, Th17/Th2 are prevalent in normal pregnancy and exclusively present at the implantation site of the embryo.

The levels of IL-4 (p = 0.00000001), IL-17A (p = 0.003), IL-17F (p = 0.00001) and IL-22 (p = 0.00002), produced by the CD4+ T cell clones at the implantation site are higher than the levels of these cytokines distant from the implantation site (Fig. 4b), indicating that there is an increase of production of Th2-type and Th17-type cytokines at the implantation site.

We confirmed these results by determining mRNA expression in Fallopian tube tissue taken at the embryo implantation site and tissue sampled distant from the implantation site of 3 women suffering from ectopic pregnancy (Fig. 4c). At the implantation site, the levels of mRNA for Th2-type molecules (IL-4 and GATA3) and for Th17-type molecules (IL-17A and RORC) were increased compared to the mRNA levels for these molecules distant from the implantation site. In contrast, distant from the implantation site mRNA production of IFN-γ is increased compared to those expressed at the embryo implantation site (Fig. 4c).

Soluble HLA-G5 mediates the development of Th17/Th2 cells by increasing IL-4 and IL-17A production of the CD4+ T helper cells

We can speculate about the origin of the factor(s) present in the uterine microenvironment that is able to induce Th17/Th2 cells by increasing the production of both IL-4 and IL-17A of the CD4+ T helper cells. Years ago, we reported that progesterone could induce Th2 responses [44]. Recently it has been shown that progesterone inhibits IL-17 production [45]. Thus, progesterone cannot be the factor responsible for Th17/Th2 cell development. Very recently, we showed that soluble HLA-G5 induces an increased production of IL-4 by CD4+ T helper cells [40]. We wondered if HLA-G5 could also induce IL-17A production by the CD4+ T cells and could be the factor responsible for the development of Th17/Th2 cells at the implantation site in normal pregnancy.

To investigate the possible influence of HLA-G5 on IL-4 and IL-17 production of antigen-specific T cells, we generated streptokinase (SK)-specific T cell lines (TCL) from 5 donors cultured in the absence or presence of HLA-G5. As a control, peripheral blood mononuclear cells from the same donors were stimulated with SK in the presence of IL-4, a powerful inducer of Th2 differentiation [46] and IL-12, a potent inducer of Th1 differentiation [47], which indicate that SK-specific TCL are modulated in our culture conditions (data not shown). When we measured the cytokines present in the supernatants of SK-specific T cell lines, we found a significant increase of IL-4 secretion (p = 0.0001) by the SK-specific T cell lines in response to IL-4, and a significant increase of IFN-γ (p = 0.006) in response to IL-12 (data not shown). This suggests that the culture conditions were satisfactory for the modulation of the T cell line cytokine profile.

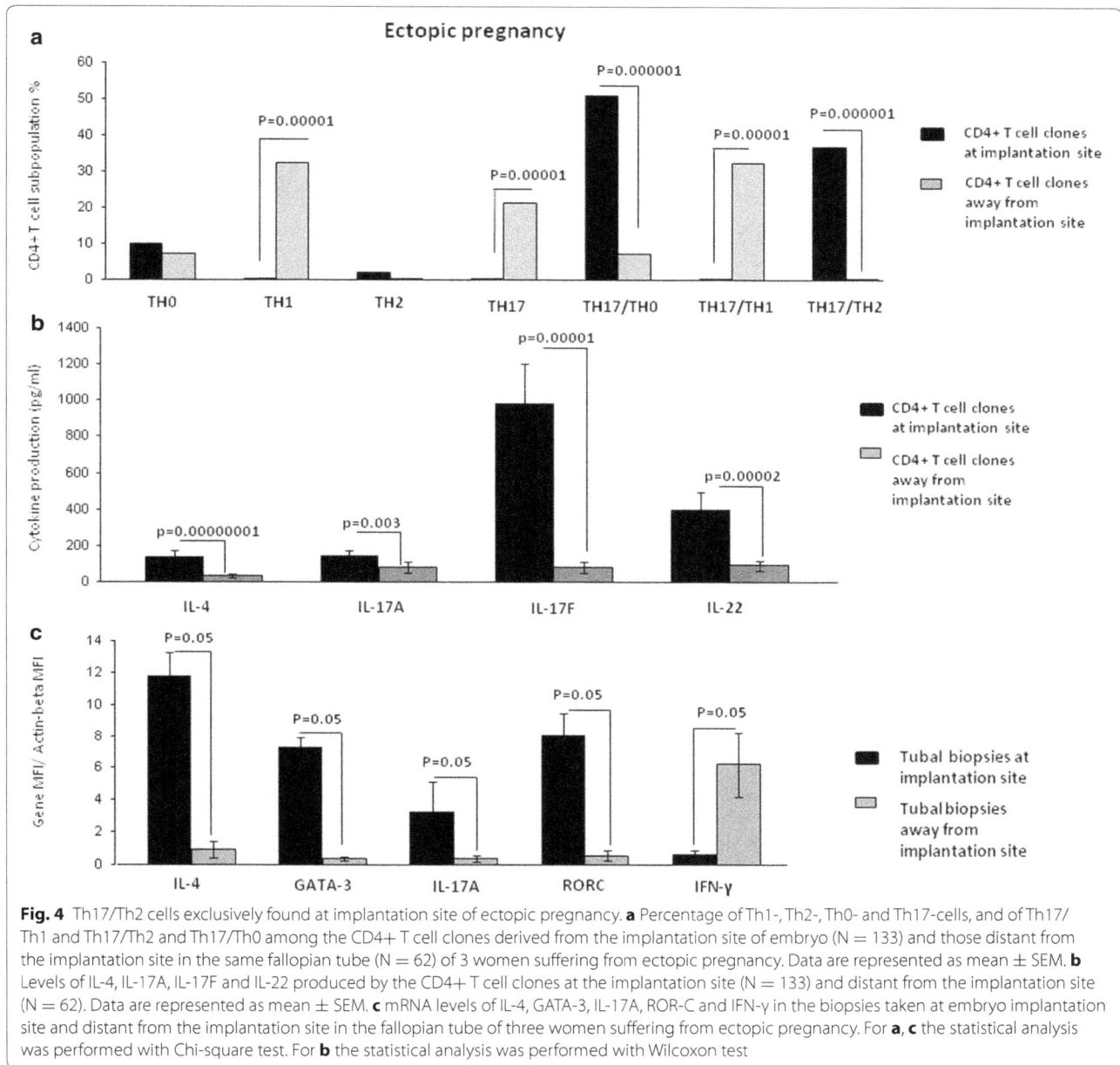

Fig. 4 Th17/Th2 cells exclusively found at implantation site of ectopic pregnancy. **a** Percentage of Th1-, Th2-, Th0- and Th17-cells, and of Th17/Th1 and Th17/Th2 and Th17/Th0 among the CD4+ T cell clones derived from the implantation site of embryo (N = 133) and those distant from the implantation site in the same fallopian tube (N = 62) of 3 women suffering from ectopic pregnancy. Data are represented as mean ± SEM. **b** Levels of IL-4, IL-17A, IL-17F and IL-22 produced by the CD4+ T cell clones at the implantation site (N = 133) and distant from the implantation site (N = 62). Data are represented as mean ± SEM. **c** mRNA levels of IL-4, GATA-3, IL-17A, ROR-C and IFN-γ in the biopsies taken at embryo implantation site and distant from the implantation site in the fallopian tube of three women suffering from ectopic pregnancy. For **a**, **c** the statistical analysis was performed with Chi-square test. For **b** the statistical analysis was performed with Wilcoxon test

A statistically significant increase of IL-4 (p = 0.0002), IL-17A (p = 0.005) and IL-17F (p = 0.028) was observed with the SK-specific T cell lines generated in the presence of HLA-G5 1 μg/ml (Fig. 5a). In contrast, IFN-γ production in response to HLA-G5 was not statistically significant (Fig. 5a). We then analyzed the cytokine mRNA levels of SK-specific T cell lines by RT-PCR (Fig. 5b). A statistically significant increase of IL-4 (p = 0.042), IL-17A (p = 0.043), IL-17F (p = 0.042) and IL-23R (receptor expressed by Th17 cells) (p = 0.043) mRNA expression was observed with the SK-specific T cell lines generated

in the presence of HLA-G5 compared to the SK-specific T cell lines generated in the absence of HLA-G5 (Fig. 5b). By contrast, no significant differences were observed for IFN-γ mRNA expression between the T cell lines generated in the presence or in the absence of HLA-G5 (Fig. 5b). These findings confirmed the results obtained at the protein level.

We derived CD4+ T cell clones from each of the SK-specific T cell lines of 4 donors (68 T cell clones in the absence of HLA-G5 and 87 T cell clones in the presence of HLA-G5). Subsequent analysis of their ability to

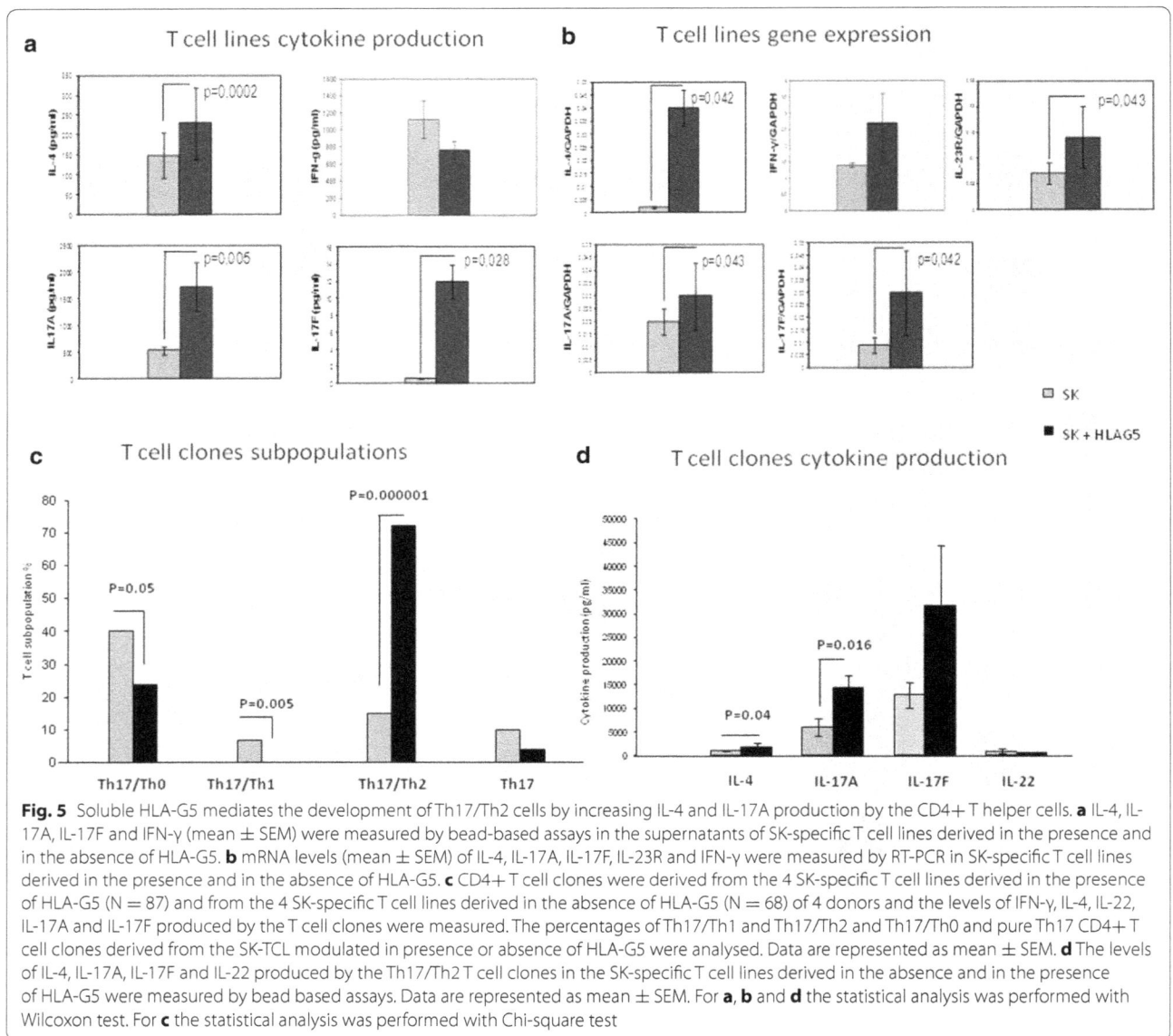

Fig. 5 Soluble HLA-G5 mediates the development of Th17/Th2 cells by increasing IL-4 and IL-17A production by the CD4+ T helper cells. **a** IL-4, IL-17A, IL-17F and IFN-γ (mean ± SEM) were measured by bead-based assays in the supernatants of SK-specific T cell lines derived in the presence and in the absence of HLA-G5. **b** mRNA levels (mean ± SEM) of IL-4, IL-17A, IL-17F, IL-23R and IFN-γ were measured by RT-PCR in SK-specific T cell lines derived in the presence and in the absence of HLA-G5. **c** CD4+ T cell lines were derived from the 4 SK-specific T cell lines derived in the presence of HLA-G5 (N = 87) and from the 4 SK-specific T cell lines derived in the absence of HLA-G5 (N = 68) of 4 donors and the levels of IFN-γ, IL-4, IL-22, IL-17A and IL-17F produced by the T cell clones were measured. The percentages of Th17/Th1 and Th17/Th2 and Th17/Th0 and pure Th17 CD4+ T cell clones derived from the SK-TCL modulated in presence or absence of HLA-G5 were analysed. Data are represented as mean ± SEM. **d** The levels of IL-4, IL-17A, IL-17F and IL-22 produced by the Th17/Th2 T cell clones in the SK-specific T cell lines derived in the absence and in the presence of HLA-G5 were measured by bead based assays. Data are represented as mean ± SEM. For **a**, **b** and **d** the statistical analysis was performed with Wilcoxon test. For **c** the statistical analysis was performed with Chi-square test

produce IFN-γ, IL-4, IL-22, IL-17A and IL-17F (Fig. 5c) was performed. We analyzed the percentages of Th17/Th1 (producing IL-17A, IL-17F, IL-22 and IFN-γ) and Th17/Th2 (producing IL-17A, IL-17F, IL-22 and IL-4) and Th17/Th0 (producing IL-17A, IL-17F, IL-22, IL-4 and IFN-γ) and pure Th17 CD4+ T cell clones derived from the SK-TCL modulated in the presence or absence of HLA-G5 (Fig. 5c, d).

The percentage of Th17/Th2 CD4+ T cell clones increases in the presence of HLA-G5 (p = 0.000001) (Fig. 5c). However, the percentage of Th17/Th1 (p = 0.005) and Th17/Th0 (p = 0.05) T cell clones is decreased in the presence of HLA-G5, but there is no

difference in the percentage of Th17 clones in the absence or in the presence of HLA-G5 (Fig. 5c).

The small percentage of Th17/Th2 T cell clones in the absence of HLA-G5 (Fig. 5c), prompted us to analyze the levels of Th2- and Th17-type cytokines produced by the Th17/Th2 T cell clones in the absence and in the presence of HLA-G5. We measured the cytokines present in the supernatants of CD4+ T cell clones derived from the SK-specific T cell lines (Fig. 5d). We found a significant increase in the secretion of IL-4 (p = 0.04) and IL-17A (p = 0.016) by the Th2/Th17 T cell clones derived from SK-TCL generated in the presence to HLA-G 5, compared to Th2/Th17 clones derived from SK-TCL without

HLA-G5. By comparison, the levels of IL-17F and IL-22 were not significantly modified (Fig. 5d).

The above findings indicate that HLA-G5 increases the production of both IL-17 and IL-4 by antigen-specific T cells in response to HLA-G5, thus upregulating the development of Th17/Th2 cells found at the site of embryo implantation (Additional file 1: Figure S1).

Discussion

Our findings seem to confirm the results reported by Wang [31] and Nakashima [33] showing that the percentage of IL-17 producing T cells in the decidua of unexplained recurrent abortion is higher than the percentage of IL-17-producing cells in the decidua of normal pregnancy. However, we did not find a significant increase of the IL-17 production by CD4+ T cell clones generated from the decidua of women with a normal pregnancy compared to the IL-17 production of CD4+ T cell clones generated from the decidua obtained of women suffering from unexplained recurrent abortion. Prior investigations [31, 33] did not make comparative measurements of IL-17 production by decidual CD4+ T cells in normal pregnancy and miscarriages and none identified Th17 subpopulations able to produce IL-4 or IFN-γ together with IL-17 (Th17/Th2 and Th17/Th1, respectively). Moreover, Th17 cells at the implantation site were never investigated. In the present study, we found that the number of IL-17-producing CD4+ T cell clones is increased in the decidua of normal pregnancy compared to peripheral blood, and more importantly, we observed an associated production of IL-4 and IL-17 by a large number of decidual CD4+ T cell clones (18 % of Th17/Th2 clones) in successful pregnancy. Accordingly, we found that freshly purified CD4+ T cells obtained from decidua of elective terminations of pregnancy, which have already been activated by trophoblast in vivo as recently demonstrated [40], can produce spontaneously and simultaneously IL-17 and IL-4 without any additional in vitro stimulation. The association of IL-17 and IL-4 production has been observed in allergic disorders known to be characterized by a Th2-type response [35], but the percentage of Th17/Th2 cells in peripheral blood of healthy subjects is very low (0.04 %) and increases only slightly in the peripheral blood of allergic patients with chronic asthma (1.3 %). To our knowledge, our study demonstrates for the first time a physiologic condition, namely successful pregnancy, in which the percentage of Th17/Th2 cells is markedly elevated. Interestingly, it was reported that in allergic disorders 0 % of Th17/Th2 T cell clones derived from purified peripheral blood CD161+CCR6+Th17 cells were obtained, but if CD161+CCR6+Th17 cells were cultured in the presence of IL-4, the percentage of Th17/Th2 cells increased to 14 % [35]. These findings suggest that Th17 cells switch toward Th17/Th2 cells, which could be modulated by the strongly Th2-type microenvironment induced in particular by high concentrations of progesterone in the decidua [44]. Thus, our findings contradict those reported by other authors [31, 32] who suggested that Th17 cells may promote miscarriage and be deleterious for pregnancy because of their capacity to induce alloantigens rejection [13]. Our data do not support a pathogenic role for IL-17 producing CD4+ T cells in pregnancy, rather we suggest that a beneficial role of Th17 cells play a beneficial role when they also produce IL-4 during the first trimester of human pregnancy. Furthermore, the Th17/Th2 cells are present only at the embryo implantation site. By contrast, Th17/Th1 cells and Th17 cells are prevalent, not only when the implantation fails but also when embryo implantation does not occur. Th17/Th1 could be involved as a potential cause of the abortion or could just be a consequence of this event. The functional activity of Th17/Th1 cells may be the result rather than the cause of pregnancy failure. Even in this case, however, the production of IFN-γ and IL-17, known to be involved in allograft rejection, may aggravate the situation and accelerate fetal allograft rejection and thus spontaneous abortion.

We have also demonstrated that HLA-G5, a factor present in the pregnant uterus microenvironment [48] and produced by both trophoblast and embryo, is responsible, at least in part, for the development of Th17/Th2 cells which in turn seem to be crucial for successful embryo implantation.

Conclusion

Infection-related immunity during gestation, responsible for a large number of miscarriages, seems to be preferentially directed towards combating extracellular microbial pathogens. During fetal development, interleukin (IL)-23, IL-10 and IL-6, as well as T-helper-17 (Th17)-mediated immune responses, are upregulated, whereas tumour necrosis factor-α (TNF-α) and IL-1β- and Th1-mediated immune responses are downregulated in the intrauterine environment (in both the fetal compartment and amniotic compartment) [49]. We hypothesize that IL-17/IL-4 producing decidual CD4+ T cells could be beneficial and useful for the maintenance of pregnancy, because they may promote an adequate response required to protect the mother against dangerous extracellular pathogens. In addition, the IL-4 produced by these cells together with the Th2 cells in the decidua [22] may induce tolerance towards paternal HLA-C expressed by the conceptus, through the production of IL-4. Moreover, IL-17 could be beneficial for successful pregnancy because it could promote the proliferation and invasion of human extravillous cytotrophoblast [50], important for gestational development.

We postulate that IL-17 could be essential for the success of pregnancy at certain stages of pregnancy but not so important or deleterious at other stages. The chronology of action of IL-17, alone or in association with other cytokines, should be further investigated to better understand the mechanisms by which pregnancy may or may not be affected by Th17 cells.

Authors' contributions

MPP conceived the study and designed the experiments, analysed all the data and wrote the manuscript. PLB supervised and analyzed flow cytometry data, participated in discussion and revision of the manuscript. DR organized handling and shipment of Fallopian tube samples, participated in the design of the ectopic pregnancy experiments. LL, FL and OK performed the multiplex bead-based assays, the T cell lines cultures, the decidual and Fallopian tube T cell clones cultures and RT-PCR. MA performed HLA-G5 purification as well as purification of decidual and peripheral blood CD4+ T cells, culture, and subsequent multicolor flow cytometry experiments. AB collected undamaged decidua basalis. FL provided input into the execution of flow cytometry studies. VD provided input into the execution of flow cytometry studies. YC performed purification of decidual and peripheral blood CD4+ T cells, their cultures, and flow cytometry experiments and analysis. HH collected ectopic pregnancy specimens. EM and SR approved and authorized all the processes. All authors read and approved the final manuscript.

Author details

[1] Department of Experimental and Clinical Medicine and DENOTHE Excellence Center, University of Florence, Largo Brambilla 3, 50134 Florence, Italy. [2] INSERM UMR1043, CNRS UMR5282, Centre de Physiopathologie Toulouse-Purpan, Université de Toulouse III, 31024 Toulouse, France. [3] Gynécologie-Obstétrique, Hôpital Paule de Viguier, Toulouse, France. [4] Department of Physiology and Immunology, Medical Faculty, University of Rijeka, 51000 Rijeka, Croatia. [5] Department of Gynecology and Obstetrics, Medical Faculty, University of Rijeka, 51000 Rijeka, Croatia.

Acknowledgements

The work performed in MPP, PLB and DR laboratories was supported by the European NoE EMBIC (LSHM-CT-2004-512040), MPP was supported by Intramural Scientific Research (ex-60 %) of the University of Florence. Work performed in PLB lab was also supported by INSERM, CNRS and Toulouse III University. DR was supported by University of Rijeka (13.06.1.1.06).

References

1. King A, Burrows TD, Hiby SE, Bowen JM, Joseph S, Verma S, et al. Surface expression of HLA-C antigen by human extravillous trophoblast. Placenta. 2000;21:376–87.
2. Colucci F, Moffett A, Trowsdale J. Medawar and the immunological paradox of pregnancy: 60 years on. Eur J Immunol. 2014;44:1883–5.
3. Romagnani S. Human Th1 and Th2 subsets: doubt no more. Immunol Today. 1991;12:256–7.
4. Harrington LE, Hatton RD, Mangan PR, Turner H, Murphy TL, Murphy KM, et al. Interleukin 17-producing CD4+ effector T cells develop via a lineage distinct from the T helper type 1 and 2 lineages. Nat Immunol. 2005;6:1123–32.
5. Acosta-Rodriguez EV, Rivino L, Geginat J, Jarrossay D, Gattorno M, Lanzavecchia A, et al. Surface phenotype and antigenic specificity of human interleukin 17-producing T helper memory cells. Nat Immunol. 2007;8:639–46.
6. Annunziato F, Cosmi L, Santarlasci V, Maggi L, Liotta F, Mazzinghi B, et al. Phenotypic and functional features of human Th17 cells. J Exp Med. 2007;204:1849–61.

7. Chen Z, Laurence A, O'Shea JJ. Signal transduction pathways and transcriptional regulation in the control of Th17 differentiation. Semin Immunol. 2007;19:400–8.
8. Santarlasci V, Maggi L, Capone M, Frosali F, Querci V, De Palma R, et al. TGF-beta indirectly favours the development of human Th17 cells by inhibiting Th1 cells. Eur J Immunol. 2009;39:207–15.
9. Murphy CA, Langrish CL, Chen Y, Blumenschein W, McClanahan T, Kastelein RA, et al. Divergent pro-and anti-inflammatory roles for IL-23 and IL-12 in joint autoimmune inflammation. J Exp Med. 2003;198:1951–7.
10. Cosmi L, De Palma R, Santarlasci V, Maggi L, Capone M, Frosali F, et al. Human interleukin-17-producing cells originate from a CD161+CD4+ T-cell precursor. J Exp Med. 2008;205:1903–16.
11. Cua DJ, Sherlock J, Chen Y, Murphy CA, Joyce B, Seymour B, et al. Interleukin-23 rather than interleukin-12 is the critical cytokine for autoimmune inflammation of the brain. Nature. 2003;421:744–8.
12. Kleinschek MA, Boniface K, Sadekova S, Grein J, Murphy EE, Turner SP, et al. Circulating and gut-resident human Th17 cells express CD161 and promote intestinal inflammation. J Exp Med. 2009;206:525–34.
13. Chen H, Wang W, Xie H, Xu X, Wu J, Jiang Z, et al. A pathogenic role of IL- 17 at the early stage of corneal allograft rejection. Transpl Immunol. 2009;21:155–61.
14. Yuan X, Paez-Cortez J, Schmitt-Knosalla I, D'Addio F, Mfarrej B, Donnarumma M, et al. A novel role of CD4 Th17 cells in mediating cardiac allograft rejection and vasculopathy. J Exp Med. 2008;205:3133–44.
15. Strom TB, Roy-Chaudury R, Manfro R, Zheng XX, Nickerson PW, Wood K, et al. The Th1/Th2 paradigm and allograft response. Curr Opin Immunol. 1996;8:688–93.
16. Suthanthiran M, Strom TB. Immunobiology and immunopharmacology of organ allograft rejection. J Clin Immunol. 1995;15:161–71.
17. Burns WR, Wang Y, Tang PC, Ranjbaran H, Iakimov A, Kim J, et al. Recruitment of CXCR3+ and CCR5+ T cells and production of interferon-gamma-inducible chemokines in rejecting human arteries. Am J Transplant. 2005;5:1226–36.
18. Waaga AM, Gasser M, Kist-van Holthe JE, Najafian N, Muller A, Vella JP, et al. Regulatory functions of self-restricted MHC class II allopeptide-specific Th2 clones in vivo. J. Clin. Invest. 2001;107:909–16.
19. Graca L, Cobbolt SP, Waldmann H. Identification of regulatory T cells in tolerated allografts. J Exp Med. 2002;195:1641–6.
20. Wegmann TG, Lin H, Guilbert L, Mossmann TR. Bidirectional cytokine interactions in the maternal-fetal relationship: is successful pregnancy a Th2 phenomenon? Immunol Today. 1993;14:353–6.
21. Chaouat G, Assal Meliani A, Martal J, Raghupathy R, Elliot JF, Mossman T, et al. IL-10 prevents naturally occurring fetal loss in the CBA x DBA/2 mating combination, and local defect in IL-10 production in this abortion-prone combination is corrected by in vivo injection of IFN-tau. J Immunol. 1995;154:4261–8.
22. Piccinni MP, Beloni L, Livi C, Maggi E, Scarselli GF, Romagnani S. Defective production of both leukemia inhibitory factor and type 2 T-helper cytokines by decidual T cells in unexplained recurrent abortions. Nat Med. 1998;4:1020–4.
23. Piccinni MP, Scaletti C, Vultaggio A, Maggi E, Romagnani S. Defective production of LIF, M-CSF and Th2-type cytokines by T cells at fetomaternal interface is associated with pregnancy loss. J Reprod Immunol. 2001;52:35–43.
24. Piccinni MP. T cell tolerance towards the fetal allograft. J Reprod Immunol. 2010;85:71–5.
25. Ruocco MG, Chaouat G, Florez L, Bensussan A, Klatzmann D. Regulatory T-cells in pregnancy: historical perspective, state of the art, and burning questions. Front Immunol. 2014;21:389–99.
26. Michaëlsson J, Mold JE, McCune JM, Nixon DF. Regulation of T cell responses in the developing human fetus. J Immunol. 2006;176:5741–8.
27. Kallikourdis M, Andersen KG, Welch KA, Betz AG. Alloantigen-enhanced accumulation of CCR5+ 'effector' regulatory T cells in the gravid uterus. Proc Natl Acad Sci USA. 2007;104:594–9.
28. Shima T, Inada K, Nakashima A, Ushijima A, Ito M, Yoshino O, Saito S. Paternal antigen-specific proliferating regulatory T cells are increased in uterine-draining lymph nodes just before implantation and in pregnant uterus just after implantation by seminal plasma-priming in allogeneic mouse pregnancy. J Reprod Immunol. 2015;108:72–82.
29. Inada K, Shima T, Nakashima A, Aoki K, Ito M, Saito S. Characterization of regulatory T cells in decidua of miscarriage cases with abnormal or

normal fetal chromosomal content. J Reprod Immunol. 2013;97:104–11.

30. Robertson SA, Prins JR, Sharkey DJ, Moldenhauer LM. Seminal fluid and the generation of regulatory T cells for embryo implantation. Am J Reprod Immunol. 2013;4:315–30.

31. Wang WJ, Hao CF, Yi-Lin Yin GJ, Bao SH, Qiu LH, Lin QD. Increased prevalence of T helper 17 (Th17) cells in peripheral blood and decidua in unexplained recurrent spontaneous abortion patients. J Reprod Immunol. 2010;84:164–70.

32. Wang WJ, Liu FJ, Qu HM, Hao CF, Qu QL, Xiong-Wang Bao HC, et al. Regulation of the expression of Th17 cells and regulatory T cells by IL-27 in patients with unexplained early recurrent miscarriage. J Reprod Immunol. 2013;99:39–45.

33. Nakashima A, Ito M, Shima T, Bac ND, Hidaka T, Saito S. Accumulation of IL-17-positive cells in decidua of inevitable abortion cases. Am J Reprod Immunol. 2010;64:4–11.

34. Lee YK, Turner H, Maynard CL, Oliver JR, Chen D, Elson CO, et al. Late developmental plasticity in the T helper 17 lineage. Immunity. 2009;30:92–107.

35. Cosmi L, Maggi L, Santarlasci V, Capone M, Cardilicchia E, Frosali F, et al. Identification of a novel subset of human circulating memory CD4(+) T cells that produce both IL-17A and IL-4. J Allergy Clin Immunol. 2010;125:222–30.

36. El Costa H, Casemayou A, Aguerre-Girr M, Rabot M, Berrebi A, Parant O, et al. Critical and differential roles of NKp46- and NKp30-activating receptors expressed by uterine NK cells in early pregnancy. J Immunol. 2008;181:3009–17.

37. Barakonyi A, Kovacs KT, Miko E, Szereday L, Varga P, Szekeres-Bartho J. Recognition of nonclassical HLA class I antigens by gamma delta T cells during pregnancy. J Immunol. 2002;168:2683–8.

38. Piccinni MP, Lombardelli L, Logiodice F, Tesi D, Kullolli O, Biagiotti R, et al. Potential pathogenetic role of Th17, Th0, and Th2 cells in erosive and reticular oral lichen planus. Oral Dis. 2014;20:212–8.

39. Fournel S, Aguerre-Girr M, Campan A, Salauze L, Berrebi A, Lone YC. Soluble HLA-G: purification from eukaryotic transfected cells and detection by a specific ELISA. Am J Reprod Immunol. 1999;42:22–9.

40. Lombardelli L, Aguerre-Girr M, Logiodice F, Kullolli O, Casart Y, Polgar B, et al. HLA-G5 induces IL-4 secretion critical for successful pregnancy through differential expression of ILT2 receptor on decidual CD4+ T cells and macrophages. J Immunol. 2013;191:3651–62.

41. Pappas J, Quan N, Ghildyal N. A single- step enrichment of Th2 lymphocytes using CCR4 microbeads. Immunol Lett. 2006;102:110–14.

42. Zingoni A, Soto H, Hedrick JA, Stoppacciaro A, Storlazzi CT, Sinigaglia F, et al. The chemokine receptor CCR8 is preferentially expressed in Th2 but not Th1 cells. J Immunol. 1998;161:547–51.

43. Syrbe U, Siveke J, Hamann A. Th1/Th2 subsets: distinct differences in homing and chemokine receptor expression? Springer Semin Immunopathol. 1999;21:263–85.

44. Piccinni MP, Giudizi MG, Biagiotti R, Beloni L, Giannarini L, Sampognaro S, et al. Progesterone favors the development of human T helper cells producing Th2-type cytokines and promotes both IL-4 production and membrane CD30 expression in established Th1 cells clones. J Immunol. 1995;155:128–33.

45. Xu L, Dong B, Wang H, Zeng Z, Liu W, Chen N, et al. Progesterone suppresses Th17 cell responses, and enhances the development of regulatory T cells, through thymic stromal lymphopoietin-dependent mechanisms in experimental gonococcal genital tract infection. Microbes Infect. 2013;15:796–805.

46. Maggi E, Parronchi P, Manetti R, Simonelli C, Piccinni MP, Rugiu FS, et al. Reciprocal regulatory effects of IFN-gamma and IL-4 on the in vitro development of human Th1 and Th2 clones. J Immunol. 1992;148:2142–7.

47. Manetti R, Parronchi P, Giudizi MG, Piccinni MP, Maggi E, Trinchieri G, et al. Natural killer cell stimulatory factor (interleukin 12 [IL-12]) induces T helper type 1 (Th1)-specific immune responses and inhibits the development of IL-4-producing Th cells. J Exp Med. 1993;177:1199–204.

48. Le Bouteiller P. HLA-G in human early pregnancy: control of uterine immune cell activation and likely vascular remodelling. Biomed J. 2015;38(1):32–8. doi:10.4103/2319-4170.131376.

49. Witkin SS, Linhares IM, Bongiovanni AM, Herway C, Skupski D. Unique alterations in infection-induced immune activation during pregnancy. BJOG. 2011;118:145–53.

50. Wu HX, Jin LP, Xu B, Liang SS, Li DJ. Decidual stromal cells recruit Th17 cells into decidua to promote proliferation and invasion of human trophoblast cells by secreting IL-17. Cell Mol Immunol. 2014;11:253–62.

14

Asthma under/misdiagnosis in primary care setting: an observational community-based study

Maria Sandra Magnoni[1*], Marco Caminati[2], Gianenrico Senna[2], Fabio Arpinelli[1], Andrea Rizzi[1], Anna Rita Dama[2], Michele Schiappoli[2], Germano Bettoncelli[3] and Gaetano Caramori[4]

Abstract

Background: Published data suggest that asthma is significantly under/misdiagnosed. The present community-based study performed in Italy aims at investigating the level of asthma under/misdiagnosis among patients referring to the General Practitioner (GP) for respiratory symptoms and undergoing Inhaled corticosteroids.

Methods: A sub-analysis of a previously published observational cross-sectional study has been provided. It included subjects registered in the GP databases with at least three prescriptions of inhaled or nebulised corticosteroids during the 12 months preceding the start of the study. All subjects, independently of the diagnosis, were invited to visit their GP's office for a standardised interview and to fill the European Community Respiratory Health Survey (ECRHS) questionnaire.

Results: The studies involved 540 GPs in most of the Italian regions and 2090 subjects (mean age 54.9 years, 54.1 % females) were enrolled. Among them 991 cases of physician-diagnosed asthma were observed while 1099 subjects received a diagnosis other than asthma (chronic obstructive pulmonary disease, chronic upper respiratory tract infections etc.). Among the lasts, the ECRHS questionnaire was suggestive for asthma diagnosis in 365 subjects (33.2 %).

Conclusions: The data suggest that there is still a large under/misdiagnosis of asthma in the Italian primary care setting, despite the spread of GINA guidelines nearly 20 years before this study. A validated tool like the ECRHS questionnaire has detected a considerable proportion of potentially asthmatic patients who should be addressed to lung function assessment to confirm the diagnosis. Further educational efforts directed to the GPs are needed to improve their diagnosis of asthma (SAM104964).

Keywords: Asthma, ECRHS questionnaire, Under diagnosis, Misdiagnosis, Primary care

Background

A significant asthma under/misdiagnosis has been highlighted by some Italian studies. Ciprandi et al. [1] investigated the epidemiological features of asthma in a homogeneous population of 18-year-old male conscripts referred to La Spezia Military Navy Hospital for a call-up visit and found a not negligible under-diagnosis and inadequate treatment of asthma. In 7.4 % of conscripts asthma had been newly diagnosed during the study and about one quarter of the asthmatic subjects received no treatment at all. Bellia et al. [2] showed that asthma in the elderly is frequently confused with chronic obstructive pulmonary disease (COPD) and that in patients with mild functional impairment asthma may be under-diagnosed. A decreased perception of dyspnoea, or the intermittent onset of asthma symptoms, may account for under/misdiagnosis or delayed diagnosis of the disease [3]. Under/delayed-diagnosis and consequent under/delayed-treatment start might be important factors contributing to asthma morbidity, whereas early detection and treatment of asthma might improve the long-term prognosis of these patients.

*Correspondence: maria-sandra.s.magnoni@gsk.com
[1] Medical and Scientific Department, GlaxoSmithKline, Verona, Italy
Full list of author information is available at the end of the article

The European Community Respiratory Health Survey (ECRHS) questionnaire has been proposed as a validated tool useful in identifying asthmatic patients [4–6]. The aim of the present community-based study was to investigate the level of asthma under/misdiagnosis in a primary care setting, by comparing physician diagnosis and the ECRHS questionnaire results. Patients undergoing inhaled corticosteroids (ICS) for a physician-diagnosed respiratory disease other than asthma were included as the study population. The results are reported as a sub-analysis of a previously published observational cross-sectional study [7].

Methods

Full details of the study design and patient population have been reported elsewhere [7] and are summarised here.

Study design

A multicentre, observational cross-sectional study involving of 540 Italian General Practitioners (GPs) has been conducted. The protocol was approved by the Ethic Committee of the Italian Society of General Medicine (SIMG; http://www.simg.it). Written informed consent was obtained by each patient before the inclusion into the study. Invitation to participate to the study was sent to all the GPs owning a computerised patient database according to the information stored in the archive of the European School of General Medicine (Scuola Europea di Medicina Generale, SEMG, Firenze, Italy).

Adult patients (≥18-years old) diagnosed with a respiratory disease and receiving at least 3 prescriptions of inhaled corticosteroids (ICS) during the previous 12 months (metered-dose inhaler -MDI-, dry powder inhaler -DPI- or nebulise) were enrolled. A concomitant prescription including long-acting beta2 agonists and/or theophylline and/or nedocromil or sodium cromoglycate, and/or anti-leukotrienes, and/or anticholinergic drugs was considered as an exclusion criterion, as usually these drugs are specifically and unequivocally prescribed for asthma or COPD.

This study was performed from September 2005 to January 2006. Every participating physician was requested to retrospectively select the last ten eligible consecutive patients since the study beginning date.

The selected patients were invited to perform a follow-up visit and to fill in an ECRHS respiratory symptom questionnaire. The first page contains validated questions on the presence of asthma and asthma-like symptoms, frequency of asthma attacks, age at onset and remission of asthma, doctor diagnosis of asthma, presence of chronic cough and phlegm, and smoking habits. The second page collects information on the last 12 months about: indirect costs (number of working days lost and number of impaired general activity days resulting from

asthma); type and frequency of doctor visits and laboratory tests performed because of asthma; frequency of hospital admissions and emergency department (ED) visits resulting from asthma; treatment; type of prescription (when needed or for daily use) [4–6]. A subject with a questionnaire positive for respiratory symptoms (wheezing, nocturnal chest tightness, attack of breathlessness after activity at rest or at night; or 1 asthma attack) was considered a subject with current asthma.

Results

Overall a response rate of 89 % was recorded corresponding to 2090 subjects (mean age 54.9 years, 54.1 % females). Among these subjects, according to the physician diagnosis 991 were affected by asthma and 1099 suffered from a respiratory disease other than asthma.

Table 1 shows demographic and clinical data of enrolled patients: comorbidities, such as cardiovascular diseases, are more frequently reported in patients with diagnosis other than asthma, whereas the prevalence of allergic disorders is higher in patients with asthma.

In patients diagnosed with a respiratory disease other than asthma, COPD was the most frequently reported (21.7 %), followed by not specified upper respiratory tract infections (12.2 %), chronic or acute bronchitis (11.5 %). Overall, upper respiratory symptoms and/or signs were present in around 40 % of these patients, classified as allergic or vasomotor rhinitis, chronic otitis/sinusitis, not specified otitis/sinusitis, not specified rhinitis, not specified acute upper respiratory tract infections and not specified upper respiratory tract infections. In 4.9 % other different respiratory diseases were reported.

Table 1 Main characteristics of the patients with diagnosis with diagnosis other than asthma [N = 1099]

	N (%)	95 % IC
Mean age [years (SD)]	58.4 (18.3)	
Mean age at diagnosis of asthma (SD)	–	–
Female [n (%)]	590 (53.7)	50.6–56.6
Smoking habits		
Non smokers [n (%)]	614 (55.9)	52.8–58.8
Past smokers [n (%)]	199 (18.1)	15.8–20.5
Current smokers [n (%)]	277 (25.2)	22.6–27.8
Smoking history, mean years (SD)	(14.1) 10.8	–
Concomitant diseases		
Cardiovascular	445 (40.5)	37.5–43.4
Respiratory	119 (10.8)	9.0–12.8
Ear nose and throat (ENT)	171 (15.6)	13.4–17.8
Allergy	103 (9.4)	7.7–11.2
Spirometry	181 (16.5)	14.3–18.7

% accounting also for missing data

Missing data: smoking habits = 20

Among patients diagnosed with a respiratory disease different from asthma (1099), the ECRHS asthma questionnaire suggested asthma diagnosis in 365 (33.2 %) of them (Fig. 1). The characteristics of this subgroup are reported in Table 2. Most diagnoses (about 60 %) were related to chronic obstructive lung diseases, bronchitis (chronic or acute bronchitis), whereas around 20 % were related to high respiratory airways (acute or chronic upper respiratory tract infections, allergic or vasomotor rhinitis, otitis/sinusitis). Of note, only 16.5 % of patients had undergone lung function assessment in the last 12 months. In particular, less than 30 % of asthmatic patients according to the ECRHS questionnaire and 38.6 % of physician-diagnosed asthmatic patients underwent spirometry (Table 1).

Discussion

Our study highlights that according to the ECRHS results, asthma should be highly suspected in 33.2 % in patients diagnosed with a respiratory disease different from asthma by their GP and undergoing ICS treatment. Furthermore only 16.5 % of the overall study population had undergone lung function assessment in the last 12 months, despite suffering from a physician-diagnosed respiratory disease.

The results of our study show a poor accordance between physician-reported and ECRHS questionnaire-related asthma diagnosis. Assuming the good sensibility and specificity of the ECRHS questionnaire, the results confirm that Italian GPs do not optimally recognise

Table 2 Diagnosis reported in the GP data base of the 365 subjects identified as asthmatics by ECRHS questionnaire

Diagnosis	Patients (n)	%
COPD	128	35.1
Chronic bronchitis or acute bronchitis	53	14.5
Respiratory symptoms or signs	47	12.9
Upper respiratory tract infections (n.s.)	21	5.8
Acute bronchitis	20	5.5
Bronchitis n.s.	15	4.1
Allergic or vasomotor rhinitis	11	3.0
Chronic upper respiratory tract infections	10	2.7
Chronic otitis/sinusitis	10	2.7
Acute upper respiratory tract infections (n.s)	10	2.7
Otitis/sinusitis (n.s.)	8	2.2
Other respiratory diseases	32	8.8
Total	365	100.0

n.s. not specified

respiratory symptoms as asthma manifestations. This finding is in agreement with previous studies, showing that 7.4 % of enrolled subjects had been newly diagnosed with asthma during the study and about one quarter of the asthmatic subjects received no treatment at all [1].

It is not surprising that in our cohort of patients, selected on the basis of ICS use, many of them had a diagnosis different from asthma. In Italy, patients with COPD, acute and chronic bronchitis, acute upper respiratory tract infections, rhinitis or not well defined respiratory symptoms are extensively treated with ICS, as also reported in other studies, including a large-scale paediatric survey [8].

Among the patients identified as asthmatics according to ECRHS questionnaire, 35 % had a diagnosis of COPD in GP database, although around 56 % of them had never smoked. Distinguishing asthma from COPD is often problematic, particularly in smokers and older adults, and in a significant proportion of patients COPD and asthma features may coexist [9]: spirometry, besides clinical history, could help to address the question of differential diagnosis, and it should always be performed in patients with respiratory symptoms. Nevertheless in our study less than 30 % of asthmatic patients according to the ECRHS questionnaire and 38.6 % of physician-diagnosed asthmatic patients underwent lung function assessment during the previous 12 months. Limited prescription of lung function tests in general practice (physicians may not be fully familiar with the interpretation of results) and poor accessibility to spirometers, which are mostly available in the hospital setting due to lack of time to perform office spirometry (in most cases GPs in Italy do not have technical or nursing support), may account

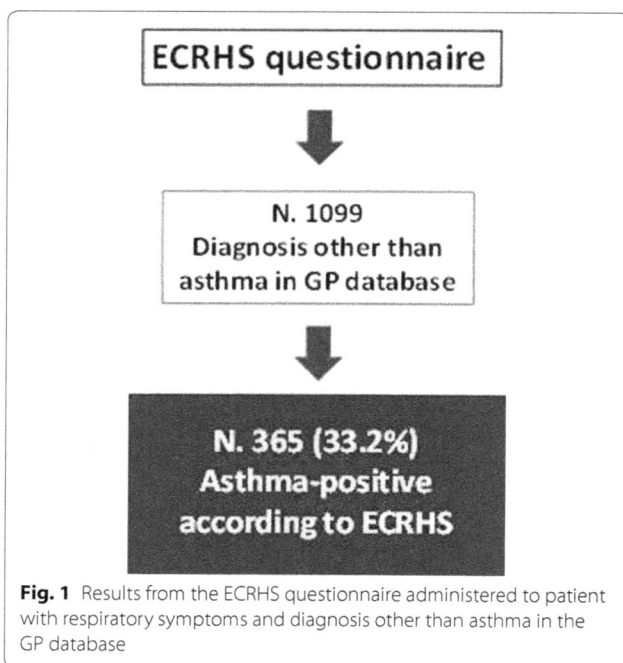

Fig. 1 Results from the ECRHS questionnaire administered to patient with respiratory symptoms and diagnosis other than asthma in the GP database

for under-utilization of spirometry in primary care [10, 11].

Around 20 % of the patients identified as asthmatics according to ECRHS questionnaire had a diagnosis of upper airway disease in the GP database (allergic or vasomotor rhinitis or otitis/sinusitis). It is well known that allergic rhinitis and sinusitis are often associated with asthma and constitute the main risk factor for its development. Another Italian study showed that subjects with allergic rhinitis show an eightfold risk of having asthma compared to subjects without allergic rhinitis [12]. Furthermore, in a large cohort study on subjects with allergic rhinitis without diagnosis of asthma, bronchial hyper-responsiveness and also bronchial obstruction were detected in a high percentage of patients, both during and outside the pollen season [13], underlining the importance of lung function assessment in patients with chronic upper airways symptoms. Nevertheless the lack of asthma identification in these patients suggests that asthma is still regarded mainly as an intermittent disease, or misrecognized as a clinical manifestation of viral infections.

Our study has some potential limitation. Firstly, only patients on ICS treatment were included in the survey, whereas those treated with other respiratory drugs were excluded. Although inhaled corticosteroids are the gold standard of asthma therapy, in general practice there is a wide range of treatments for patients with respiratory symptoms. Thus, the rate of mis/underdiagnosis of asthma observed in this study presumably affects milder patients. As regards patients treated with various anti-asthmatic agents, such as combinations of ICS and bronchodilators, recent evidence suggests a considerable amount of overdiagnosis of asthma [14]. Secondly, untreated patients were excluded from the study population, thus patients with milder disease have been potentially lost.

Our data suggest that there is still a considerable under/misdiagnosis of asthma in the Italian primary care settings, and that the use of a validated questionnaire could be of helpful in identifying patients to address to lung function assessment.

Conclusions
Asthma under/misdiagnosis and consequent inappropriate pharmacological treatment still affect asthma management. Furthermore they represent important factors contributing to asthma morbidity and mortality, whereas early detection and management might improve the long-term prognosis of affected patients. Educational efforts should be directed to improve the capability of primary care professionals, particularly GPs, to recognise asthma symptoms and to address patients to the correct diagnostic work-up and proper treatment. The use of a validated questionnaire could be of help for patients' identification.

Abbreviations
GP: General Practitioner; ECRHS: European Community Respiratory Health Survey; COPD: chronic obstructive pulmonary disease; ICS: inhaled corticosteroids; MDI: metered-dose inhaler; DPI: dry powder inhaler; ED: emergency department.

Authors' contributions
MSM, FA and AR designed the study. GB and GC coordinated the data collection. MC, GS, AR and MS contributed to data analysis and interpretation. MSM, MC and GS prepared the final version of the manuscript. All authors read and approved the final manuscript.

Authors' information
MC is the current Junior Members Chairperson of the Italian Society of Allergy, Asthma and Clinical Immunology (SIAAIC). GS is the current vice-President of the Italian Society of Allergy, Asthma and Clinical Immunology (SIAAIC).

Author details
[1] Medical and Scientific Department, GlaxoSmithKline, Verona, Italy. [2] Allergy Unit, Verona University and General Hospital, Piazzale Stefani 1, 37126 Verona, Italy. [3] Società Italiana di Medicina Generale, Florence, Italy. [4] Dipartimento di Scienze Mediche, Sezione di Medicina Interna e Cardiorespiratoria, Centro Interdipartimentale per lo Studio delle Malattie Infiammatorie delle Vie Aeree e Patologie Fumo-Correlate (CEMICEF, formerly termed Centro), Università di Ferrara, Ferrara, Italy.

Acknowledgements
We would like to warmly thank all the Italian General Practitioners involved in the present study. The present study has been supported by an unrestricted educational grant from GlaxoSmithKline spa, Verona, Italy.

References
1. Ciprandi G, Vizzaccaro A, Cirillo I, Tosco M, Passalacqua G, Canonica GW. Underdiagnosis and undertreatment of asthma: a 9-year study of Italian conscripts. Int Arch Allergy Immunol. 2001;125:211–5.
2. Bellia V, Battaglia S, Catalano F, Scichilone N, Incalzi RA, Imperiale C, et al. Aging and disability affect misdiagnosis of COPD in elderly asthmatics. The SARA Study. Chest. 2003;123:1066–72.
3. van Weel C. Underdiagnosis of asthma and COPD: is the general practitioner to blame? Monaldi Arch Chest Dis. 2002;57:65–8.
4. de Marco R, Cerveri I, Bugiani M, Ferrari M, Verlato G. An undetected burden of asthma in Italy: the relationship between clinical and epidemiological diagnosis of asthma. Eur Respir J. 1998;11:599–605.
5. de Marco R, Zanolin ME, Accordini S, Signorelli D, Marinoni A, Bugiani M, et al. A new questionnaire for the repeat of the first stage of the European Community Respiratory Health Survey: a pilot study. Eur Respir J. 1999;14:1044–8.
6. de Marco R, Bugiani M, Cazzoletti L, Carosso A, Accordini S, Buriani O, et al, for ISAYA study Group. The control of asthma in Italy. A multicentre descriptive study on young adults with doctor diagnosed current asthma. Allergy. 2003; 58:221–228.
7. Caminati M, Bettoncelli G, Magnoni MS, Rizzi A, Testi R, Passalacqua G, et al. The level of control of mild asthma in general practice: an observational community-based study. J Asthma. 2014;51:91–6.
8. Clavenna A, Rossi E, Berti A, Pedrazzi G, De Rosa M. Bonati M; ARNO Working Group. Inappropriate use of antiasthmatic drugs in the Italian paediatric population. Eur J Clin Pharmacol. 2003;59:565–9.

9. The Global Strategy for Asthma Management and Prevention Report 2015. http://www.ginasthma.org/local/uploads/files/GINA_Report_2015_May19.pdf. Accessed 30 May 2015.

10. Lusuardi M, De Benedetto F, Paggiaro P, Sanguinetti CM, Brazzola G, Ferri P, et al. A randomised controlled trial on office spirometry in asthma and COPD in standard general practice: data from spirometry in asthma and COPD. A comparative evaluation Italian Study. Chest. 2006;129:844–52.

11. Caramori G, Bettoncelli G, Tosatto R, Arpinelli F, Visonà G, Invernizzi G, et al. Underuse of spirometry by general pratictioners for the diagnosis of COPD in Italy. Monaldi Arch Chest Dis. 2005;63:6–12.

12. Bugiani M, Carosso A, Migliore E, Piccioni P, Corsico A, Olivieri M, et al. Allergic rhinitis and asthma comorbidity in a survey of young adults in Italy. Allergy. 2005;60:165–70.

13. Cirillo I, Vizzaccaro I, Tosca MA, Negrini S, Negrini AC, Marseglia GL, et al. Bronchial hyperreactivity and spirometric impairment in patients with allergic rhinitis. Monaldi Arch Chest Dis. 2005;63:79–83.

14. Heffler E, Pizzimenti S, Guida G et al. Prevalence of over-/misdiagnosis of asthma in patients referred to an allergy clinic. J Asthma. 2015;1–4.

15

Unmet diagnostic needs in contact oral mucosal allergies

Paola Lucia Minciullo[1*], Giovanni Paolino[2], Maddalena Vacca[3], Sebastiano Gangemi[1,4] and Eustachio Nettis[3]

Abstract

The oral mucosa including the lips is constantly exposed to several noxious stimuli, irritants and allergens. However, oral contact pathologies are not frequently seen because of the relative resistance of the oral mucosa to irritant agents and allergens due to anatomical and physiological factors. The spectrum of signs and symptoms of oral contact allergies (OCA) is broad and a large number of condition can be the clinical expression of OCA such as allergic contact stomatitis, allergic contact cheilitis, geographic tongue, oral lichenoid reactions, burning mouth syndrome. The main etiological factors causing OCA are dental materials, food and oral hygiene products, as they contain flavouring agents and preservatives. The personal medical history of the patient is helpful to perform a diagnosis, as a positive history for recent dental procedures. Sometimes histology is mandatory. When it cannot identify a direct cause of a substance, in both acute and chronic OCA, patch tests can play a pivotal role in the diagnosis. However, patch tests might have several pitfalls. Indeed, the presence of metal ions as haptens and specifically the differences in their concentrations in oral mucosa and in standard preparation for patch testing and in the differences in pH of the medium might result in either false positive/negative reactions or non-specific irritative reactions. Another limitation of patch test results is the difficulty to assess the clinical relevance of haptens contained in dental materials and only the removal of dental materials or the avoidance of other contactant and consequent improvement of the disease may demonstrate the haptens' responsibility. In conclusion, the wide spectrum of clinical presentations, the broad range of materials and allergens which can cause it, the difficult interpretation of patch-test results, the clinical relevance assessment of haptens found positive at patch test are the main factors that make sometimes difficult the diagnosis and the management of OCA that requires an interdisciplinary approach to the patient.

Keywords: Contact oral mucosal allergy, Stomatitis, Cheilitis, Geographic tongue, Oral lichenois lesions, Burning mouth syndrome, Unmet needs, Hypersensitivity reaction, Diagnosis, Patch test

Background

The oral mucosa including the lips is constantly exposed to several noxious stimuli, irritants and allergens. However, oral contact pathologies are not frequently seen because of the relative resistance of the oral mucosa to irritant agents and allergens due to anatomical and physiological factors such as the high vascularization that favors absorption and prevents prolonged contact with allergens, the low density of Langerhans cells and T lymphocytes and the dilution of irritants and allergens by saliva that also buffers alkaline compounds [1].

When the reaction caused by the contact of a substance with the oral mucosa is mediated by immunological mechanisms, predominantly Th1 lymphocytes, it can be assimilated to contact dermatitis of allergic physiopathology and should be called allergic contact reaction. If there is no immune mechanism involved, the proper term is nonallergic contact reaction, but terms like irritant/toxic contact reaction could be used to describe the disease [2].

The spectrum of signs and symptoms of oral contact allergies (OCA) is broad. No single pathognomonic or specific clinical picture of OCA exists; the usual elementary lesions comprise: erythema, edema, desquamation,

*Correspondence: pminciullo@unime.it
[1] School and Division of Allergy and Clinical Immunology, Department of Clinical and Experimental Medicine, University Hospital "G. Martino", Messina, Italy
Full list of author information is available at the end of the article

vesicle formation and ulceration, leukoplakia-like lesions, and lichenoid reactions [3].

Clinical signs are frequently less pronounced than subjective symptoms, and patients commonly experience severe functional problems despite only mild mucosal alterations [3].

Patients with no clinically evident lesions may experience burning or paresthesia, whereas other patients may have pain attributable to lichenoid tissue changes or frank oral ulceration [4].

A large number of condition can be the clinical expression of OCA and it is often very difficult or even impossible to distinguish OCA from chronic physical or chemical irritations, irritative contact dermatitis/stomatitis and other types of stomatitis, chronic trauma produced by teeth or fillings in poor condition, irritation caused by the wearing of dentures, parafunctional habits or other types of trauma and signs of disease with oral manifestations [5].

Clinical entities associated to contact oral mucosal allergies

Different clinical entities may be associated to an OCA. In some of these the allergic origin is established and the relationship with well known allergenic substances has been clearly demonstrated. Other entities recognize a multi factorial origin and a delayed hypersensitivity reaction may be one of the etiological factors involved (Table 1).

Allergic contact stomatitis is a contact allergic reaction caused by different substances, which cause inflammation of the entire oral mucosa. Lesions are found in the form of erythema, edema, vesicles, bullae, erosions and ulcerations. Oral flavorings, preservatives, and dental materials are common allergens [4, 6]. When the reaction is caused by prosthetic material, we speak of *prosthetic allergic stomatitis* [7]. Allergic contact stomatitis can be associated with cheilitis.

Allergic contact cheilitis is a superficial inflammation of the lip that can occur either alone or be associated with stomatitis or perioral eczema. Usually, allergic contact cheilitis is caused by cosmetic and hygiene products. Less frequently, it is caused by dental material contact

with musical instruments, topical medicines or food allergens [4, 8].

Geographic tongue is a benign, usually asymptomatic disorder involving dorsal surface of the tongue which appears as depapillated areas with leading and folded edges in yellowish or grayish white color and sometimes with unclear borders. The disorder is characterized by exacerbations and remissions with recovering in one area and the appearance in other areas very quickly; thus, it is also called *benign migratory glossitis* [9, 10]. Allergy has been suggested as a major etiologic factor in geographic tongue and nickel sulphate is the most frequent apten found positive at patch test [9, 11].

Oral lichenoid reactions (OLRs) are clinical and histological contemporaries of Oral Lichen Planus (OLP) often indistinguishable in manifestations. In contrast to the idiopathic nature of OLP, OLRs are often associated with a known identifiable inciting factor [12]. The presentation of OLR, in the same way as OLP, can be with reticular white patches, papules, plaques, erosions, or ulceration [13]. The etiology of OLRs may represent the oral manifestation of a chronic irritation in some patients or be the clinical result of a delayed hypersensitivity reaction in others. OLRs have been described in response to numerous culprit factors, including antimalarial drugs, oral antidiabetic medication, antihypertensive agents and nonsteroidal antiinflammatory drugs, as well as acrylic resins and metals used in dental practice [5]. Dental amalgam has been the most implicated restorative material in the induction of OLLs, due to the release of mercury [12, 14].

Burning mouth syndrome (BMS) is a complex disorder characterized by warm or burning sensation in the oral mucosa without any visible changes or lesions. This condition is probably of multi-factorial origin and can be classified into two forms: primary (essential/idiopathic), the organic causes (local/systemic) cannot be identified, but the peripheral and central neuropathic pathways are involved, and secondary form, determined by local factors, systemic or psychological. A number of triggers, local or systemic, which may be responsible for the sensation of burning mouth have been identified. Local factors include also contact allergens such as dental material and alloys, allergenic foods in hygienic/cosmetic, antiseptics [4, 15–17].

Etiological factors

The human oral mucosa is subjected to many pathogens potentially causing a contact allergy. Three types of contact allergy in the oral mucosa can be labelled: dental materials, food and oral hygiene products. The last two factors are involved as they contain flavouring agents and preservatives (Fig. 1).

Table 1 Classification of pathologies of secure or suspected allergic origin

Pathologies of secure allergic origin	Pathologies of suspected allergic origin
Allergic contact stomatitis	Geographic tongue
Allergic contact cheilitis	Oral lichenoid reactions
	Burning mouth syndrome

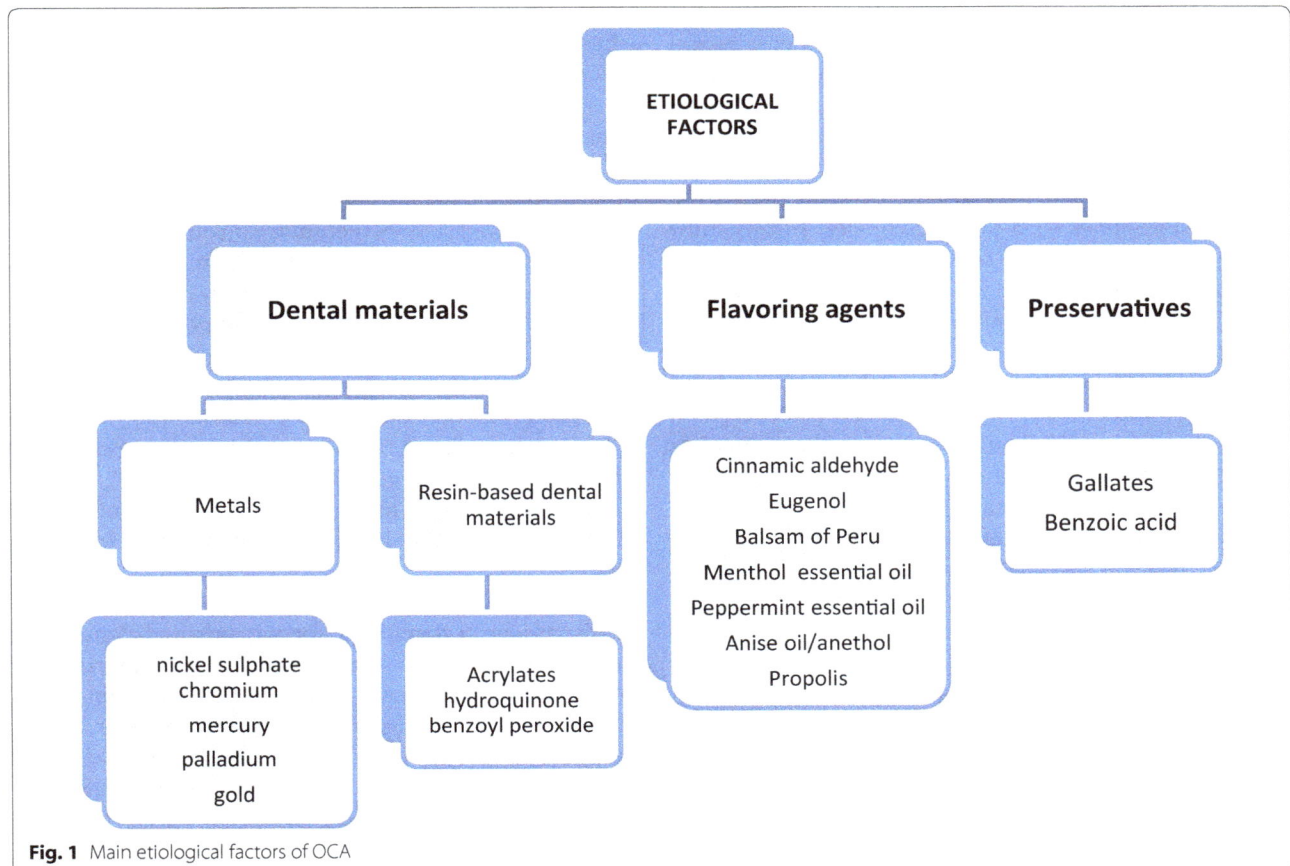

Fig. 1 Main etiological factors of OCA

Dental materials

Dental products may cause acute, as well sometimes chronic, reactions and problems also to dental personnel because of their occupational exposure. Base-metal dental alloys mainly involved in contact allergy are nickel sulphate, chromium, mercury, palladium and gold. Other materials commonly used in dental restorations including filling, bridges and crowns are (meth) acrylates, composite resins and ethylene amines. Mercury is held in amalgam, a dental alloy used frequently for restoration of teeth for well over 100 years. Mercury can be released as vapour or salt dissolved in saliva during the normal mouth activity like eating or drinking or chewing and the quantity handed out is directly proportional to the one present in the restoration. The others components of amalgam are silver, tin, copper and trace of other metals like zinc. Therefore, the amalgam can locally cause tongue and buccal mucosa lesions like an OLR and the free mercury contained in this type of restoration can cause rise to hypersensitivity reaction [13, 18, 19]. Further, in the work by Raap et al. [20], 28 of the patients have shown allergy reactions to metals used in dentistry. In particular, four patients had positive patch test reactions to mercury. From the study of Dunsche et al. [21] it results that after 20 days of exposition to dental amalgam 96 % of all animals suffered mucosa lesions: 25 % of those had positive patch test to mercury. Also Koch and Bahmer [22] report that 78.9 % patients with OLL were sensitized to mercury.

Nickel is one of the most important metal involved in contact dermatitis and unfortunately its use is very wide in everyday life. Nickel ions, released from nickel-containing alloys used frequently in dentistry, may induce OCA. In a study by Khamaysi et al. [23] in patients who had undergone dental treatment whit oral contact lesions, nickel sulphate was the metal mainly involved with a rate of 13.2 %. On the contrary, in an important meta-analysis that involved thirty studies, it was clear that orthodontic treatment with nickel-containing alloys had no significant effect on nickel hypersensitivity. However, in dentistry it is a base-metal alloy largely used. In the medical literature you also find studies of biocompatibility effects of exposure to base metal dental alloys. One of them employed a three dimensional human derived oral mucosa model to asses this biocompatibility [24]. In another study, it was hypothesized that this kind of human model would provide insights into the mechanism of nickel-induced toxicity. The oral mucosa model treated with nickel–chromium alloy has been compared with one treated with cobalt–chromium alloy and one untreated. The adverse effects increased for the Ni–Cr alloy, proving a Co–Cr enhanced biocompatibility [25]. Lastly, was also studied the release of nickel ions from stainless steel alloys used in dental braces. In this study [26] in 31 nickel-sensitive individuals that were treated with four different stainless steel alloys were searched the amount of nickel ions in saliva and sweet and patch test reactivity for all the alloys. The results showed that small amount of ions were present both in saliva and sweet and none of the nickel-sensitive subjects had positive patch test with the four alloys, indicating that these stainless steel alloys would be safe also in patients with nickel sensitivity. There are also hints in the literature about titanium dental implants. In a study by Flatebo et al. [27], the objective was the histological evaluation of a non-perforated mucosa covered by a maxillary titanium implant with regard to its tissue reaction.

The study included thirteen patients without previous implants. From the histological analysis of the tissues, any sensitivity reaction to titanium implant was proved.

Gold is another metal that can cause a contact hypersensitivity. It is widely used in dentistry as well as in piercing. In dentistry, it is mainly used for the restoration of rear dental arches because in that site the strength is more important than the esthetics. The gold alloys are composed by 80 % of this metal. In several studies it resulted the most common allergen after the nickel [28]. In a study by Vamnes et al. [29], 25 % of patients showed a positive reaction to gold at the patch test and there was a statistically significant correlation between positive tests and presence of dental gold.

Also in Ahlgren's study [30] there was a statistically significant correlation between positive patch testing to gold in a rate of 30.4 % among the patients involved in the study and the presence of dental gold in a rate of 74.2 % among the previous rate.

In the palladium alloy this metal is present at 75 % and it is known that palladium, in ionic form and at sufficiently high concentrations, has toxic and allergic effects on biological systems.

The allergy to palladium almost always occurs in individuals who are sensitive to nickel [31]. In a recent study by Muris et al. on patients with oral disease, 24.3 % reacted to palladium and 25.2 % to nickel. The patients with palladium sensitization was associated with oral restoration like dental crows and they had lamented OLRs, xerostomia, and metal taste. In conclusion of this study, it was evinced that patients with dental restoration with palladium and oral disease should get themselves checked [32].

Resin-based dental materials are synthetic resins. More precisely, they are self-curing acrylic resins based on polymathic methacrylate.

There may be OCA caused by this kind of dental materials used for fillings or restoration. Tillberg and al. [33], have conducted a study recording time to onset, duration and any reactions after exposition to resin-based dental substances. Of 618 patients observed, 36 were affected by oral lesions, intra and extra-oral, appeared within 24 h after treatment. The patients mainly showed skin problems, oral ulcers and burning mouth. The conclusion of this study was that immediate reactions were more frequently than delayed reactions and they established that such events were not allergic reactions.

Also Kaaber et al. have published 12 cases of allergic reaction to dental resin like burning mouth and stomatitis [34].

It has been studied the potential toxicity of methyl methacrylate in dental use for patients and dental personnel and at least in vitro it is possible to evaluate cells toxicity from this dental material. The observable reactions could be asthmatic symptoms, local neurological symptoms, irritant and local dermatological reactions [35]. As shown by several studies reported in medical literature by authors like Kanerva, contact allergy to (meth) acrylates is most commonly observed in dental personnel. In contrast, this type of contact allergy in patients is less frequent and indeed only case reports can be found in literature [36].

Flavoring agents

While many studies investigated the role of metals and dental materials in patients with OCA, the involvement of flavoring agents and preservatives were rarely examined.

Flavoring agents involved in OCA are usually used in food products, skin care products and oral hygiene products as toothpaste and mouthwash. Torgerson et al. found that the most allergenic flavoring was fragrance mix, with a rate of positive reactions of 9.8 %. However, eugenol tested as a single allergen was positive in 0.7 % of cases [4]. Other studies showed eugenol-induced positive reactions in 0, 0.6, and 2 % of patients [37–40]. Balsam of Peru was the second most reactive flavouring agent reported in the study of Torgerson with a rate of 7.2 % [4]. Also cinnamon products can cause oral hypersentivity reactions [41]. However, the real incidence of OCA to cinnamic aldehyde is not known. This oral contact allergy is a rare condition also known as *cinnamon contact stomatitis* [42, 43]. Other flavouring substances, such as menthol or peppermint essential oil, can cause oral contact reactions [44–47].

Cases of stomatitis and cheilitis sometimes combined with loss of taste, have been worldwide associated with exposure to anise oil and/or anethole used as flavoring agents [reviewed in 47].

Propolis also, used as lozenges, solutions or sprays, toothpastes and mouthwashes may cause stomatitis, cheilitis and ulcerations. It can cause also an occupational contact allergy in musicians and people who make stringed musical instruments [48–53].

Preservatives

The three main gallates are octyl, propyl and dodecyl are responsible of OCA, mainly cheilitis and stomatitis, due to the ingestion of gallates-containig food (such as bakery products) and the use of cosmetics, in particular lipstick [4, 39, 54–56].

Another preservative responsible of oral OCA is benzoic acid, with a rate of positive reactions reported between 3 and 11 % [4, 38, 41, 56].

Diagnostic tools

Objective examination

The personal medical history of the patient is helpful to perform a correct diagnosis, as a positive history for recent dental procedures. In this regard, also the specific anatomic region of the oral mucosa can help the clinician in a correct diagnostic orientation. The involvement of the lateral tongue and buccal mucosa are more suggestive for OLRs, rather other diseases; for this reason, the sidedness of the lesions (rather than symmetry) favor the diagnosis of OLRs [57]. Furthermore, rarely, OLRs involves gingivae and palate, being less involved by the dental restorations.

In OCA the main diagnostic patterns are the chronic lichenoid pattern and the erythematous/patch pattern; other rare clinical presentations are urticarial lesions, edematous lesions, ulceration and vesicular lesions [58]. In acute contact mucositis, at first, the area is swelling and vesicular, associated with an itching and burning sensation, while in the later stages the mucosa becomes whitish with the clinical findings reported above. The main causes of acute contact mucositis are gloves, latex, toothpastes, and every possible allergen, that came into contact with the mucosa [13]. In these cases, the diagnosis is often clinical and objective (due to the direct relationship between the allergen and the mucosal reaction), without the necessity to perform a biopsy. Finally, sudden rashes involving both the oral cavities and lips associated with itching and burning, are often suggestive of an allergy to chemicals toothpastes, dental floss and

chewing gum, because these products act on a wider anatomical area [57].

Histology

Histology in the more uncertain lesions is mandatory. In this latter case, the presence of eosinophils together with spongiosis, exocytosis of lymphocytes with occasional neutrophils, thickening of the basement membrane region, keratinocyte apoptosis, plasma cells and perivascular infiltrate, allow the diagnosis of OCA, excluding lichen planus and/or other disorders. While, a singular histology is seen only in dermatitis due to cinnamon, where a chronic interface mucositis is mixed with lymphocytes, plasma cells, and histiocytes with a peri-vascular lymphoid infiltrate [59]. However in several cases the pathology is not diriment and the correct diagnosis may be made only with the clinical examination and/or with the use of cutaneous patch tests.

Patch tests

Up to date there is not a standardized consensus regarding the allergen used for the test, however there are series of allergens (under the European consensus), which include several dental materials, as well as other additional allergens [13]. Usually skin testing is preferable to mucosal testing, due to a higher specificity and sensitivity, as well as to the simplicity of the procedure [60]. Besides, in order to perform a test, the concentration of the allergen should be 5–12 times higher in the oral mucosa, if compared to the skin, resulting in more adverse events [13].

Homstrup et al. [60], trying to avoid the routine use of patch tests for all patients with lichen planus like lesions and threatening unnecessary sensitizations in this class of patients, he listed the required points to perform patch tests in contact oral dermatitis, as follows: (1) OLRs or mucositis resistant to treatments; (2) objective and clinical evident relationship between the mucosal lesions and the suspected allergen; (3) absence of symmetry in the lesions. However patch tests can show false positivity and for this reason they are not reliable in the 100 % of cases [13]. In this regard, a careful clinical examination remains the main diagnostic orientation.

The baselines allergens used during the clinical practice regards in Italy about 28 substances, while targeted testing is designated exclusively by the specialist and thus applied to allergens according to profession (according to the sample of the material brought along). Specifically for dental materials, dermatologist conducts epicutaneous testing for certain substances, in cooperation with the dentist. According to Khamaysi et al. the most common contact allergens in OCA are gold sodium thiosulfate (14 %), nickel sulfate (13.2 %), mercury (9.9 %), palladium–chloride (7.4 %), cobalt–chloride (5 %) and 2-hydroxyethyl methacrylate (5.8 %) [7, 23]. At the same time, most common allergens for specific oral diseases are summarized on Table 2.

Unaccepted methodologies

Finally, still unaccepted methodologies in this area, that have been used without real evidence are oral patch tests. Indeed, their effectiveness in the clinical practice is not yet accepted and there are no objective evidence about this diagnostic tool [37].

Unmet needs

Nowadays the diagnosis of OCA relies, aside an accurate clinical examination, on patch testing and histology [61]. Even though largely used for contact dermatitis, with regards to contact allergies of the oral mucosa, patch testing might have several pitfalls. Indeed, in OCA, the haptens triggering the activation of T cells are often metal ions constantly eroded from metallic materials present in the oral mucosa. These metal ions, under neutral pH conditions, are normally at low concentrations. An ideal patch test should reproduce the metal erosion that occurs in the metal equipment. However, a standard preparation for patch testing for metals typically contains a metal salt with higher metal ions concentrations compared to the condition of the oral mucosa. Moreover, the metal salt is dissolved into an acidic medium, whereas the oral saliva pH is normally neutral [40]. These latter two conditions, in terms of diagnosis, might result in either false positive/negative reactions or non-specific irritative reactions. To overcome these limitations it has been recently proposed, with encouraging results, on mouse models, to use metal nanoballs for patch testing. These metal nanoballs are indeed conceived to mimic the ions release happening in vivo in patients [62].

Another limitation of patch test results is the difficulty to assess the clinical relevance of positive haptens and only the clearance of a reaction after avoiding a

Table 2 Most common allergens for specific oral diseases

Disease	Allergen
Burning mouth syndrome	Potassium dicyanoaurate
Lichenois reactions	Potassium dicyanoaurate
Cheilitis	Aroma mixtures
Stomatitis	Mercury
Gingivitis	Potassium dicyanoaurate
Orofacial granulomatosis	Nickel sulfatehexahydrate
Perioral dermatitis	Cobalt–chloride
Recurrent stomatitis aphtosa	Vanillin

contactant may demonstrate the haptens' responsibility. However, the number of contactants encountered in daily life, particularly in oral mucosa, and the wide chemical complexity of these contactants makes avoidance challenging. [4, 63].

Histology is another important diagnostic tool that can help diagnosis in the case of unclear clinical presentation of OCA. As for patch testing this latter technique can be further improved. The T cell infiltration present in delayed hypersensitivity reactions can be also observed in other chronic clinical conditions. Therefore, in the case of OCA it would be useful to know whether at the site of the lesion, T cells specific for a given hapten are present. To this aim it would be useful to analyse the TCR repertoire of the infiltrating T cells. In pre-clinical models of metal allergy, this has been done with promising results showing that during chromium-induced allergic contact dermatitis, chromium-specific T cells accumulate at the site of inflammation [64].

A recent work by Di Tola et al. using flow cytometry technique demonstrate that in nickel sensitive patients, after oral exposure to nickel, circulating Th and Cytotoxic T cells are significantly increased [65]. With regards to OCA the analysis of peripheral blood population using flow cytometry would be a useful as complementary tool for diagnosis. This would help to characterize the T cell subtypes involved in the allergic reaction and, thereby, find a more personalized and efficient treatment.

Conclusions

Although not so frequent, OCA might be observed in the daily practice, causing non-rare diagnostic pitfalls. The spectrum of clinical presentations is very wide and delayed hypersentivity mechanism has been demonstrated in only few entities such as allergic contact stomatitis and cheilitis, whereas in the other diseases as geographic tongue, OLRs and BMS contact allergy is one of the possible triggering factors.

The range of materials which can cause an OCA is very broad. In addition to the dental materials that remain for long time in the oral cavity, numerous are the substances that daily come in contact with the oral mucosa though food and oral hygiene products. Therefore, is very difficult to find the culprit substance. The knowledge of patient's habits and an accurate clinical examination together with patch testing with the suspected allergens are the major point in the management of contact oral mucosal allergies. However, the clinical relevance assessment of haptens found positive at patch test are the main factors that make sometimes difficult the diagnosis and the management of OCA, since the avoidance of the responsible substances is arduous and not even possible and requires an interdisciplinary approach to the patient.

Abbreviations

OCA: oral contact allergies; OLRs: oral lichenoid reactions; OLP: oral lichen planus; BMS: burning mouths syndrome.

Authors' contributions

PLM and EN made substantial contributions to conception and design of this review and participated in critical revision and drafting of final version of the manuscript. GP and MV participated in literature search, acquisition of data and manuscript writing. SG participated in critical revision and drafting of final version of the manuscript and gave final approval of the version to be published. All authors read and approved the final manuscript.

Author details

[1] School and Division of Allergy and Clinical Immunology, Department of Clinical and Experimental Medicine, University Hospital "G. Martino", Messina, Italy. [2] Unit of Dermatology, "Sapienza" University of Rome, Rome, Italy. [3] Section of Allergology and Clinical Immunology, Department of Internal Medicine and Infectious Diseases, University of Bari Medical School, Bari, Italy. [4] Institute of Applied Sciences and Intelligent Systems (ISASI), Messina Unit, Messina, Italy.

References

1. Tosti A, Piraccini BM, Pazzaglia M. Contact stomatitis. Emedicine. 2002. http://www.emedicine.com/derm/topic647.htm.
2. Johansson SG, Bieber T, Dahl R, Friedmann PS, Lanier BQ, Lockey RF, et al. Revised nomenclature for allergy for global use: report of the nomenclature review committee of the World Allergy Organization, October 2003. J Allergy Clin Immunol. 2004;113:832–6.
3. Tosti A, Piraccini BM, Peluso AM. Contact and irritant stomatitis. Semin Cutan Med Surg. 1997;16:314–9.
4. Torgerson RR, Davis MD, Bruce AJ, Farmer SA, Rogers RS 3rd. Contact allergy in oral disease. J Am Acad Dermatol. 2007;57:315–21.
5. Mallo Pérez L, DíazDonado C. Intraoral contact allergy to materials used in dental practice. a critical review. Med Oral. 2003;8:334–47.
6. LeSueur BW, Yiannias JA. Contact stomatitis. Dermatol Clin. 2003;21:105–14.
7. Bakula A, Lugović-Mihić L, Situm M, Turcin J, Sinković A. Contact allergy in the mouth: diversity of clinical presentations and diagnosis of common allergens relevant to dental practice. Acta Clin Croat. 2011;50:553–61.
8. Collet E, Jeudy G, Dalac S. Cheilitis, perioral dermatitis and contact allergy. Eur J Dermatol. 2013;23:303–7.
9. Honarmand M, Farhad Mollashahi L, Shirzaiy M, Sehhatpour M. Geographic tongue and associated risk factors among Iranian dental patients. Iran J Public Health. 2013;42:215–9.
10. Assimakopoulos D, Patrikakos G, Fotika C, Elisaf M. Benign migratory glossitis or geographic tongue: an enigmatic oral lesion. Am J Med. 2002;113:751–5.
11. Goregen M, Melikoglu M, Miloglu O, Erdem T. Predisposition of allergy in patients with benign migratory glossitis. Oral Surg Oral Med Oral Pathol Oral Radiol Endodontol. 2010;110:470–4.
12. Kamath VV, Setlur K, Yerlagudda K. Oral lichenoid lesions—a review and update. Indian J Dermatol. 2015;60:102.
13. McParland H, Warnakulasuriya S. Oral lichenoid contact lesions to mercury and dental amalgam—a review. J Biomed Biotechnol. 2012;2012:589569.
14. Thanyavuthi A, Boonchai W, Kasemsarn P. Amalgam contact allergy in oral lichenoid lesions. Dermatitis. 2016;27(4):215–21.

15. Jimson S, Rajesh E, Krupaa RJ, Kasthuri M. Burning mouth syndrome. J Pharm Bioallied Sci. 2015;7(Suppl 1):S194–6.
16. Coculescu EC, Tovaru S, Coculescu BI. Epidemiological and etiological aspects of burning mouth syndrome. J Med Life. 2014;7:305–9.
17. Steele JC, Bruce AJ, Davis MD, Torgerson RR, Drage LA, Rogers RS 3rd. Clinically relevant patch test results in patients with burning mouth syndrome. Dermatitis. 2012;23:61–70.
18. McCullough MJ, Tyas MJ. Local adverse effects of amalgam restoration. Int Dent J. 2008;58:3–9.
19. Vimy MJ, Lorscheider FL. Serial measurements of intraoral air mercury: estimation of daily dose from dental amalgam. J Dent Res. 1985;64:1072–5.
20. Raap U, Stiesch M, Reh H, Kapp A, Werfel T. Investigation of contact allergy to dental metals in 206 patients. Contact Dermat. 2009;60:339–43.
21. Dunsche A, Frank MP, Lüttges J, Acil Y, Brasch J, Christophers E, Springer IN. Lichenoid reactions of murine mucosa associated with amalgam. Br J Dermatol. 2003;148:741–8.
22. Koch P, Bahmer FA. Oral lesions and symtomps related to metals used in dental restorations: a clinical, allergological and histologic study. J Am Acad Dermatol. 1999;41:422–30.
23. Khamaysi Z, Bergman R, Weltfriend S. Positive patch test reactions to allergens of the dental series and the relation to the clinical presentations. Contact Dermat. 2006;55:216–8.
24. McGinley EL, Moran GP, Fleming GJ. Biocompatibility effects of indirect exposure of base-metal dental casting alloys to a human-derived three-dimensional oral mucosa model. J Dent. 2013;41:1091–100.
25. McGinley EL, Moran GP, Fleming GJ. Base-metal dental casting alloy biocompatibility assessment using a human-derived three-dimensional oral mucosa model. Acta Biomater. 2012;8:432–8.
26. Jensen CS, Lisby S, Baadsgaard O, Byrialsen K, Menné T. Release of nickel ions from stainless steel alloys used in dental braces and their patch test reactivity in nickel-sensitive individuals. Contact Dermat. 2003;48:300–4.
27. Flatebø RS, Johannessen AC, Grønningsaeter AG, Bøe OE, Gjerdet NR, Grung B, et al. Host response to titanium dental implant placement evaluated in a human oral model. J Periodontol. 2006;77:1201–10.
28. Björkner B, Bruze M, Möller H. High frequency of contact allergy to gold sodium thiosulfate An indication of goldallergy? Contact Dermat. 1994;30:144–51.
29. Vamnes JS, Morken T, Helland S, Gjerdet NR. Dental gold alloys and contact hypersensitivity. Contact Dermat. 2000;42:128–33.
30. Ahlgren C, Ahnlide I, Björkner B, Bruze M, Liedholm R, Möller H, et al. Contact allergy to gold is correlated to dental gold. Acta Derm Venereol. 2002;82:41–4.
31. Wataha JC, Hanks CT. Biological effects of palladium and risk of using palladium in dental casting alloys. J Oral Rehabil. 1996;23:309–20.
32. Muris J, Goossens A, Goncalo M, Bircher AJ, Giménez-Arnau A, Foti C, et al. Sensitization to palladium and nickel in Europe and the relationship with oral disease and dental alloys. Contact Dermat. 2015;72:286–96.
33. Tillberg A, Stenberg B, Berglund A. Reactions to resin-based dental materials in patients—type, time to onset, duration, and consequence of the reaction. Contact Dermat. 2009;61:313–9.
34. Kaaber S, Thulin H, Nielsen E. Skin sensitivity to denture base materials in the burning mouth syndrome. Contact Dermat. 1999;40:50–1.
35. Leggat PA, Kedjarune U. Toxicity of methyl methacrylate in dentistry. Int Dent J. 2003;53:126–31.
36. Kanerva L, Alanko K, Estlander T. Allergic contact gingivostomatitis from a temporary crown made of methacrylates and epoxy diacrylates. Allergy. 1999;54:1316–21.
37. Alanko K, Kanerva L, Jolanki R, Kannas L, Estlander T. Oral mucosal diseases investigated by patch testing with a dental screening series. Contact Dermat. 1996;34:263–7.
38. Kanerva L, Rantanen T, Aalto-Korte K, Estlander T, Hannuksela M, Harvima RJ, et al. A multicenter study of patch test reactions with dental screening series. Am J Contact Dermat. 2001;12:83–7.
39. Shah M, Lewis FM, Gawkrodger DJ. Contact allergy in patients with oral symptoms: a study of 47 patients. Am J Contact Dermat. 1996;7:146–51.
40. Kim TW, Kim WI, Mun JH, Song M, Kim HS, Kim BS, Kim MB, Ko HC. Patch testing with dental screening series in oral disease. Ann Dermatol. 2015;27:389–93.
41. Wray D, Rees SR, Gibson J, Forsyth A. The role of allergy in oral mucosal diseases. QJM. 2000;93:507–11.

42. Isaac-Renton M, Li MK, Parsons LM. Cinnamon spice and everything not nice: many features of intraoral allergy to cinnamic aldehyde. Dermatitis. 2015;26:116–21.

43. Calapai G, Miroddi M, Mannucci C, Minciullo P, Gangemi S. Oral adverse reactions due to cinnamon-flavoured chewing gums consumption. Oral Dis. 2014;20:637–43.

44. Morton C, Garioch J, Todd P, Lamey P, Forsyth A. Contact sensitivity to menthol and peppermint in patients with intra-oral symptoms. Contact Dermat. 1995;32:281–4.

45. Sainio EA, Kanerva L. Contact allergens in toothpastes and a review of their hypersensitivity. Contact Dermat. 1995;33:100–5.

46. Herro E, Jacob SE. Menthapiperita (peppermint). Dermatitis. 2010;21:327–9.

47. Calapai G, Minciullo PL, Miroddi M, Chinou I, Gangemi S, Schmidt RJ. Contact dermatitis as an adverse reaction to some topically used European herbal medicinal products—part 3: mentha × piperita–*Solanum dulcamara*. Contact Dermat. 2015. doi:10.1111/cod.12483.

48. de Groot AC. Propolis: a review of properties, applications, chemical composition, contact allergy, and other adverse effects. Dermatitis. 2013;24:263–82.

49. Brailo V, Boras VV, Alajbeg I, Juras V. Delayed contact sensitivity on the lips and oral mucosa due to propolis-case report. Med Oral Patol Oral Cir Bucal. 2006;11:E303–4.

50. Fernandez SG, Luaces EL, Madoz SE, Aleman EA, Apinaniz MA, Purroy Al. Allergic contact stomatitis due to therapeutic propolis. Contact Dermat. 2004;50:321.

51. Pasolini G, Semenza D, Capazera R, Sala R, Zane C, Rodell R, et al. Allergic contact cheilitis induced by contact with propolis-enriched honey. Contact Dermat. 2004;50:322–3.

52. Hay KD, Greig DE. Propolis allergy: a cause of oral mucositis with ulceration. Oral Surg Oral Med Oral Pathol. 1990;70:584–6.

53. Budimir V, Brailo V, Alajbeg I, Vučićević Boras V, Budimir J. Allergic contact cheilitis and perioral dermatitis caused by propolis: case report. Acta Dermatovenerol Croat. 2012;20:187–90.

54. Gamboni SE, Palmer AM, Nixon RL. Allergic contact stomatitis to dodecyl-gallate? a review of the relevance of positive patch test results to gallates. Australas J Dermatol. 2013;54:213–7.

55. García-Melgares ML, de la Cuadra J, Martín B, Laguna C, Martínez L, Alegre V. Sensitization to gallates: review of 46 cases. Actas Dermosifiliogr. 2007;98:688–93.

56. O'Gorman SM, Torgerson RR. Contact allergy in cheilitis. Int J Dermatol. 2016;55:e386–91.

57. Sheehan MP, Huynh M, Chung M, Zirwas M, Feldman SR. Clinical handbook of contact dermatitis: diagnosis and management by body region. New York: CRC Press; 2015.

58. Vivas AP, Migliari DA. Cinnamon-induced oral mucosal contact reaction. Open Dent J. 2015;9:257–9.

59. Lewis R. Shelton Conn: clinical outline of oral pathology. New York: People's Medical Pub; 2011.

60. Holmstrup P. Oral mucosa and skin reactions to amalgam. Adv Dent Res. 1992;6:120–4.

61. Mowad CM. Patch testing: pitfalls and performance. Curr Opin Allergy Clin Immunol. 2006;6:340–4.

62. Sugiyama T, Uo M, Wada T, Hongo T, Omagari D, Komiyama K, et al. Novel metal allergy patch test using metal nanoballs. J Nanobiotechnol. 2014;12:51.

63. Minciullo PL, Galati P, Isola S, Lombardo G, Gangemi S, Di Leo E, et al. The role of dental series patch tests in oral mucosal diseases. Dermatitis. 2010;21:123–4.

64. Shigematsu H, Kumagai K, Kobayashi H, Eguchi T, Kitaura K, Suzuki S, et al. Accumulation of metal-specific T cells in inflamed skin in a novel murine model of chromium-induced allergic contact dermatitis. PLoS ONE. 2014;9:e85983.

65. Di Tola M, Marino M, Amodeo R, Tabacco F, Casale R, Portaro L, et al. Immunological characterization of the allergic contact mucositis related to the ingestion ofnickel-rich foods. Immunobiology. 2014;219:522–30.

16

Choosing wisely in Allergology: a Slow Medicine approach to the discipline promoted by the Italian Society of Allergy, Asthma and Clinical Immunology (SIAAIC)

Enrico Heffler[1*], Massimo Landi[2], Silvana Quadrino[3,6], Cristoforo Incorvaia[4], Stefano Pizzimenti[5], Sandra Vernero[6], Nunzio Crimi[1], Giovanni Rolla[7] and Giorgio Walter Canonica[8]

Abstract

Background: One of the main problem health care systems are facis is the mis-use and over-use of medical resources (including useless exams, surgical interventions, medical treatments, screening procedures…) which may lead to high health care related costs without increased patients' benefit and possible harm to the patients themselves. The "Choosing wisely" campaign, in Italy denominated "Doing more does not mean doing better", tries to educate doctors and citizens at a correct use of medical resources.

Methods: the Italian Society of Allergy, Asthma and Clinical Immunology (SIAAIC) adhered to the "Doing more does not mean doing better" campaing and made a list of the 5 allergological procedures with the highest evidence of inappropriateness.

Results: the 5 recommendations were: "Do not perform allergy tests for drugs (including anhestetics) and/or foods when there are neither clinical history nor symptoms suggestive of hypersensitivity reactions"; "Do not perform the so-called "food intolerance tests" (apart from those which are validated for suspect celiac disease or lactose enzymatic intolerance)"; "Do not perform serological allergy tests (i.e.: total IgE, specific IgE, ISAC) as first-line tests or as "screening" assays"; "Do not treat patients sensitized to allergens or aptens if there is not a clear correlation between exposure to that specific allergen/apten and symptoms suggestive of allergic reaction"; "Do not diagnose asthma without having performed lung function tests".

Conclusions: An important role scientific societies should play is to advise on correct diagnostic and therapeutical pathways. For this reason SIAAIC decided to adhere to the Slow Medicine Italy campaign "Doing more does not mean doing better" with the aim of warning the scientific community and the citizens/patients about some allergological procedures, which, when performed in the wrong clinical setting, may be not only useless, but unnecessarily expensive and even harmful for patients' health.

Keywords: Allergy, Slow medicine, Chossing wisely, Appropriateness, Asthma, Food allergy

Background

The concept of "Slow Medicine" has been coined by Dr. Alberto Dolara, an Italian cardiologist that in 2002 invited his colleagues to give the deserved value to the time spent in improving the patient-doctor relationship, implementing a more "human and thoughtful medicine" [1], but these underlying ideas were somehow anticipated from some phylosophers such as Ivan Illich that, with his "Medical nemesis" published in 1974, argued that the medicalization in recent decades of so many of life's vicissitudes—including birth and death—and the so called "hubris of medicine" frequently caused more harm than

*Correspondence: heffler.enrico@gmail.com
[1] Department of Clinical and Experimental Medicine, Respiratory Medicine and Allergy, University of Catania, Catania, Italy
Full list of author information is available at the end of the article

good and rendered many people in effect lifelong patients [2].

In the last few years, we assisted to a worldwide dramatic increase in interest in the "Slow Medicine" concept, and this was also endorsed by the former British Medical Journal (BMJ) editor in chief, professor Richard Smith, which wrote: "slow medicine—like slow food and slow lovemaking—is the best kind of medicine for the 21st century" [3].

One of the main problem the "Slow Medicine" approach is trying to face to promote possible solutions, is the mis-use and over-use of medical resources (including useless exams, surgical interventions, medical treatments, screening procedures…) which is well known to lead to both high health care related costs without increased patients' benefit [4] and possible harm to the patients themselves [5, 6].

Into this context, the "Choosing wisely" campaign started in the USA in 2012 [7, 8] and then spread in several other countries, including Italy with the name "Doing more does not mean doing better" ("Fare di più non significa fare meglio" in Italian) [9–11], has the main goal of identifying the most probable inappropriate medical procedures for each specialty, protecting patients' interests through a partnership between health professionals and patients and users [12].

In order to create an accurate list of the five medical procedures with the highest probability of inappropriateness for each specialty, Slow Medicine Italy [13] invited the most relevant Italian scientific societies to adhere to the "Doing more does not mean doing better" campaign. The Italian Society of Allergy, Asthma and Clinical Immunology (SIAAIC), the largest Italian scientific society in the field with more than 700 active members, enthusiastically adhered to the campaign. In this article we will described and discuss the methodology used and the obtained results to make the list of five allergological procedures with the highest probability of inappropriateness.

Methods

After formal adhesion of SIAAIC to the "Doing more does not mean doing better" campaign, a working group of senior and junior members of the Society and experts in the field of Allergology has been established. The board discussed and identified a first list of allergological procedures with a possible high degree of inappropriateness. The board members performed an extensive search on PubMed and Cochrane Database, without any limit of age, gender or time of publication, in order to find enough evidence of inappropriateness for each identified allergological procedure (search keywords were depending on the subjects of the identified allergologica procedures; all types of articles were included into the evaluation), selecting the five with the highest evidence of inappropriateness taking also in consideration the frequency and the social impact of each of them, and reporting them as a "do not" suggestion. The list of the identified 5 most inappropriate allergological procedures is reported in Table 1.

This list has been approved by both the Executive Committees of SIAAIC and Slow Medicine Italy, published on their websites [14, 15] and spread as a poster sent to all SIAAIC members.

Results and discussion

We here briefly discuss each of the identified 5 most inappropriate allergological procedures.

Do not perform allergy tests for drugs (including anhestetics) And/or foods when there are neither clinical history nor symptoms suggestive of hypersensitivity reactions

In absence of clinical history or symptoms suggestive of hypersensitivity reactions (i.e.: urticaria, angioedema, other typical muco-cutaneous manifestations, hypotension, respiratory symptoms, contemporary involvement of two or more organs, or any other consisting organ damage) allergometric tests do not have any clinical value and have a poor predictive value of future allergic reactions [16]. In this context, a positive allergometric test indicates only an immunological sensitization to the tested antigen.

Table 1 The list of identified 5 most inappropriate allergological procedures

Do not perform allergy tests for drugs (including anhestetics) and/or foods when there are neither clinical history nor symptoms suggestive of hypersensitivity reactions

Do not perform the so-called "food intolerance tests" (apart from those which are validated for suspect celiac disease or lactose enzymatic intolerance)

Do not perform serological allergy tests (i.e.: total IgE, specific IgE, component-resolved diagnosis) as first-line tests or as "screening" of inhalant & food immediate hypersensitivity assays

Do not treat patients sensitized to allergens or aptens if there is not a clear correlation between exposure to that specific allergen/apten and symptoms suggestive of allergic reaction. This recommendation is particularly strong for allergen immunotherapy and elimination diets

Do not diagnose asthma without having performed lung function tests (including bronchodilating test and/or bronchial challenge)

On the other hand, a negative test is indicative only of the current absence of sensitization but it does not exclude the possibility of future allergic reactions.

The harms connected to this procedure are:

1. Non adequate therapeutical approaches (including diets [16]) which are potentially harmful because they may preclude the use of drugs or the assumption of foods the patient is not allergic to;
2. it has been described, in two small non randomized controlled trials and therefore with low quality of evidence, the possibility of new sensitizations to the tested antigens induced by the tests themselves [17, 18].

Do not perform the so-called "food intolerance tests" (apart from those which are validated for suspect celiac disease and lactose enzymatic intolerance)

Several assays and techniques are constantly proposed to many patients to identify supposed food intolerance. These methods include, for example, VEGA-test, Cytotoxic test, serum specific IgG4 dosage, chemical analysis of hair, applied kinesiology, iridology, and "bioresonance" analysis. None of these methods reached sufficient evidence of efficacy, accuracy and repeatability in diagnosis food allergy/intolerance [19–28].

The use of these methods, giving unreliable and not clinically relevant results, put the patient at risk of inappropriate diets which are potentially harmful for health, without finding a solution to the symptoms reported by the patient [29, 30].

This recommendation is particularly important in a context of non adequate perception and knowledge of food allergy/intolerance symptoms by both patients and general practitioners [31].

Do not perform serological allergy tests (i.e.: total ige, specific ige, component-resolved diagnosis) as first-line tests or as "screening" of inhalant and food immediate hypersensitivity assays

Cutaneous allergometric tests, if possible, should be considered as the first diagnostic tests in case of consisting clinical history and symptoms with a suspect allergic reaction, as they give faster results, they are less invasive and cheaper than serological tests. Moreover, there is a moderate evidence that, at least for food allergies, that skin tests have at least the same diagnostic accuracy of serological tests [32, 33].

Exceptions to this recommendations are:

1. Situations in which cutaneous tests are not feasible, such as hypo- or hyper-reactive cutaneous states (i.e.: chronic assumption of antihistamines or systemic corticosteroids, or the presence of frank dermographism);
2. Non availability of any accurate extracts to perform skin tests against the availability of serological tests for the same allergen [16, 34].
3. When the clinical history suggests an unusually greater risk of anaphylaxis from skin testing [35].

Total IgE assessment is of limited clinical utility in most of the cases, as it is not necessarily indicative of allergic sensitization: allergic patients may have both normal or elevated total IgE levels, and patients with high total IgE levels are not necessarily atopic subjects [16, 34, 36].

Measuring total IgE is otherwise indicated for the diagnosis of allergic bronchopulmonary aspergillosis, hyper IgE syndrome, as well for verification that the patient with severe allergic asthma is a suitable candidate for anti-IgE therapy with total serum IgE levels between 30 and 1500 IU/ml.

Moreover, all serum allergological tests should be interpreted by specialists/experts in Allergy and Clinical Immunology as a wrong interpretation can lead a non expert doctor to offer therapeutical and/or dietetical inappropriate approaches which may be harmful for the patient's health.

Do not treat patients sensitized to allergens or aptens if there is not a clear correlation between exposure to that specific allergen/apten and symptoms suggestive of allergic reaction. This recommendation is particularly strong for allergen immunotherapy and elimination diets

The finding of a positive allergometric test for an allergen or apten whose exposure is not associated with symptoms compatible with allergic reaction is only indicative of immunological sensitization and not necessarily of clinical manifestations related to hypersensitivity reaction [16, 34]. Therefore, there is no indication to treat these patients.

Moreover, as far as food allergy, given the limitation of cutaneous and serological tests, oral food challenges (ideally Double-Blind Placebo-Controlled Food-Challenges) are still the gold standard in IgE and non IgE mediated food allergy in order to establish a firm diagnosis, determine threshold reactivity, assess tolerance and the response to immuno-modulation [37].

Suggesting a treatment (including immunotherapic or dietetic strategies) to these patients may expose them to the risk of useless and potentially harmful therapies [38–40].

In particular, elimination diets, when they are not indicated, may expose the patient to nutritional deficiencies with no improvement of symptoms for which the allergometric investigations had been carried out [39, 40].

Do not diagnose asthma without having performed lung function tests (including bronchodilating test and/or bronchial challenge)

To rely only upon asthma-like symptoms (i.e.: dyspnea, chest tightness, cough, wheezing) is not sufficient to make a correct diagnosis of asthma, as these symptoms may be from alternate causes, such as chronic obstructive pulmonary disease (COPD), congestive heart failure, extrathoracic airway hyperresponsiveness syndromes (e.g. vocal cord dysfunction, VCD), gastroesophageal reflux disease, hyperventilation syndrome etc. [41–44]. This behavior can be harmful for patients as they may be receive a wrong treatment for their complaints; this is particularly important when patients are affected by other relevant comorbidities as it happens in elderly [45].

International asthma guidelines stress the need of performing complete lung function assessment to identify bronchial hyperreactivity and/or reversibility of bronchial obstruction [46]. Patients with asthma-like symptoms and normal spirometry should underwent to an aspecific bronchial challenge (i.e.: with methacholine) while those with an obstructive spirometric pattern should be evaluated for the degree of reversibility during a bronchodilating test (i.e.: with salbutamol). Beyond the increased costs of care, the consequences of misdiagnosing asthma include delaying a correct diagnosis and treatment [43].

Conclusions

In this article we described the methodology used and the obtained results to make the list of five allergological procedures with the highest probability of inappropriateness [14, 15], in the context of the "Doing more does not mean doing better" campaign proposed by Slow Medicine Italy [9–11]. The five selected procedures were identified by an expert panel of senior and junior Italian allergologists.

The modern medicine is imbued with inappropriate medical procedures, wastes, conflicts of interest and fraud deriving from the economic and financial interactions between prescribers, purchasers of health technologies and the industry [13]. Another important cause which may induce the doctors to order inappropriate procedures lies in malpractice claims from patients (defensive medicine). This behavior is often encouraged by the message, which comes from the "media" and easily received by patients, that in medicine "more is always better" and that "doing less is always an index of medical malpractice" [47].

An important role scientific societies should play is to produce and disseminate Diagnostic-Therapeutic-Healthcare Protocols/Pathways, based on the best evidence based scientific knowledge, to guarantee the patients receive the correct diagnosis and the appropriate treatment. For this reason SIAAIC decided to adhere to the Slow Medicine Italy campaign "Doing more does not mean doing better" with the aim of warning the scientific community and the citizens/patients about some allergological procedures, which, when performed in the wrong clinical setting, may be not only useless, but unnecessarily expensive and even harmful for patients' health.

We think that doctors and patients should take more time to define together the most appropriate pathway which lead to the right diagnosis and to the most appropriate treatment. Doctors should always explain the patients what the exams they order mean in case they turned normal or altered and why some exams are not useful at all for the specific diagnosis the patients are looking for. An open and trustful patient-physician relationship appears to be important to avoid useless exams and to achieve more accurate diagnoses .

Abbreviations

SIAAIC: Italian Society of Allergy, Asthma and Clinical Immunology; COPD: chronic obstructive pulmonary disease; VCD: vocal cord dysfunction.

Authors' contributions

EH, SP, CI, GR, NC, ML and GWC were part of the SIAAIC experts board that defined the 5 procedures with high probability of inappropriateness, contributed in writing these procedures and this manuscript, and in critically revision the drafts of both the 5 selected procedures and the present article. SQ and SV gave their contribution supporting the SIAAIC working group with information on Slow Medicine and the "Choosing wisely" international project, writing part of the manuscript and critically revising it. All authors read and approved the final manuscript.

Author details

[1] Department of Clinical and Experimental Medicine, Respiratory Medicine and Allergy, University of Catania, Catania, Italy. [2] Pediatrician Primary Care, Turin, Italy. [3] "Change" Institute, Turin, Italy. [4] Allergy/Pulmonary Rehabilitation, ICP Hospital, Milan, Italy. [5] ASL-TO3, Allergy Outpatients' Clinic, "Edoardo Agnelli" Hospital, Pinerolo, TO, Italy. [6] "Slow Medicine Italy", Turin, Italy. [7] Department of Medical Sciences, Allergy and Clinical Immunology, University of Torino, Turin, Italy. [8] Allergy and Respiratory Diseases Clinic, DIMI-Department of Internal Medicine, IRCCS AOU S.Martino-IST, Genoa, Italy.

References

1. Dolara A. Invitation to "slow medicine". Ital Heart J Suppl. 2002;3(1):100–1.
2. Illich I. Medical nemesis. London: Calder & Boyars; 1974.
3. Smith R. The case for slow medicine. 2012. http://blogs.bmj.com/bmj/2012/12/17/richardsmith-the-case-for-slow-medicine.
4. Himmelstein DU, Woolhandler S. Cost without benefit. Administrative waste in U.S. health care. N Engl J Med. 1986;314(7):441–5.
5. BMJ Evidence Center: Clinical evidence Handbook. BMJ Publishing Group. 2012. http://clinicalevidence.bmj.com/x/set/static/cms/ce-handbook.html.

6.	Krogsbøll LT, Jørgensen KJ, Larsen CG, Gøtzsche PC. General health checks in adults for reducing morbidity and mortality from disease: Cochrane systematic review and meta-analysis. BMJ. 2012;345:e7191.

7.	http://www.choosingwisely.org/.

8.	Levinson W, Kallewaard M, Bhatia RS, Wolfson D, Shortt S, Kerr EA, Choosing Wisely International Working Group Wisely International Working Group. 'Choosing Wisely': a growing international campaign. BMJ Qual Saf. 2015;24(2):167–74.

9.	Vernero S. Choosing wisely and Italy's "Doing more does not mean doing better" project. Rev Allergy Clin Immunol. 2014;24:1–3.

10.	Vernero S, Domenighetti G, Bonaldi A. Italy's "Doing more does not mean doing better" campaign. BMJ. 2014;349:g4703.

11.	http://www.slowmedicine.it/fare-di-piu-non-significa-fare-meglio/pratiche-arischio-di-inappropriatezza-in-italia.html.

12.	Hurley R. Can doctors reduce harmful medical overuse worldwide? BMJ. 2014;349:g4289.

13.	Bonaldi A, Vernero S. Italy's slow medicine: a new paradigm in medicine. Recenti Prog Med. 2015;106(2):85–91.

14.	http://www.siaaic.eu/source-siaaic/Segreteria/Eventi/Slow_Medicine_in%20allergologia.pdf.

15.	http://www.slowmedicine.it/pdf/Pratiche/Societ%C3%A0%20Italiana%20di%20Allergologia,%20Asma%20e%20Immunologia%20Clinica%20(SIAAIC)-%20allergologia.pdf.

16.	Boyce JA, Assa'ad A, Burks AW, Jones SM, Sampson HA, Wood RA, Plaut M, Cooper SF, Fenton MJ, Arshad SH, Bahna SL, Beck LA, Byrd-Bredbenner C, Camargo CA Jr, Eichenfield L, Furuta GT, Hanifin JM, Jones C, Kraft M, Levy BD, Lieberman P, Luccioli S, McCall KM, Schneider LC, Simon RA, Simons FE, Teach SJ, Yawn BP, Schwaninger JM. Guidelines for the diagnosis and management of food allergy in the United States: report of the NIAID-sponsored expert panel. J Allergy Clin Immunol. 2010;126(6 Suppl):S1–58.

17.	Nugent JS, Quinn JM, McGrath CM, Hrncir DE, Boleman WT, Freeman TM. Determination of the incidence of sensitization after penicillin skin testing. Ann Allergy Asthma Immunol. 2003;90(4):398–403.

18.	Uter W, Hillen U, Geier J. Is incident sensitization to p-phenylenediamine related to particular exposure patterns? Results of a questionnaire study. Contact Dermat. 2007;56(5):266.

19.	Stapel SO, Asero R, Ballmer-Webwe BK. Testing for IgG4 against foods is not recommended as a diagnostic tool. EAACI Task Force Report. Allergy. 2008;63:793–6.

20.	Carr S, Chan E, Lavine E, Moote W. CSACI Position statement on the testing of food-specific IgG. Allerg Asthma Clin Imunol. 2012;8(1):12.

21.	Senna G, Bonadonna P, Schiappoli M, Leo G, Lombardi C, Passalacqua G. Pattern of use and diagnostic value of complementary/alternative tests for adverse reactions to food. Allergy. 2005;60(9):1216–7.

22.	Semizzi M, Senna G, Crivellaro M, Rapacioli G, Passalacqua G, Canonica WG, Bellavite P. A double-blind, placebo-controlled study on the diagnostic accuracy of an electrodermal test in allergic subjects. Clin Exp Allergy. 2002;32(6):928–32.

23.	Garron JS. Kinesiology and food allergy. Br Med J Clin Res Ed. 1988;296(6636):1573–4.

24.	Lüdtke R, Kunz B, Seeber N, Ring J. Test-retest-reliability and validity of the Kinesiology muscle test. Complement Ther Med. 2001;9(3):141–5.

25.	Ernst E. Iridology: not useful and potentially harmful. Arch Ophthalmol. 2000;118(1):120–1.

26.	Barrett S. Commercial hair analysis. Science or scam? JAMA. 1985;254(8):1041–5.

27.	Sethi TJ, Lessof MH, Kemeny DM, Lambourn E, Tobin S, Bradley A. How reliable are commercial allergy tests? Lancet. 1987;1(8524):92–4.

28.	Lewith GT, Kenyon JN, Broomfield J, Prescott P, Goddard J, Holgate ST. Is electrodermal testing as effective as skin prick tests for diagnosing allergies? A double blind, randomised block design study. BMJ. 2001;322(7279):131–4.

29.	Senna G, Gani F, Leo G, Schiappoli M. Alternative tests in the diagnosis of food allergies. Recenti Prog Med. 2002;93(5):327–34.

30.	Senna G, Passalacqua G, Crivellaro M, Bonadonna P, Gani F, Dorizzi R, Dama A, Canonica GW, Lombardi C. Unconventional medicine: a risk of undertreatment of allergic patients. Allergy. 1999;54(10):1117–9.

31.	Heffler E, Minciullo PL, Fassio F, Rossi FW, Patafi M, Mondino M, Badiu I, Guida G on the behalf of Junior Members working group of Italian Society of Allergy and Clinical Imunology (SIAIC). Pertinence of requested allergy consultations for suspected food allergy/intolerance. A Junior Members working group of Italian Society of Allergy and Clinical Immunology (SIAIC) multicenter study. Ital J Allergol Clin Immunol 2011;21:18–24.

32.	Chafen JJ, Newberry SJ, Riedl MA, Bravata DM, Maglione M, Suttorp MJ, Sundaram V, Paige NM, Towfigh A, Hulley BJ, Shekelle PG. Diagnosing and managing common food allergies: a systematic review. JAMA. 2010;303(18):1848–56.

33.	Schneider Chafen JJ, Newberry S, Riedl M, Bravata DM, Maglione M, Suttorp M, Sundaram V, Paige NM, Towfigh A, Hulley BJ, Shekelle PG. Prevalence, Natural History, Diagnosis, and Treatment of Food Allergy. A Systematic Review of the Evidence. RAND Corporation. 2010. http://www.rand.org/content/dam/rand/pubs/working_papers/2010/RAND_WR757-1.pdf.

34.	Sicerer SH, Wood RA, American Academy of Pediatrics Section On Allergy And Immunology. Allergy testing in childhood: using allergen-specific IgE tests. Pediatrics. 2012;129(1):193–7.

35.	Bernstein IL, Li JT, Bernstein DI, Hamilton R, Spector SL, Tan R, Sicerer S, Golden DB, Khan DA, Nicklas RA, Portnoy JM, Blessing-Moore J, Cox L, Lang DM, Oppenheimer J, Randolph CC, Schuller DE, Tilles SA, Wallace DV, Levetin E, Weber R, American Academy of Allergy, Asthma and Immunology, American College of Allergy, Asthma and Immunology. Allergy diagnostic testing: an updated practice parameter. Ann Allergy Asthma Immunol. 2008;100(3 Suppl 3):S1–148.

36.	Kerkhof M, Dubois AE, Postma DS, Schouten JP, de Monchy JG. Role and interpretation of total serum IgE measurements in the diagnosis of allergic airway disease in adults. Allergy. 2003;58(9):905–11.

37.	Muraro A, Werfel T, Hoffmann-Sommergruber K, Roberts G, Beyer K, Bindslev-Jensen C, Cardona V, Dubois A, duToit G, Eigenmann P, Fernandez Rivas M, Halken S, Hickstein L, Høst A, Knol E, Lack G, Marchisotto MJ, Niggemann B, Nwaru BI, Papadopoulos NG, Poulsen LK, Santos AF, Skypala I, Schoepfer A, Van Ree R, Venter C, Worm M, Vlieg-Boerstra B, Panesar S, de Silva D, Soares-Weiser K, Sheikh A, Ballmer-Weber BK, Nilsson C, de Jong NW, Akdis CA; EAACI Food Allergy and Anaphylaxis Guidelines Group. EAACI food allergy and anaphylaxis guidelines: diagnosis and management of food allergy. Allergy. 2014;69(8):1008–25.

38.	Passalacqua G, Compalati E, Canonica GW. Sublingual Immunotherapy: clinical indications in the WAO-SLIT Position Paper. World Allergy Organ J. 2010;3(7):216–9.

39.	NICE Diagnosis and assessment of food allergy in children and young people in primary care and community settings. 2011. http://guidance.nice.org.uk/CG116/Guidance.

40.	Guidance on food allergy in children. Editorial. The Lancet. 2011;377:691.

41.	Luks VP, Vandemheen KL, Aaron SD. Confirmation of asthma in an era of overdiagnosis. Eur Respir J. 2010;36:255–60.

42.	Aaron SD, Vandemheen KL, Boulet LP, et al. Overdiagnosis of asthma in obese and nonobese adults. CMAJ. 2008;179:1121–31.

43.	Heffler E, Pizzimenti S, Guida G, Bucca C, Rolla G. Prevalence of over-/misdiagnosis of asthma in patients referred to an allergy clinic. J Asthma. 2015;19:1–4. doi: 10.3109/02770903.2015.1026442. (Epub ahead of print).

44.	Goldstein MF, Veza BA, Dunsky EH, et al. Comparisons of peak diurnal expiratory flow variation, postbronchodilator FEV(1) responses, and methacholine inhalation challenges in the evaluation of suspected asthma. Chest. 2001;119:1001–10.

45.	Scichilone N, Ventura MT, Bonini M, Braido F, Bucca C, Caminati M, Del Giacco S, Heffler E, Lombardi C, Matucci A, Milanese M, Paganelli R, Passalacqua G, Patella V, Ridolo E, Rolla G, Rossi O, Schiavino D, Senna G, Steinhilber G, Vultaggio A, Canonica G. Choosing wisely: practical considerations on treatment efficacy and safety of asthma in the elderly. Clin Mol Allergy. 2015;13(1):7.

46.	Global Initiative for Asthma (GINA). Global strategy for asthma mangement and prevention. 2011. http://www.ginasthma.org.

47.	Toraldo DM, Vergari U, Toraldo M. Medical malpractice, defensive medicine and role of the "media" in Italy. Multidiscip Respir Med. 2015;10(1):12.

17

Effects of specific allergen immunotherapy on biological markers and clinical parameters in asthmatic children

I. Djuric-Filipovic[1], Marco Caminati[2*], D. Filipovic[3], C. Salvottini[4] and Z. Zivkovic[5,6]

Abstract

Background: Allergen-specific immunotherapy (AIT) is the only treatment able to change the natural course of allergic diseases. We aimed at investigating the clinical efficacy of SLITOR (Serbian registered vaccine for sublingual allergen specific immunotherapy).

Methods: 7–18 years old children with allergic asthma and rhinitis were enrolled and addressed to the active (AIT plus pharmacological treatment) or control (standard pharmacological treatment only) group. Clinical and medications scores, lung function and exhaled FeNO were measured at baseline and at every follow-up.

Results: There was a significant improvement in both nasal and asthma symptom scores as well as in medication score in SLIT group. SLIT showed an important influence on lung function and airway inflammation.

Conclusions: Our data showed that SLITOR was effective not only in terms of patient reported outcomes but an improvement of pulmonary function and decrease of lower airway inflammation were also observed.

Keywords: Allergen specific immunotherapy, Asthma, Childhood, exhaled NO

Background

Asthma is a chronic disease of the airways characterized by inflammation and bronchial remodeling. With a global prevalence of 9.4% in 6–7 years old patients and 12.6% in 13–14 years old patients asthma is one of the most common chronic diseases in childhood age [1, 2]. The growing medical and social burden of asthma is often described as the 'allergy epidemic' [3]. Allergen-specific immunotherapy (AIT) holds a great promise in the management of allergic conditions, as it is the only treatment able to change the natural course of respiratory allergic diseases [4]. The disease modifying effect assumes a special relevance in the pediatric age, when the plasticity of the immune system is maximal, and the preventive effects can

be reasonably expected [5]. During the last three decades sublingual immunotherapy (SLIT) impressively developed, offering patients an excellent safety and acceptance profile, and a similar efficacy profile when compared with subcutaneous immunotherapy (SCIT) [6, 7]. Although the clinical efficacy of SLIT in children with asthma and allergic rhinitis has been proved in many double blind placebo control randomized clinical trials (DBPC-RCT) and meta-analysis, there is a lack of objective measures related to SLIT efficacy, besides patients reported outcomes [8]. Most of the published studies have considered clinical scores as the main efficacy parameter, whilst immunological and inflammatory parameters have been only occasionally investigated [9]. Recent research has been more focused on identifying objective biomarkers. They can be helpful in early detection of subjects at risk of asthma development as well as in asthma management, from the diagnosis to follow-up, and in treatment tailoring [10]. Up to now several immunological changes related to AIT

*Correspondence: ma.caminati@gmail.com
[2] Allergy Unit and Asthma Center, Verona University and General Hospital, Piazzale Stefani 1, 37126 Verona, Italy
Full list of author information is available at the end of the article

mechanisms of action have been described: allergen specific IgE, allergen-specific blocking IgG4, eosinophil reactivity, FeNO, eosinophil cationic protein (ECP), allergen specific suppressor T cells as well as the deviation of type 2 T helper cells (Th2) response in favor of Th1 response [11, 12]. FeNO measurement is currently the only validated non-invasive method for assessing asthma-related eosinophilic inflammation in clinical practice. Literature data has already shown that treatment with inhaled or oral corticosteroids as well as with biological treatment such as monoclonal humanized anti-IgE antibody is able to decrease the level of FeNO in children with asthma and allergic rhinitis [13].

The aims of our study were:

1. To prove the clinical efficacy of SLITOR (registered vaccine for sublingual allergen specific immunotherapy) produced by the local Serbian Institute for virology, vaccines and serum (Torlak, Belgrade, Serbia) in terms of improvement of clinical symptoms (nasal and bronchial symptoms) and decrease of medication usage.
2. To show the impact of SLIT on the improvement of pulmonary function
3. To investigate the influence of SLIT on eosinophil airway inflammation—measured with the concentration of exhaled NO (FeNO)

Methods

Our study was a real life controlled observational study. The study was conducted in the Children's Hospital for Lung Diseases and Tuberculosis, Medical Centre "Dr Dragiša Mišović", Belgrade, Serbia. The protocol was approved by the Ethical Committee of the hospital. Informed consent was obtained from all parents or caregivers of the participants. The active group was addressed to SLIT plus standard pharmacotherapy, whereas the control group undertook standard pharmacological treatment only.

Patients were considered eligible for SLIT according to the following factors: diagnosis of allergic rhinitis, diagnosis of asthma under control with standard pharmacological treatment (without acute exacerbation in the last 6 months, without systemic corticosteroids in the last 6 months, without hospitalisation due to acute asthma attacks in the last 6 months, FEV1 $\geq$80%), positive skin prick tests with inhaled allergens, positive in vitro tests (CAP-RAST immunoassay, minimum IgE class III), age range between 7 and 18 years old. Hypersensitivity to any of the vaccines components, presence or suspect of malignancies, autoimmune systemic diseases as well as immunodeficiency were considered exclusion criteria.

Skin prick tests (SPT) were performed according to published guidelines with a standard battery of glycerinated extracts (Institute of Virology, Vaccines and Sera TORLAK, Belgrade, Serbia). The following allergens were tested: house dust, dust mite (*Dermatophagoides* spp.), cockroach, mold, animal dander, pollens (tree, grass and weed). Histamine and saline were used as positive and negative controls, respectively. A drop of each allergen extract was placed on the volar surface of the forearm and was penetrated with a separate lancet. After 15 min, the wheal reaction was measured as the mean of the longest diameter and the diameter perpendicular to it. Reactions (mean wheal diameter $\geq$3 mm) were considered positive [17]. Serum specific IgE to allergens extract were assayed with an automated immuno-fluorimetric method (ImmunoCAP 100; Phadia, Upsalla, Sweden). The results were expressed as CAP scores from class 0–6, according to the manufacture's instruction, ($\geq$class 3 was accepted as relevant).

SLITOR (registered vaccine for sublingual allergen specific immunotherapy) produced by the local Serbian Institute for virology, vaccines and serum Torlak, Belgrade, Serbia was used in the study. The allergen extracts were used for the preparation of sublingual-swallow "vaccines" in phosphate-buffered saline with 50% glycerol. Quality of allergen extract was tested with sodium dodecyl sulphate polyacrylamide gel electrophoresis (SDS-PAGE) and western blot technique (Fig. 1). The potency of the solution was expressed as protein nitrogen unit (PNU)/ml and prepared in three strengths: 16, 125 and 1000 PNU/ml.

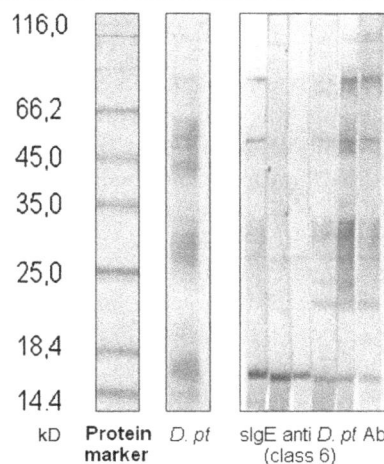

Fig. 1 Pre-treatment SDS-PAGE analysis of *Dermatophagoides pteronyssinus* extract and IgE-binding profiles class 6 from six sIgE positive patients from SLIT group. *SDS-PAGE* sodium dodecyl sulfate–polyacrylamide gel electrophoresis, *D. pt Dermatophagoides pteronyssinus*, *Ab* antibody, *sIgE* specific immunoglobulin E, *SLIT* sublingual immunotherapy

According to manufacturer's recommendations, in the build-up phase (45 days), patients received increasing doses of the extract, starting with one drop of 16 PNU/ml and increasing to 15 drops in 15 days. Daily dose was taken sublingually, applied on a sugar cube in the morning, half an hour before breakfast. This process was repeated also for the 125 and 1000 PNU/ml. Finally, patient was switched to maintenance phase regimen, using 15 drops of the 1000 PNU/ml twice a week for the following 24 months. Allergen proteins concentration in maintenance therapy was equivalent to 19.9 µg/ml i.e. 0.995 µg of allergen proteins in one drop of extract. Calculated mean cumulative monthly dose of allergen proteins was 119.4 µg, while the mean cumulative dose per year was about 1.4 mg.

Patients from both groups (irrespective to SLIT) received an appropriate pharmacological treatment according to ARIA and GINA guidelines depending on symptoms: oral antihistamines, intranasal corticosteroid, inhaled corticosteroid and inhaled bronchodilator.

Clinical evaluation

All patients were followed up during the 2 years from the beginning of the protocol. Patients were asked to fill in the symptom and medication score diary on a daily base twice a day (in the morning and in the evening) during 1-month period or during the pollen season for patients who were sensitized to seasonal allergens. Older children were also asked to calculate the mean values, usually with parents help.

The following symptoms of AR were scored: rhinorrhea, sneezing, nasal itching and blocked nose. In addition, for the AR with AA patients, next symptoms were scored: chest tightness, shortness of breath, cough and wheezing. Each symptom was scored as 0 (absent), 1 (mild), 2 (moderate), 3 (severe) and the mean monthly symptom score (SS) was calculated. The use of symptomatic medications was also recorded daily, during the same period. Anti-allergic medication requirement was evaluated as the monthly mean medication score (MS). Airways eosinophilic inflammation measurement was performed with NIOX MINO (Aerocrine, Solna, Sweden). The data were interpreted according to the recommendations of American Thoracic Society (ATS) [14–17] (Table 1). Conditions potentially influencing FeNO values

(anxiety, cardiac disease, chronic obtrusive disease, GERB, non eosionophilic asthma, rhinosinusitis, voice cord dysfunction, cyctic fibrosis, primary ciliary dyskinesia infection and asthma exacerbation) were excluded.

Lung function test was performed at each visit using Jaeger, Pneumo Screen spirometry. Subjects were advised to avoid the use of the short-acting bronchodilator at least 12 h before the test. FEV1 values were expressed as a percentage of predicted values.

The patients receiving SLIT were required to record and give their report on a specific diary card, in the case of side effects: local (oral itching/burning, swelling, oedema of the uvula or tongue) or systemic adverse reactions (asthma, rhinitis, urticaria, angioedema, generalized itching, gastrointestinal symptoms—abdominal pain, nausea, vomiting, shock).

Statistical analysis

The sample size was calculated with the software package G power. A sufficient number of observation units for the error level $\alpha = 0.05$ and power of the study $1-\beta = 0.8$ is 0.72 were considered. Descriptive and analytical statistical methods were used. The following descriptive variables were described: measures of central tendency (mean, median), measure of dispersion (standard deviation, interval of variation). Analytical statistical methods were used to test differences, parametric and nonparametric variables. Student's t test and analysis of variance of repeated measurements were used. Chi square test, McNemar test, Mann–Whitney test, Wilcoxon test, Friedman test were also included. All data were analyzed in SPSS 15.0 software package. (SPSS Inc., Chicago, Illinois, USA).

Results

Overall 59 patients (mean age, 13.18 ± 3.433 range 7–20 years; 50.8% boys; 49.2% girls) were included: 34 (20 girls and 14 boys) received SLIT as an add-on to drug therapy and 25 (10 girls and 15 boys) received anti-allergic and asthmatic drug therapy alone. Patients from SLIT and control group were homogenous for all demographic and clinical characteristics.

We found clinical improvement in the SLIT group, demonstrated by statistically significant decrease of all rhinitis symptoms after 2 years of SLIT vs. baseline for both groups (Table 2).

According to our statistical analysis 75% of patients on SLIT didn't complain about nasal congestion after 2 years of treatment; 80% of the patients in the same group didn't have nasal pruritus, whereas SLIT was effective in treating rhinorrhea and sneezing in 75% patients. On the other side standard pharmacotherapy didn't have such a significant impact on nasal symptoms. We also

Table 1 FeNO interpretation

Asthma	FeNO (>12 years) (ppb)	FeNO(<12 years) (ppb)
Control asthma	<25	<20
Intermediate	25–30	25–30
Non-control asthma	>50	>35

Table 2 The distribution of values for a patient rhinitis symptom scores

Nasal congestion	$\chi^2 = 37,783$; p < 0.001
Nasal pruritus	$\chi^2 = 38,346$; p < 0.001
Rhinorrhea	$\chi^2 = 42,012$; p < 0.001
Sneezing	$\chi^2 = 44,831$; p < 0.001

found a statistically significant inter-group difference for all rhinitis symptom scores, after 1st year with a further improvement of symptoms in the group on SLIT during the 2nd year of follow up period.

A similar clinical improvement SLIT expressed on asthma symptom scores. Our results demonstrated decrease of all asthma symptom scores during the follow up period for all participants with a statistical significant influence of SLIT group on that improvement. The results are showed in Table 3. After 2 years of SLIT treatment more than 80% of the patients didn't complain about cough, night cough, and chest breathless and wheezing. We also found a statistically significant inter-group difference for all asthma symptom scores, after 1st year with a further improvement of symptoms in the group on SLIT during the 2nd year of follow up period. All data are summarized in Table 4.

χ^2 test showed statistical significant differences for all rhinitis and asthma scores in all of three periods. At the beginning of the follow up period children in SLIT group had more severe symptoms in comparison with children on standard pharmacotherapy. Even after a 1-year follow

Table 3 The distribution of values for asthma symptom scores

Cough	$\chi^2 = 62,384$; p < 0.001
Night cough	$\chi^2 = 47,743$; p < 0.001
Chest breathless	$\chi^2 = 49,622$; p < 0.001
Wheezing	$\chi^2 = 49,078$; p < 0.001

up we, a significant improvement was registered. Similar results were observed at 2nd year, especially for patients with more severe symptoms.

The data from our study showed that after 2 years the use of inhaled corticosteroids, intranasal corticosteroids, $\beta2$ agonists was significantly reduced in the group of patients on SLIT (Z = − 4311 p < 0.001, $\chi^2 = 30,785$; p < 0.001, Q = 28,783; p < 0.001 respectively), in comparison with the control group (Fig. 2). The patients in the experimental group also used statistically less antihistamines ($\chi^2 = 32,774$; p < 0.001) and leukotrienes ($^*\chi^2 = 30,785$; p < 0.001) in comparison with the patients in non-SLIT group, but only after 2 years of AIT.

Although at the beginning of the study all patients had FEV1 ≥80% of predicted value, SLIT showed a significant improvement of FEV1 just after 1 year with a further improvement in the 2nd year of follow up period (F = 3514; p = 0.036), while at the same time FEV1 remain without any improvement in children on standard pharmacotherapy (F = 3199; p = 0.048) (Fig. 3).

The level of FeNO decreased significantly in all the three measurements during SLIT course ($\chi^2 = 52,220$; p < 0.001). During the follow up period significant differences between the groups in all three measurements were observed. Patients in the experimental group had significantly higher values of FeNO in all measurements. When we compared the values in each group independently, we found only significant reduction in the experimental group. We observed both significant reduction between FeNO1 and FeNO2 (p < 0.001) and between FeNO2 and FeNO3. Throughout the treatment period there was a sustained significant reduction between FeNO2 and FeNO3. Max value for FeNO1 was 111 ppb, while MaxFeNO2 and FeNO3 were 78 and 56 ppb consecutively. Here we showed that there is an influence of SLIT on the FeNO values in children in experimental group, whereas no reduction in FeNO values were registered in the control group (Table 5, Fig. 4).

Table 4 χ^2 test symptoms scores during SLIT course

Symptoms	At the beginning χ^2	After 1 year χ^2	After 2 year χ^2
Nasal congestion	10,299	8732	10,835
Nasal pruritus	5601	8877	8737
Rhinorrhea	8119	10,001	12,464
Sneezing	6407	10,605	9821
Cough	8100	5322	16,028
Night cough	9114	5177	12,666
Chest breathless	5656	2154	9680
Wheezing	10,664	12,294	12,362

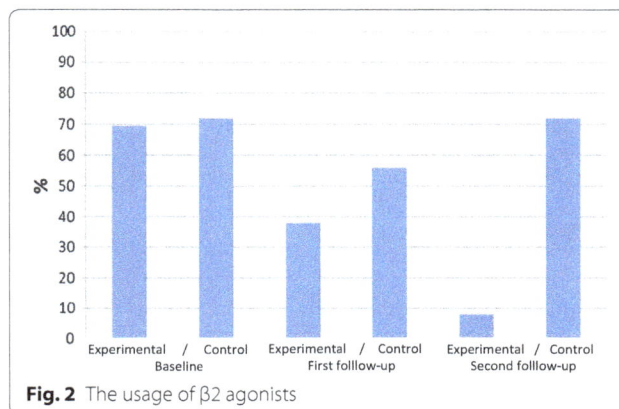

Fig. 2 The usage of $\beta2$ agonists

Table 5 The level of FeNO (Legend FeNO I baseline. FeNO II–1st year of follow-up period, FeNO III-2nd year of follow-up period)

	N	Mean value	SD	Median	Minimum	Maximum
No 1	34	60.65	20.467	56.00	31	111
No 2	34	43.18	8.990	43.00	31	78
No 3	34	34.15	6.985	32.00	22	56

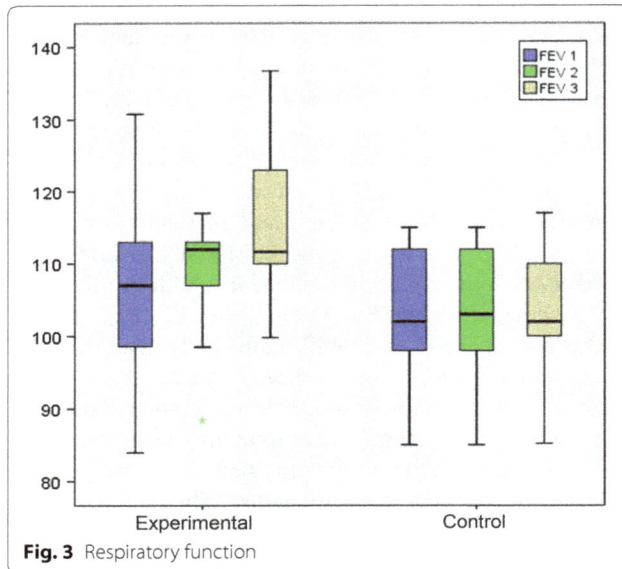
Fig. 3 Respiratory function

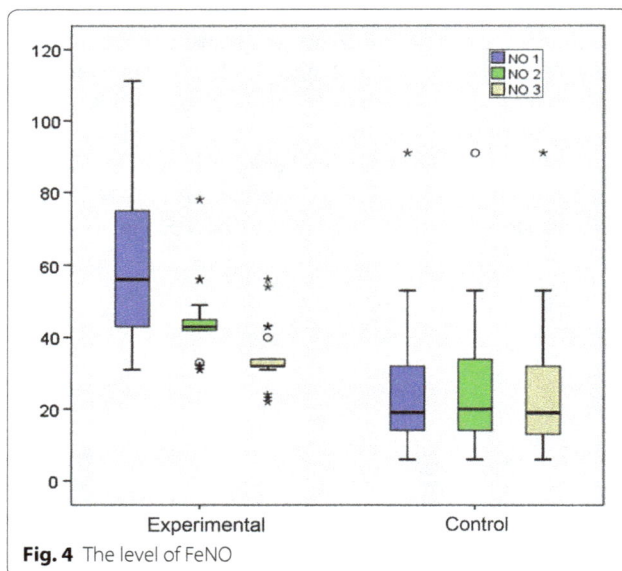
Fig. 4 The level of FeNO

Safety assessment

There were no local side effects that required treatment. Three side effects were reported. All of them involved mild to moderate gastrointestinal complaints (mouth burning or itching and stomachache and nausea) and self- resolve in a few days without any intervention. It is noteworthy that no serious adverse events were reported in the present survey, and the incidence of side-effects appeared to be lower than that reported for injective immunotherapy.

Discussion

This is one of the first studies evaluating clinical efficacy, pulmonary function, FeNO and safety in children with both allergic rhinitis and asthma undergoing SLIT or drug treatment. In the current study we found: (a) statistically significant improvement in nasal and asthma symptom scores after 1 year of treatment in SLIT group, with further improvement in the 2nd year of follow up (75 and 80% respectively) compared with control group; (b) only three patients reported mild local and systemic adverse reactions; (c) statistically significant improvement of pulmonary function; (d) statistically significant decrease of eosinophilic inflammation of lower airways measured with FeNO. Since SLIT was first introduced for treatment of respiratory allergies in children and later accepted as a viable alternative to SCIT, need for an assessment of its efficacy and safety in respiratory allergy has emerged [18]. Consequently, many randomized double blind placebo controlled and open controlled trials [19–27], as well as a number of systematic reviews and meta-analyses have been carried out to determine the efficacy and safety of SLIT [28–36]. Data from literature suggested overall clinical effectiveness of SLIT in patients with AR and AA, although the conclusions were restricted by heterogeneity of the studies, especially concerning the manufacturer's variability of allergen content in commercial extracts. In our study the only available SLIT extracts in Serbia was used, and the exact dose in micrograms of major allergen was calculated.

The comparison between immunotherapy and standard pharmacological treatment is still a matter of debate. Clinical effects of SLIT can be appreciated only in the long term period (months), whereas traditional drugs act immediately. Data from literature showed that efficacy of SLIT is dose-dependent and sufficient duration of treatment is essential to elicit the immunologic changes underlying its clinical effectiveness. According to our results, SLIT seems to be a beneficial therapeutic strategy. In our study, after 12 months of treatment, reduction in all clinical scores was observed in the SLIT group (in up to 75% of the patients). Reduction of drug intake indicates that pharmacological treatment does not prime SLIT efficacy. Comparison between groups showed statistically significant reduction of drug scores and symptoms scores in SLIT group.

Exhaled NO has been shown to reflect the levels of airway inflammation in asthmatic patients [37, 38]. In addition, it has also been reported that asthmatic patients show higher levels of NO in peripheral blood and that serum levels can be used as an additional inflammatory marker in asthma [39]. No study has yet investigated the effect of AIT on NO concentration, although AIT with *D. pteronyssinus* and *D. farinae* extracts has been found to reduce exhaled NO in asthmatic children with mite allergy [40]. However the results from the studies are controversial and a clear demonstration of a reduction in exhaled NO in asthmatic patients taking SLIT is lacking [41]. According to our data NO levels decreased after SLIT, possibly reflecting a reduction in systemic allergic inflammation.

Some potential limitations of our study have to be pointed out. Patients were not stratified according to sensitizations, which could have an impact on SLIT effectiveness and results of clinical scores. The small study population sample did not allow a proper subanalysis by sensitization profile. Furthermore the quality of SLIT extract is questionable, but the extract we used is the only available product in Serbian market.

Conclusions

Our data showed that SLITOR is an effective treatment, decreasing both symptom and medication scores in the active group. These findings suggest that SLIT may have preventive effects, showing in children with intermittent asthma and AR a lower occurrence of persistent airway inflammation. Combining clinical outcomes with respiratory function and FeNO values, we could be able to phenotype the most adequate patients who will benefit from SLIT. When evaluating the effect of AIT, it is appropriate to consider results affecting both the upper and the lower airways, whereas measurement of FeNO is of a great importance.

Abbreviations

AIT: allergen-specific immunotherapy; DBPC-RCT: double blind placebo control randomized clinical trials; ECP: eosinophil cationic protein; FeNO: exhaled nitric oxide; FEV1: forced expiratory volume in 1 s; GERD: gastro-esophageal reflux disease; GINA: Global initiative for asthma; ICS: inhaled corticosteroids; INCS: intranasal corticosteroids; ITT: intent-to-treat; LABA: long acting beta agonists; RAST: radioimmunoassay allergen specific test; SCIT: subcutaneous immunotherapy; SLIT: sublingual immunotherapy; SPT: skin prick test.

Authors' contributions

IDF and ZZ conceived and designed the study, and coordinated the data collection. IDF and MC revised the study results and drafted the manuscript. DF and CS contributed to data interpretation and manuscript preparation. All authors read and approved the final manuscript.

Author details

[1] Faculty of Medical Science, University of Kragujevac, Svetozara Markovica 64, 34000 Kragujevac, Serbia. [2] Allergy Unit and Asthma Center, Verona University and General Hospital, Piazzale Stefani 1, 37126 Verona, Italy. [3] Institution for Emergency Medical Care, Bulevar Franša Depera 5, 11000 Belgrade, Serbia. [4] Department of Internal Medicine and Therapeutics, University of Pavia, Strada Nuova 65, Pavia, Italy. [5] Children's Hospital for Lung Diseases and Tuberculosis, Medical Center "Dr. Dragiša Mišović", Belgrade, Pilota Mihajla Tepica 1, 11000 Belgrade, Serbia. [6] Faculty of Pharmacy, University Business Academy in Novi Sad, Trg Mladenca 5, 2100, Novi Sad, Serbia.

References

1. Gough H, Grabenhenrich L, Reich A, et al. Allergic multimorbidity of asthma, rhinitis and eczema over 20 years in the German birth cohort MAS. Pediatr Allergy Immunol. 2015;26:431–7.
2. Caminati M, Duric-Filipovic I, Arasi S, Peroni DG, Zivkovic Z, Senna G. Respiratory allergies in childhood: recent advances and future challenges. Pediatr Allergy Immunol. 2015;26:702–10.
3. Alduraywish SA, Lodge CJ, Campbell B, et al. The march from early life food sensitization to allergic disease: a systematic review and meta-analyses of birth cohort studies. Allergy. 2015. doi:10.1111/all.1278.
4. Arasi S, Passalacqua G, Caminiti L, Crisafulli G, Fiamingo C, Pajno GB. Efficacy and safety of sublingual immunotherapy in children. Expert Rev Clin Immunol. 2016;12(1):49–56.
5. Živković Z, Cerović S, Djurić-Filipović I, Vukašinović Z, Jocić-Stojanović J, Bajec-Opančina A. (2012). Clinical implications and facts about allergic rhinitis (AR) in children, allergic rhinitis, Prof. Marek Kowalski (Ed.), ISBN: 978-953-51-0288-5, InTech, http://www.intechopen.com/books/allergic-rhinitis/allergic-rhinitis-in-childhood-clinical-implications-and-allergen-specific-immunotherapy.
6. Caminati M, Dama AR, Djuric I, Montagni M, Schiappoli M, Ridolo E, Senna G, Canonica GW. Incidence and risk factors for subcutaneous immunotherapy anaphylaxis: the optimization of safety. Expert Rev Clin Immunol. 2015;11(2):233–45.
7. Đurić-Filipović I, Caminati M, Kostić G, Filipović Đ, Živković Z. Allergen specific sublingual immunotherapy in children with asthma and allergic rhinitis. World J Pediatr. 2016;12(3):283–90.
8. Živković Z, Djurić-Filipović I, Živanović S. Current issues on sublingual allergen-specific immunotherapy in children with asthma and allergic rhinitis. Srp Arh Celok Lek. 2016;144(5–6):345–50.
9. Passalacqua G, Canonica GW. Allergen immunotherapy: history and future developments. Immunol Allergy Clin North Am. 2016;36(1):1–12. doi:10.1016/j.iac.2015.08.001.
10. Jutel M, Agache I, Bonini S, Burks AW, Calderon M, Canonica W, et al. International consensus on allergy immunotherapy. J Allergy Clin Immunol. 2015;136(3):556–68. doi:10.1016/j.jaci.2015.04.047.
11. Bannier MA, van de Kant KD, Jobsis Q, Dompeling E. Biomarkers to predict asthma in wheezing preschool children. Clin Exp Allergy. 2015;45:1040–50.
12. Moschino L, Zanconato S, Bozzetto S, Baraldi E, Carraro S. Childhood asthma biomarkers: present knowledge and future steps. Paediatr Respir Rev. 2015;12:S1526–42.
13. Payne DN, Adcock IM, Wilson NM, Oates T, Scallan M, Bush A. Relationship between exhaled nitric oxide and mucosal eosinophilic inflammation in children with difficult asthma, after treatment with oral prednisolone. Am J Respir Crit Care Med. 2001;164:1376–81.
14. American Thoracic Society, European Respiratory Society. ATS/ERS recommendations for standardized procedures for the online and offline measurement of exhaled lower respiratory nitric oxide and nasal nitric oxide. Am J Respir Crit Care Med. 2005;171:912–30.

15. Dweik RA, Boggs PB, Erzurum SC, on behalf of the American Thoracic Society Committee on Interpretation of Exhaled Nitric Oxide Levels (FeNO) for Clinical Applications, et al. An official ATS clinical practice guideline: interpretation of exhaled nitric oxide levels (FeNO) for clinical applications. Am J Respir Crit Care Med. 2011;184:602–15.

16. Cristescu SM, Mandon J, Harren FJ, Meriläinen P, Högman M. Methods of NO detection in exhaled breath. J Breath Res. 2013;7:017104.

17. Kovesi T, Kulka R, Dales R. Exhaled nitric oxide concentration is affected by age, height, and race in healthy 9- to 12-year-old children. Chest. 2008;133:169–75.

18. Tari MG, Mancino M, Monti G. Efficacy of sublingual immunotherapy in patients with rhinitis and asthma due to house dust mite. A double blind study. Allergol Immunopathol. 1990;18:277–84.

19. Hirsch T, Sahn M, Leupold W. Double blind placebo controlled study of sublingual immunotherapy with house dust mite extracts in children. Pediatr Allergy Immunol. 1997;8(1):21–7.

20. Vourdas D, Syrigou E, Potamianou P, Carat F, Batard T. Double -blind, placebo-controlled evaluation of sublingual immunotherapy with standardized olivepollen extract in pediatric patients with allergic rhino-conjunctivitis and mild asthma due to olive pollen sensitization. Allergy. 1998;53:662–72.

21. La Rosa M, Ranno C, Andre´ C, Carat F, Tosca MA, Canonica GW. Double-blind placebo-controlled evaluation of sublingual swallow immunother-apy with standardized *Parietaria judaica* extract in children with allergic rhinoconjunctivitis. J Allergy Clin Immunol. 1999;104:425–32.

22. Pajno GB, Morabito L, Barberio G, Parmiani S. Clinical and immunologic effects of long-term sublingual immunotherapy in asthmatic children sensitized to mites: a double-blind, placebo-controlled study. Allergy. 2000;55:842–9.

23. Caffarelli C, Sensi LG, Marcucci F, Cavagni C. Preseasonal local allergoid immunotherapy to grass pollen in children: a double-blind, placebo-controlled, randomized trial. Allergy. 2000;55:1142–7.

24. Yuksel H, Tanac R, Gousseinov A, Demir E. Sublingual immunotherapy and influence on urinary leukotrienes in season al pediatric allergy. J Investig Allergol Clin Immunol. 1999;9:305–13.

25. Bahceciler NN, Isik U, Barlan IB, Basaran MM. Efficacy of sublingual immu-notherapy in children with asthma and rhinitis: a double-blind, placebo-controlled study. Pediatr Pulmonol. 2001;32:49–55.

26. Bufe A, Ziegler-Kirbach E, Stoeckmann E, Heidemann P, Gehlhar K, Holland-Letz T, et al. Efficacy of sublingual swallow immunotherapy in children with severe grass pollen allergic symptoms: a double-blind placebo-controlled study. Allergy. 2004;59:498–504.

27. Rolinck-Werninghaus C, Wolf H, Liebke C, Baars JC, Lange J, Kopp MV, et al. A pros pective, randomized, double-blind, placebo-controlled multi-centre study on the efficacy and safety of sublingual immunother-apy (SLIT) in children with seasonal allergic rhinoconjunctivitis to grass pollen. Allergy. 2004;59:1285–93.

28. Stelmach I, Kaczmarek-Woz´niak J, Majak P, Olszowiec-Chlebna M, Jerzynska J. Efficacy and safety of high-doses sublingual immunotherapy in ultra-rush scheme in children allergic to grass pollen. Clin Exp Allergy. 2009;39:401–8.

29. Penagos M, Compalati E, Tarantini F, Baena-Cagnani R, Huerta J, Passal-acqua G, et al. Efficacy of sublingual immunotherapy in the treatment of allergic rhinitis in pediatric patients 3 to 18 years of age: a meta-analysis of randomized, placebo-controlled, double-blind trials. Ann Allergy Asthma Immunol. 2006;97:141–8.

30. Radulovic S, Wilson D, Calderon M, Durham S. Systematic reviews of sublingual immunotherapy (SLIT). Allergy. 2011;66:740–52.

31. Wilson DR, Torres LI, Durham SR. Sublingual immunotherapy for allergic rhinitis. Cochrane Database Syst Rev. 2003;2:CD002893.

32. Calamita Z, Saconato H, Pelá AB, Atallah AN. Efficacy of sublingual immu-notherapy in asthma: systematic review of randomized-clinical trials using the Cochrane Collaboration method. Allergy. 2006;10:1162–72.

33. Penagos M, Passalacqua G, Compalati E, Baena-Cagnani CE, Orozco S, Pedroza A, et al. Metaanalysis of the efficacy of sublingual immunother-apy in the treatment of allergic asthma in pediatric patients, 3 to 18 years of age. Chest. 2008;133:599–609.

34. Nelson H, Blaiss M, Nolte H, Wu¨rtz SØ, Andersen JS, Durham SR. Efficacy and safety of the SQ-standardized grass allergy immunotherapy tablet in mono- and polysensitized subjects. Allergy. 2013;68:252–5.

35. Malling HJ, Montagut A, Melac M, Patriarca G, Panzner P, Seberova E, et al. Efficacy and safety of 5-grass pollen sublingual immunotherapy tablets in patients with different clinical profiles of allergic rhinoconjunctivitis. Clin Exp Allergy. 2009;39(3):387–93.

36. Marogna M, Spadolini I, Massolo A, Canonica GW, Passalacqua G. Long-lasting effects of sublingual immunotherapy according to its duration: a 15-year prospective study. J Allergy Clin Immunol. 2010;126(5):969–75.

37. Kharitonov SA, Yates D, Robbins RA, Logan-Sinclair R, Shinebourne E, Barnes PJ. Increased nitric oxide in exhaled air of asthmatic patients. Lancet. 1994;343:133–5.

38. Massaro AF, Mehta S, Lilly CM, Kobzik L, Reilly JJ, Drazen JM. Elevated nitric oxide concentrations in isolated lower airway gas of asthmatic subjects. Am J Respir Crit Care Med. 1996;153:1510–4.

39. de Arruda-Chaves E, De Conti D, Tebaldi T. Nitric oxide sera levels as an inflammatory marker in asthma. J Investig Allergol Clin Immunol. 2002;12(2):120–3.

40. Hung CH, Lee MY, Tsai YG, Cheng SN, Yang KD. Hyposensitization therapy reduced exhaled nitric oxide in asthmatic children with corticosteroid dependency. Acta Paediatr Taiwan. 2004;45:89–93.

41. Inci D, Altintas DU, Kendirli SG, Yilmaz M, Karakoc GB. The effect of specifi c immunotherapy on exhaled breath condensate nitrite levels. Allergy. 2006;61:899–900.

18

Biological clocks: their relevance to immune-allergic diseases

Roberto Paganelli[1,2*], Claudia Petrarca[1,2] and Mario Di Gioacchino[1,2]

Abstract

The 2017 Nobel Prize for Physiology or Medicine, awarded for the discoveries made in the past 15 years on the genetic and molecular mechanisms regulating many physiological functions, has renewed the attention to the importance of circadian rhythms. These originate from a central pacemaker in the suprachiasmatic nucleus in the brain, photoentrained via direct connection with melanopsin containing, intrinsically light-sensitive retinal ganglion cells, and it projects to periphery, thus creating an inner circadian rhythm. This regulates several activities, including sleep, feeding times, energy metabolism, endocrine and immune functions. Disturbances of these rhythms, mainly of wake/sleep, hormonal secretion and feeding, cause decrease in quality of life, as well as being involved in development of obesity, metabolic syndrome and neuropsychiatric disorders. Most immunological functions, from leukocyte numbers, activity and cytokine secretion undergo circadian variations, which might affect susceptibility to infections. The intensity of symptoms and disease severity show a 24 h pattern in many immunological and allergic diseases, including rheumatoid arthritis, bronchial asthma, atopic eczema and chronic urticaria. This is accompanied by altered sleep duration and quality, a major determinant of quality of life. Shift work and travel through time zones as well as artificial light pose new health threats by disrupting the circadian rhythms. Finally, the field of chronopharmacology uses these concepts for delivering drugs in synchrony with biological rhythms.

Keywords: Circadian rhythm, Biological clock, Immune system, Allergy, Chronopharmacology, Shift work

Background

The 2017 Nobel Prize for Physiology or Medicine has been awarded to three of the principal scientists who contributed to the discovery of the network of genes and proteins regulating the circadian rhythms based on the light/dark 24 h cycle ("The 2017 Nobel Prize in Physiology or Medicine—Press Release") [1–3].

Circadian clocks are present in unicellular organisms, in plants, insects and vertebrates [4]. The first gene encoding a critical component of a circadian clock (Period) was discovered in Drosophila by Konopka and Benzer in 1971 [5], showing that circadian clocks are genetically encoded. In mammals, circadian clocks are found in nearly all cells and tissues. They regulate and control physiological processes at the cellular, organ and organismal level, integrating signals received from outside and generated by the normal metabolism. The purpose of different levels of control is to adjust for possible local perturbations, while maintaining a circadian rhythm able to optimize energy allocation for the most likely scenario (which differs during activity and rest periods). For example, the liver clock should be synchronized to rhythms in food intake, but it should also respond to changes in energy demands or variations in oxygen supply. The organization of the mammalian multi-clock system allows for better adaptation to changing environments. This may represent a compromise between flexible adaptation to extremely unpredictable events and circadian stability, which can distinguish also the changes of light–dark hours (and temperature, humidity etc.) with the different seasons [4, 6].

Time keeping signals ("zeitgeber") in natural conditions are tied to the day-night cycle imposed by the 24 h rotation cycle of the Earth. Light, this very potent zeitgeber, regulates the 24 h sleep–wake rhythm. Sleep precludes

*Correspondence: roberto.paganelli@unich.it
[1] Dipartimento di Medicina e Scienze dell'invecchiamento, Università "G. d'Annunzio" of Chieti-Pescara, Via dei Vestini, 5, 66013 Chieti, Italy
Full list of author information is available at the end of the article

both food intake and locomotor activity. Thus, the sleep–wake rhythm governed by sunlight indirectly drives food intake and body temperature cycles. However light and food can be uncoupled (e.g. in the case of jetlag or when food intake is restricted to the natural sleeping phase as in shift work), causing misalignment of these clocks with the daily light–dark cycle of our environment [7, 8]. The field was stimulated by the finding of an intrinsically photosensitive small subgroup of retinal ganglion cells which regulate the circadian rhythms on the light–dark cycle [9, 10] and project to the suprachiasmatic nuclei (SCN) [11], the non-visual brain centers where the mammalian master biological clock is located; this has prompted the search for the molecular clock(s) driving this essential component of all living organisms. A handful of genes and proteins accounting for this complex regulatory central network has been identified.

Biological clocks

The mammalian core molecular clock consists of two feedback loops [12] connected by a central pair of transcription factors which regulate reciprocally to induce the rhythm of gene expression. The mammalian circadian clock fundamentally depends on two master genes (CLOCK and BMAL1) to drive gene expression and regulate biological functions [6]. CLOCK:BMAL1 heterodimers promote rhythmic chromatin opening and this mediates the binding of other transcription factors adjacent to CLOCK:BMAL1 [13]. Among their targets there is a group of regulatory proteins [PERIOD (PER1, 2 and 3), CRYPTOCHROME (CRY1 and 2), REV-ERB (REV-ERBa and b) and RAR-Related Orphan Receptor (RORa, b and c)]; REV-ERBs and RORs regulate BMAL1 transcription, whereas PER and CRY dimerize to inhibit the BMAL1–CLOCK dimer. PER, the protein encoded by *period* [14, 15] accumulates during the night and is degraded during the day, while other components allow nuclear translocation of PER [16, 17]. Both sleep–wake cycles and many 24-h rhythms persist in the absence of environmental cues and are controlled by internal molecular clocks [18].

Several loops dictate the production of these proteins, including steps of acetylation and phosphorylation, as well as secondary clock-regulated genes which can also feed back on central clock genes [6, 19]. In fact many different organs and tissues express functional molecular clock circuits [20]. None of the mammalian clock components is directly photoreceptive; instead, light signals from the retina are transmitted neuronally to transcription factors that regulate *period* expression. Transcriptional feedback loops are central to the generation and maintenance of circadian rhythms [21, 22]. Clocks in peripheral tissues use essentially the same molecular components as in the SCN; clocks have been detected in different hematopoietic cell lineages, including macrophages and lymphocytes [22, 23].

The origin of circadian rhythms

In humans, circadian rhythms of 24 h must be synchronized to coincide with the daily rotational cycle of the earth. The alignment of this autonomous circadian rhythm to an external rhythm is defined as entrainment. The light patterns represent the principal environmental stimulus for the rest/activity and sleep/wake cycles [24]. It is also indirectly responsible for timing of food intake, another powerful entrainer of rhythm [24, 25].

Circadian photoentrainment is the process by which the internal clock in the deep brain becomes synchronized with the daily external cycle of solar light and dark [4, 9, 26]. The clocks in most mammalian cells are not directly photoreceptive, unlike those of most other organisms, but instead are entrained indirectly to the environmental light–dark cycle via photoreception in the retina, the retino-hypothalamic tract, and a central pacemaker tissue in the suprachiasmatic nucleus (SCN) of the hypothalamus [19]. This process is initiated by a type of retinal ganglion cells that send axonal projections to the SCN, the region of the circadian pacemaker (Fig. 1). In contrast to retinal cells mediating vision, these cells are intrinsically sensitive to light, independent of synaptic input from rod and cone photoreceptors [27]. Photoentrainment of the master pacemaker needs signaling from retinal ganglion cells containing the photopigment melanopsin and intrinsically photosensitive [10]. The cryptochrome/photolyase family of photoreceptors mediates adaptive responses to ultraviolet and blue light exposure in all life forms [28]. The SCN subsequently synchronizes peripheral clocks via mediators including hormones and neuronal signals, primarily using the hypothalamic–pituitary–adrenal (HPA) axis and the autonomic nervous system [6]. The principal hormones i.e. glucocorticoids and catecholamines (epinephrine and norepinephrine), are released by the adrenal gland via the HPA axis [29], but norepinephrine is also derived from sympathetic nerve endings. The HPA is controlled by the SCN which projects to the paraventricular nucleus of the hypothalamus, and this in turn induces the release of adrenocorticotropic hormone by the pituitary, thus regulating the adrenal gland [20, 30]. Catecholamines act via adrenergic receptors, which have many effects on immune cells, as well as increasing the humoral immune responses [24].

The integrated circadian system

The central biological CLOCK system, influenced by light/dark changes, 'creates' the internal circadian rhythms, and the organism 'feels' these changes to put in

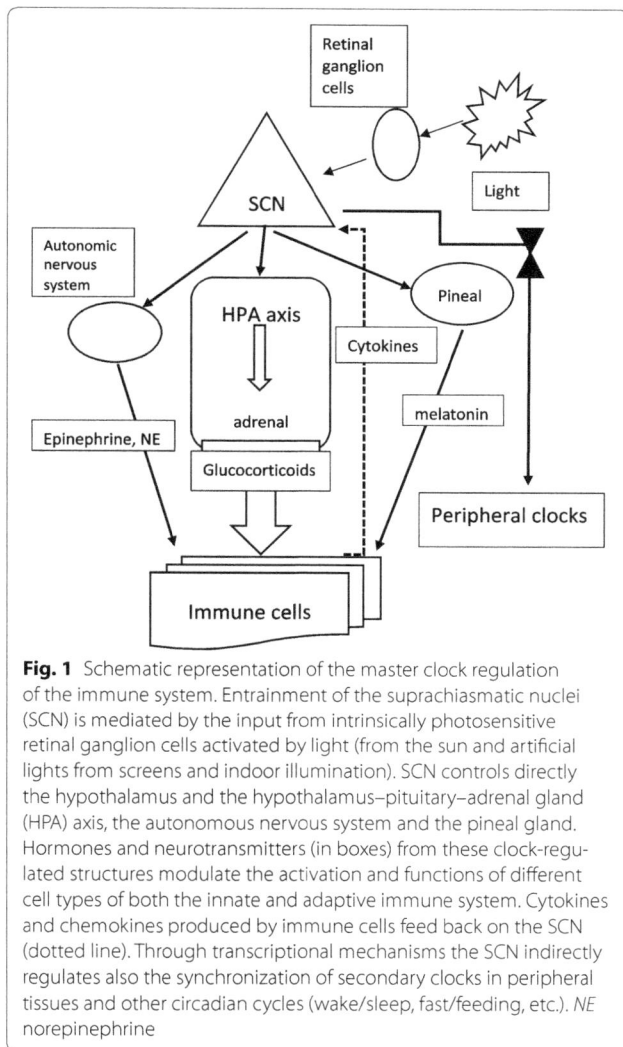

Fig. 1 Schematic representation of the master clock regulation of the immune system. Entrainment of the suprachiasmatic nuclei (SCN) is mediated by the input from intrinsically photosensitive retinal ganglion cells activated by light (from the sun and artificial lights from screens and indoor illumination). SCN controls directly the hypothalamus and the hypothalamus–pituitary–adrenal gland (HPA) axis, the autonomous nervous system and the pineal gland. Hormones and neurotransmitters (in boxes) from these clock-regulated structures modulate the activation and functions of different cell types of both the innate and adaptive immune system. Cytokines and chemokines produced by immune cells feed back on the SCN (dotted line). Through transcriptional mechanisms the SCN indirectly regulates also the synchronization of secondary clocks in peripheral tissues and other circadian cycles (wake/sleep, fast/feeding, etc.). *NE* norepinephrine

frame physical activities, including energy metabolism, sleep, and immune function.

A recent review [31] listed the following pathological conditions showing diurnal or 24 h patterning, by the organ/tissue/system affected, skin: atopic dermatitis, urticaria, psoriasis, and palmar hyperhidrosis; gastrointestinal: esophageal reflux, peptic ulcer, biliary colic, hepatic variceal hemorrhage, and proctalgia; infection: susceptibility, fever, and mortality; neural: frontal, parietal, temporal, and occipital lobe seizures, Parkinson's and Alzheimer's disease, hereditary progressive dystonia, and pain (cancer, post-surgical, diabetic neuropathy, burning mouth and temporomandibular syndromes, fibromyalgia, sciatalgia, and migraine, headache); renal: colic and nocturnal enuresis and polyuria; ocular: conjunctival redness, keratoconjunctivitis sicca, intraocular pressure, anterior ischemic optic neuropathy, and

recurrent corneal erosion syndrome; psychiatric/behavioral: major and seasonal affective depressive disorders, bipolar disorder, suicide, and addictive alcohol, tobacco, and heroin cravings and withdrawal phenomena; plus autoimmune and musculoskeletal: rheumatoid arthritis, osteoarthritis, axial spondylarthritides, gout, Sjogren's syndrome, and systemic lupus erythematosus. Some are directly linked to disruption of circadian rhythms, others result in disturbed sleep with loss of rhythmicity; the peripheral clocks in different tissues become out of phase with the central regulator and other physiologic functions, and this in turn aggravates the symptoms and alters the clinical picture.

Relevance to immunological functions

A wide range of immune parameters, such as the number of peripheral blood mononuclear cells as well as the level of cytokines, undergo daily fluctuations [32]. Total numbers of hematopoietic stem cells and most mature leukocytes peak in the circulation during the resting phase (during the night for humans) and decrease during the day [24]. Most immune cells express circadian clock genes and present a wide array of genes expressed with a 24-h rhythm. In addition to their functions in the cellular clock, circadian oscillators also participate in the development and specification of immune cell lineages. This has profound impacts on cellular functions, including a daily rhythm in the synthesis and release of cytokines, chemokines and cytolytic factors, the daily gating of the response occurring through pattern recognition receptors, circadian rhythms of cellular functions such as phagocytosis, migration to inflamed or infected tissue, cytolytic activity, and proliferative response to antigens [33]. A pioneering contribution to this area was made by Halberg [34] who discovered a diurnal susceptibility pattern in mice challenged with bacterial endotoxin. The migration of hematopoietic cells to tissues preferentially occurs during the daytime, directed by the circadian expression of cell adhesion molecules and chemokines. During the active phase it is more likely to encounter and detect pathogens and leukocyte trafficking into tissues occurs at the beginning of this phase (early morning). The increased cytokine release at this time point therefore may exacerbate any ongoing local inflammation [24]. One of the mechanisms through which the central clock entrains peripheral tissues is by the production of glucocorticoids in the adrenal gland. Many other circadian signal transduction mediators also regulate the immune response, as melatonin and the autonomic nervous system (Fig. 1).

Perturbation of the redox rhythm (linked to the circadian clock) induced by pathogen challenge triggers immune defense genes without compromising the circadian clock [35]. Activation of innate immunity via TLR4 induces systemic inflammation by eliciting neuroendocrine and leukocyte transcriptional responses, which are regulated by the circadian clock, imposing diurnal rhythm of the inflammatory response [36]. The central clock is sensitive to immune challenge and the brain receives inflammatory signals from the periphery in response to injury/infection. This in turn is thought to exacerbate sickness, develop symptoms like depression, and impair diurnal rhythms of temperature and melatonin secretion [36]. Melatonin, secreted by the pineal gland under SCN control, plays an important role in immune regulation; pinealectomy causes extensive immunosuppression, likely mediated by the decrease in lymphocytes and cytokines such as IL-2, IL-12, and TNF-α [35].

Sleep and light influences

The time and duration of sleep is tightly controlled by central mechanisms. These may be disrupted by disease processes, but also by other external conditions, such as night shifts, long range flight travels (jet-lag) and social nocturnal activity (social jet-lag). Pro-inflammatory cytokines are generally indicated as sleep-inducing, and basal plasma levels of these cytokines appear higher during the rest phase. Infection-associated sleepiness has been attributed to increased pro-inflammatory cytokine plasma levels [6].

Long-term sleep restriction leads to a gradual increase of circulating leukocytes and subpopulations (neutrophils, monocytes and lymphocytes) with alterations of the number and rhythm of neutrophils persisting after 1 week recovery of sleep [37]; also absolute sleep deprivation alters the rhythmicity of granulocytes [38]. Sleep disorders are one of the most common symptoms in patients with HIV/AIDS [39], but despite the circadian rhythm alteration induced by tat [40] HIV-infected patients with higher HIV Tat protein concentrations had better sleep quality, probably because it increases melatonin production, thus counteracting poor sleep quality induced by HIV [41]. On the opposite spectrum of sleep disorders, narcolepsy, which is generally considered an immune-mediated neurological disease characterized by excessive daytime sleepiness, has been recently characterized by increased inflammatory cytokine production and B and T cell activation markers [42] at variance with other hypersomnia patients who were immunologically distinct and did not present increased plasma cytokines. Many immunological functions depend on the influence of sleep on circadian rhythms, and loss of sleep, in turn, alters the production of glucocorticoids during the night [43]. The neuroendocrine immune response of the HPA axis and sympathetic nervous system, which is activated

in response to an antigenic challenge, with a transient inflammatory activity, can lead to metabolic diseases when chronically activated [44], since in all inflammatory conditions high amounts of energy have to be provided for the activated immune system. Experimental animal models and epidemiological data indicate that chronic circadian rhythm disruption increases the risk of metabolic diseases [8].

In patients with rheumatoid arthritis (RA), inflammation is an important covariate for the crosstalk of sleep and the HPA axis. Moreover the interrelation between sleep parameters, inflammation as objectified by C-reactive protein and serum cortisol and adrenocorticotropic hormone levels [45]. Knowledge of circadian rhythms and the influence of glucocorticoids in rheumatology is important [46]: beside optimizing treatment for the core symptoms (e.g. morning stiffness in RA), chronotherapy might also relieve important comorbid conditions such as depression and sleep disturbances [47]. Sleep and circadian disturbances are a frequent complaint of Alzheimer's disease patients, appearing early in the course of disease, and disruption of many circadian rhythms are present also in Parkinson's disease [48].

Physiological studies show that aging affects both sleep quality and quantity in humans, and sleep complaints increase with age [49]. Moreover, also feeding/fasting rhythms are compromised.

Circadian expression of secreted signaling molecules transmits timing information between cells and tissues. Such daily rhythms optimize energy use and temporally segregate incompatible processes.

Patients suffering from neuropsychiatric disorders often exhibit a loss of regulation of their biological rhythms which leads to alterations of sleep/wake, feeding, body temperature and hormonal rhythms. Increasing evidence indicates that the circadian system may be directly involved in the etiology of these disorders [50].

Light, especially short wavelength blue light, is the most potent environmental cue in circadian photoentrainment and lens aging is thought to influence this event by acting as a filter for shorter blue wavelengths [51]; light conditions during indoor activities as well as sunlight exposure are of paramount importance to preserve the circadian rhythmicity and avoid a risk factor for several chronic diseases. These considerations impact on the comorbidities of aged subjects, and the importance of the choice of the differential light-filtering properties of intraocular lenses after cataract removal [52].

Biological clocks and allergic diseases

As an important addendum to the many health consequences of abnormalities of the integrated circadian rhythms, one must just mention disorders in glucose and lipid metabolism as inducers of obesity and the development of Type 2 diabetes [53] and the multifaceted effects of the circadian control of the immune system and its activation [6, 24]. These findings highlight an integrative role of circadian rhythms in physiology [7].

Most studies have dealt with asthma, where symptoms undergo circadian variations with exacerbations occurring more frequently at night (Table 1). Nocturnal asthma is a common presentation and is associated with a more severe form of the disease [54]. Airway diseases are associated with abnormal circadian rhythms of lung function, reflected in daily changes of airway caliber, airway resistance, respiratory symptoms, and abnormal immune-inflammatory responses [55]. The molecular clock is altered by cigarette smoke, LPS, and bacterial and viral infections in mouse and human lungs and in patients with chronic airway diseases. In patients with nocturnal asthma, the difference in FEV1 (and peak expiratory flow rate) between daytime and night may be > 15%. Also diurnal FeNO variation in uncontrolled asthmatics was significantly greater than in controlled asthmatics [56]. Degree of asthma control strongly correlated with sleep quality. Individuals whose asthma was not well controlled took longer to fall asleep, awoke more often, and spent more time awake during the night compared to those with well controlled asthma. Poor asthma control, use of rescue medications, and asthma symptoms were associated with daytime sleepiness and limitations in physical activity and emotional function [57]. In a field study subdividing patients according to preferential time for activity (chronotypes), 35% of asthmatics presented nocturnal symptoms [58] and the morning chronotype was underrepresented when compared to asthmatics without nocturnal symptoms. The timing of drug treatments in asthma (chronotherapeutics) is governed by the circadian nature of asthma. The peripheral clock within the lung is localized in the Clara cell of the mouse bronchial epithelium [59]. Cyclic oscillations in the expression of genes associated with extracellular matrix, cytoskeleton, cell cycle and apoptosis [60], suggest that the repair and turnover of these components in lung are directly

or indirectly under the regulation of the lung molecular clock. There is no animal model of asthma with alterations of circadian rhythms due to mutations of components of the molecular clock. However, recently in mice lacking BMAL1 expression in myeloid cells, the induction of asthma caused markedly increased inflammation in the lungs, with higher numbers of eosinophils and increased IL-5 levels in the lung and serum [61]. Moreover, Granulocyte-macrophage colony-stimulating factor mRNA, expressed by activated eosinophils, increased threefold in early morning compared with afternoon in circulating eosinophils from asthma patients with nocturnal symptoms but not in those without [62]. Taken together all data indicate that chronotherapy of asthma offers higher chances of achieving symptoms control, and in particular those developing at night, as in most other allergic diseases [63].

Also in allergic rhinitis symptoms are commonly most severe during the night or early in the morning, and allergen-induced surface CD203c expression on basophils of seasonal allergic rhinitis patients exhibit a time-of-day-dependent variation [64]. Basophil reactivity shows daily variations depending on the circadian clock activity in basophils, which could partly explain temporal symptomatic variations in allergic rhinitis. The circadian rhythms of salivary melatonin and cortisol were found to be disrupted in patients with allergic rhinitis [65]. Sleep impairment is very common in allergic rhinitis patients and has a significant impact on disease-specific measures of general health and quality of life. The degree of sleep disturbance is directly related to the severity of the disease [66]. Intranasal steroids caused a time shift of PER2 rhythm in the mouse nasal mucosa around the peak of serum glucocorticoids, suggesting that the circadian rhythm of endogenous glucocorticoids regulates the nasal peripheral clock [67] (Table 1). This should imply that in humans steroids should be administered when no time shift can be induced, that is in the early evening.

In the case of atopic eczema, sleep disturbance affects up to 60% of children, rising even higher during exacerbations [68]. This may affect daytime activities and lead

Table 1 Circadian rhythm of symptoms in immuno-allergic diseases and acute myocardial infarction as example. Modified from Scheiermann et al. [23]

Disease	Peak time (h)	Symptom	Peak of cytokine/hormone
Asthma	Early morning	Bronchoconstriction	IL5 07 a.m.
Allergic rhinitis	Early morning	Congestion, sneezing	Cortisol 08–11 a.m.
Rheumatoid arthritis	Early morning 05–08 a.m.	Stiffness, pain	TNF+ IL6 06–08 a.m.
Myocardial infarction	Morning 09 a.m.	Pain	Epinephrine + NE 08–11 a.m.

Time when symptoms are more usually presenting is indicated (peak time) and the time of the highest circadian blood level of cytokines and hormones regulated by biological clocks

to behavioral alterations. The assessment of sleep quality should represent the relevant parameter for control of disease activity, particularly in patients suffering from worsening of symptoms at night [69]. In mice, disruption of biological rhythm causes exacerbation of contact hypersensitivity [70] probably due to altered glucocorticoid rhythmicity. Sleep and daily activity interference are considered important indicators for assessing disease activity and quality of life in chronic spontaneous urticarial [71], and a recent international observational study on quality of life concluded that chronic spontaneous urticaria markedly interfered with sleep and daily activities [72]. Previous studies had revealed circadian variations of histamine levels, peaking at 2 a.m. in mastocytosis [73], but no diurnal changes in basophil numbers [74], although basopenia is often found in chronic urticaria.

It has been shown that the circadian clocks drive the daily rhythms of IgE-mediated allergic reactions in the skin of mice. Also systemic anaphylactic reactions show a diurnal variation, which relies on the circadian clocks [75]; briefly, the circadian clock is a potent regulator the strength of IgE-dependent allergic reactions [63] in the skin but also in other target organs. A mechanistic link is still missing, whereas experimental findings suggest that Clock is a regulator of psoriasis-like skin inflammation in mice via direct modulation of IL-23R [76]. Representative examples of circadian rhythms of symptoms and molecular mediators of immune-allergic diseases are shown in Table 1.

Conclusion

The 2017 Nobel Prize for Physiology or Medicine has focused the attention on the importance of homeostasis and balanced distribution of energy resources ensured by the presence of circadian rhythms. These are centrally controlled by the master clock in the SCN and photoentrained to the light–dark cycle through inputs from melanopsin-containing retinal ganglion cells. The circadian clocks are not built in a rigid top-down scheme, allowing for oscillations of peripheral clocks in different cells and tissues, thus maximizing flexibility and adaptation to changes in the environment and in the organism. At the biochemical level, they consist of coupled feedback loops that establish a self-sustained, adjustable molecular oscillator that controls, via transcriptional programs, a wide spectrum of cellular and organismal processes. Many physiological events, from sleep to feeding, as well as immune responsiveness, are interlinked to the circadian rhythms. Their disruption can have profound effects on physiology, and modern society and way of life puts increasing pressures to push activity and sleep out of sync with circadian rhythmicity, as in working and eating habits [6]. This poses additional threats to health conditions

of workers on night shift, or subjected to long distance travel through many time zones (jet-lag) or working in artificial light conditions mimicking solar light, but with the danger deriving from blue-enriched emitting LEDs and LED screens [51]. Finally, the emerging importance of chrono-feeding (to avoid the epidemics of obesity and associated cardio-metabolic disorders) and chronopharmacology impose changes in current standard practices which have little regard for circadian rhythms.

Abbreviations

AIDS: acquired immunodeficiency syndrome; CD: cluster of differentiation; FeNO: fractional exhaled nitric oxide; FEV: forced expiratory volume; HIV: human immunodeficiency virus; HPA: hypothalamic pituitary adrenal; Ig: immunoglobulin; IL: interleukin; IL-23R: interleukin-23 receptor; LED: light emitting diode; LPS: lipopolysaccharide; NE: norepinephrine; RA: rheumatoid arthritis; SCN: suprachiasmatic nuclei; TNF: tumor necrosis factor.

Authors' contributions

RB and MDG made substantial contributions to conception and design of this review. CP participated in critical revision and drafting of final version of the manuscript. RB and MDG participated in literature search, acquisition of data and manuscript writing. All authors read and approved the final manuscript.

Author details

[1] Dipartimento di Medicina e Scienze dell'invecchiamento, Università "G. d'Annunzio" of Chieti-Pescara, Via dei Vestini, 5, 66013 Chieti, Italy. [2] *Ce.S.I.-Me.T., Chieti, Italy.

References

1. http://www.nobelprize.org/nobel_prizes/medicine/laureates/2017/press.html?utm_source=twitter&utm_medium=social&utm_campaign=twitter_tweet. Accessed 30 Oct 2017.
2. Callaway E, Ledford H. Medicine Nobel awarded for work on circadian clocks. Nature. 2017;550(7674):18.
3. Burki T. Nobel Prize awarded for discoveries in circadian rhythm. Lancet. 2017;390(10104):e25.
4. Husse J, Eichele G, Oster H. Synchronization of the mammalian circadian timing system: light can control peripheral clocks independently of the SCN clock: alternate routes of entrainment optimize the alignment of the body's circadian clock network with external time. BioEssays. 2015;37(10):1119–28.
5. Konopka RJ, Benzer S. Clock mutants of *Drosophila melanogaster*. Proc Natl Acad Sci USA. 1971;68(9):2112–6.
6. Geiger SS, Fagundes CT, Siegel RM. Chrono-immunology: progress and challenges in understanding links between the circadian and immune systems. Immunology. 2015;146(3):349–58.
7. Panda S. Circadian physiology of metabolism. Science. 2016;354(6315):1008–15.
8. Zarrinpar A, Chaix A, Panda S. Daily eating patterns and their impact on health and disease. Trends Endocrinol Metab. 2016;27(2):69–83.
9. Van Gelder RN, Buhr ED. Ocular photoreception for circadian rhythm entrainment in mammals. Annu Rev Vis Sci. 2016;2:153–69.
10. Kofuji P, Mure LS, Massman LJ, Purrier N, Panda S, Engeland WC. Intrinsically photosensitive retinal ganglion cells (ipRGCs) are necessary for light entrainment of peripheral clocks. PLoS ONE. 2016;11(12):e0168651.

11. Hall JC. Cryptochromes: sensory reception, transduction, and clock functions subserving circadian systems. Curr Opin Neurobiol. 2000;10(4):456–66.

12. Cyran SA, Buchsbaum AM, Reddy KL, Lin MC, Glossop NR, Hardin PE, et al. vrille, Pdp1, and dClock form a second feedback loop in the Drosophila circadian clock. Cell. 2003;112(3):329–41.

13. Menet JS, Pescatore S, Rosbash M. CLOCK: BMAL1 is a pioneer-like transcription factor. Genes Dev. 2014;28(1):8–13.

14. Young MW, Jackson FR, Shin HS, Bargiello TA. A biological clock in Drosophila. In: Cold Spring Harbor symposia quantitative biology, vol. 50; 1985. p. 865–75.

15. Rosbash M, Hall JC. Biological clocks in Drosophila: finding the molecules that make them tick. Cell. 1985;43(1):3–4.

16. Hardin PE, Hall JC, Rosbash M. Circadian oscillations in period gene mRNA levels are transcriptionally regulated. Proc Natl Acad Sci USA. 1992;89(24):11711–5.

17. Hardin PE, Hall JC, Rosbash M. Feedback of the Drosophila period gene product on circadian cycling of its messenger RNA levels. Nature. 1990;343(6258):536–40.

18. Young MW. Life's 24-hour clock: molecular control of circadian rhythms in animal cells. Trends Biochem Sci. 2000;25(12):601–6.

19. Wijnen H, Young MW. Interplay of circadian clocks and metabolic rhythms. Annu Rev Genet. 2006;40:409–48.

20. Dibner C, Schibler U, Albrecht U. The mammalian circadian timing system: organization and coordination of central and peripheral clocks. Annu Rev Physiol. 2010;72:517–49.

21. Menet JS, Abruzzi KC, Desrochers J, Rodriguez J, Rosbash M. Dynamic PER repression mechanisms in the Drosophila circadian clock: from on-DNA to off-DNA. Genes Dev. 2010;24(4):358–67.

22. Boivin DB, James FO, Wu A, Cho-Park PF, Xiong H, Sun ZS. Circadian clock genes oscillate in human peripheral blood mononuclear cells. Blood. 2003;102(12):4143–5.

23. Bollinger T, Leutz A, Leliavski A, Skrum L, Kovac J, Bonacina L, et al. Circadian clocks in mouse and human CD4+ T cells. PLoS ONE. 2011;6(12):e29801.

24. Scheiermann C, Kunisaki Y, Frenette PS. Circadian control of the immune system. Nat Rev Immunol. 2013;13(3):190–8.

25. Green CB, Takahashi JS, Bass J. The meter of metabolism. Cell. 2008;134(5):728–42.

26. Young MW. The molecular control of circadian behavioral rhythms and their entrainment in Drosophila. Annu Rev Biochem. 1998;67:135–52.

27. Brown RL, Robinson PR. Melanopsin—shedding light on the elusive circadian photopigment. Chronobiol Int. 2004;21(2):189–204.

28. Zoltowski BD, Vaidya AT, Top D, Widom J, Young MW, Crane BR. Structure of full-length Drosophila cryptochrome. Nature. 2011;480(7377):396–9.

29. Spies CM, Hoff P, Mazuch J, Gaber T, Maier B, Strehl C, et al. Circadian rhythms of cellular immunity in rheumatoid arthritis: a hypothesis-generating study. Clin Exp Rheumatol. 2015;33(1):34–43.

30. Dickmeis T. Glucocorticoids and the circadian clock. J Endocrinol. 2009;200(1):3–22.

31. Smolensky MH, Portaluppi F, Manfredini R, Hermida RC, Tiseo R, Sackett-Lundeen LL, et al. Diurnal and twenty-four hour patterning of human diseases: acute and chronic common and uncommon medical conditions. Sleep Med Rev. 2015;21:12–22.

32. Cermakian N, Lange T, Golombek D, Sarkar D, Nakao A, Shibata S, et al. Crosstalk between the circadian clock circuitry and the immune system. Chronobiol Int. 2013;30(7):870–88.

33. Labrecque N, Cermakian N. Circadian clocks in the immune system. J Biol Rhythms. 2015;30(4):277–90.

34. Halberg F, Johnson EA, Brown BW, Bittner JJ. Susceptibility rhythm to E. coli endotoxin and bioassay. Proc Soc Exp Biol Med. 1960;103:142–4.

35. Zhou M, Wang W, Karapetyan S, Mwimba M, Marques J, Buchler NE, et al. Redox rhythm reinforces the circadian clock to gate immune response. Nature. 2015;523(7561):472–6.

36. Mavroudis PD, Scheff JD, Calvano SE, Androulakis IP. Systems biology of circadian-immune interactions. J Innate Immun. 2013;5(2):153–62.

37. Lasselin J, Rehman JU, Akerstedt T, Lekander M, Axelsson J. Effect of long-term sleep restriction and subsequent recovery sleep on the diurnal rhythms of white blood cell subpopulations. Brain Behav Immun. 2015;47:93–9.

38. Ackermann K, Revell VL, Lao O, Rombouts EJ, Skene DJ, Kayser M. Diurnal rhythms in blood cell populations and the effect of acute sleep deprivation in healthy young men. Sleep. 2012;35(7):933–40.

39. Gamaldo CE, Spira AP, Hock RS, Salas RE, McArthur JC, David PM, et al. Sleep, function and HIV: a multi-method assessment. AIDS Behav. 2013;17(8):2808–15.

40. Clark JP 3rd, Sampair CS, Kofuji P, Nath A, Ding JM. HIV protein, transactivator of transcription, alters circadian rhythms through the light entrainment pathway. Am J Physiol Regul Integr Comp Physiol. 2005;289(3):R656–62.

41. Wang T, Jiang Z, Hou W, Li Z, Cheng S, Green LA, et al. HIV Tat protein affects circadian rhythmicity by interfering with the circadian system. HIV Med. 2014;15(9):565–70.

42. Hartmann FJ, Bernard-Valnet R, Queriault C, Mrdjen D, Weber LM, Galli E, et al. High-dimensional single-cell analysis reveals the immune signature of narcolepsy. J Exp Med. 2016;213(12):2621–33.

43. Cutolo M, Buttgereit F, Straub RH. Regulation of glucocorticoids by the central nervous system. Clin Exp Rheumatol. 2011;29(5 Suppl 68):S-19–22.

44. Spies CM, Straub RH, Buttgereit F. Energy metabolism and rheumatic diseases: from cell to organism. Arthritis Res Ther. 2012;14(3):216.

45. Straub RH, Detert J, Dziurla R, Fietze I, Loeschmann PA, Burmester GR, et al. Inflammation is an important covariate for the crosstalk of sleep and the HPA axis in rheumatoid arthritis. NeuroImmunoModulation. 2017;24(1):11–20.

46. Spies CM, Straub RH, Cutolo M, Buttgereit F. Circadian rhythms in rheumatology—a glucocorticoid perspective. Arthritis Res Ther. 2014;16(Suppl 2):S3.

47. Buttgereit F, Smolen JS, Coogan AN, Cajochen C. Clocking in: chronobiology in rheumatoid arthritis. Nat Rev Rheumatol. 2015;11(6):349–56.

48. La Morgia C, Ross-Cisneros FN, Sadun AA, Carelli V. Retinal ganglion cells and circadian rhythms in Alzheimer's disease, Parkinson's disease, and beyond. Front Neurol. 2017;8:162.

49. Vienne J, Spann R, Guo F, Rosbash M. Age-related reduction of recovery sleep and arousal threshold in Drosophila. Sleep. 2016;39(8):1613–24.

50. Menet JS, Rosbash M. When brain clocks lose track of time: cause or consequence of neuropsychiatric disorders. Curr Opin Neurobiol. 2011;21(6):849–57.

51. Hatori M, Gronfier C, Van Gelder RN, Bernstein PS, Carreras J, Panda S, et al. Global rise of potential health hazards caused by blue light-induced circadian disruption in modern aging societies. NPJ Aging Mech Dis. 2017;3:9.

52. Yan SS, Wang W. The effect of lens aging and cataract surgery on circadian rhythm. Int J Ophthalmol. 2016;9(7):1066–74.

53. Schwartsburd PM. Catabolic and anabolic faces of insulin resistance and their disorders: a new insight into circadian control of metabolic disorders leading to diabetes. Future Sci OA. 2017;3(3):FSO201.

54. Levin AM, Wang Y, Wells KE, Padhukasahasram B, Yang JJ, Burchard EG, et al. Nocturnal asthma and the importance of race/ethnicity and genetic ancestry. Am J Respir Crit Care Med. 2014;190(3):266–73.

55. Sundar IK, Yao H, Sellix MT, Rahman I. Circadian clock-coupled lung cellular and molecular functions in chronic airway diseases. Am J Respir Cell Mol Biol. 2015;53(3):285–90.

56. Saito J, Gibeon D, Macedo P, Menzies-Gow A, Bhavsar PK, Chung KF. Domiciliary diurnal variation of exhaled nitric oxide fraction for asthma control. Eur Respir J. 2014;43(2):474–84.

57. Krouse HJ, Yarandi H, McIntosh J, Cowen C, Selim V. Assessing sleep quality and daytime wakefulness in asthma using wrist actigraphy. J Asthma. 2008;45(5):389–95.

58. Ferraz E, Borges MC, Vianna EO. Influence of nocturnal asthma on chronotype. J Asthma. 2008;45(10):911–5.

59. Durrington HJ, Farrow SN, Loudon AS, Ray DW. The circadian clock and asthma. Thorax. 2014;69(1):90–2.

60. Sukumaran S, Jusko WJ, Dubois DC, Almon RR. Light-dark oscillations in the lung transcriptome: implications for lung homeostasis, repair, metabolism, disease, and drug action. J Appl Physiol (1985). 2011;110(6):1732–47.

61. Zaslona Z, Case S, Early JO, Lalor SJ, McLoughlin RM, Curtis AM, et al. The circadian protein BMAL1 in myeloid cells is a negative regulator of allergic asthma. Am J Physiol Lung Cell Mol Physiol. 2017;312(6):L855–60.

62. Esnault S, Fang Y, Kelly EA, Sedgwick JB, Fine J, Malter JS, et al. Circadian changes in granulocyte-macrophage colony-stimulating factor message in circulating eosinophils. Ann Allergy Asthma Immunol. 2007;98(1):75–82.

63. Nakao A, Nakamura Y, Shibata S. The circadian clock functions as a potent regulator of allergic reaction. Allergy. 2015;70(5):467–73.

64. Ando N, Nakamura Y, Ishimaru K, Ogawa H, Okumura K, Shimada S, et al. Allergen-specific basophil reactivity exhibits daily variations in seasonal allergic rhinitis. Allergy. 2015;70(3):319–22.

65. Fidan V, Alp HH, Gozeler M, Karaaslan O, Binay O, Cingi C. Variance of melatonin and cortisol rhythm in patients with allergic rhinitis. Am J Otolaryngol. 2013;34(5):416–9.

66. Gonzalez-Nunez V, Valero AL, Mullol J. Impact of sleep as a specific marker of quality of life in allergic rhinitis. Curr Allergy Asthma Rep. 2013;13(2):131–41.

67. Honma A, Yamada Y, Nakamaru Y, Fukuda S, Honma K, Honma S. Glucocorticoids reset the nasal circadian clock in mice. Endocrinology. 2015;156(11):4302–11.

68. Camfferman D, Kennedy JD, Gold M, Martin AJ, Lushington K. Eczema and sleep and its relationship to daytime functioning in children. Sleep Med Rev. 2010;14(6):359–69.

69. Fishbein AB, Vitaterna O, Haugh IM, Bavishi AA, Zee PC, Turek FW, et al. Nocturnal eczema: review of sleep and circadian rhythms in children with atopic dermatitis and future research directions. J Allergy Clin Immunol. 2015;136(5):1170–7.

70. Takita E, Yokota S, Tahara Y, Hirao A, Aoki N, Nakamura Y, et al. Biological clock dysfunction exacerbates contact hypersensitivity in mice. Br J Dermatol. 2013;168(1):39–46.

71. Stull D, McBride D, Tian H, Gimenez Arnau A, Maurer M, Marsland A, et al. Analysis of disease activity categories in chronic spontaneous/idiopathic urticaria. Br J Dermatol. 2017;177:1093–101.

72. Maurer M, Abuzakouk M, Berard F, Canonica W, Oude Elberink H, Gimenez-Arnau A, et al. The burden of chronic spontaneous urticaria is substantial: real-world evidence from ASSURE-CSU. Allergy. 2017;72:2005–16.

73. Friedman BS, Steinberg SC, Meggs WJ, Kaliner MA, Frieri M, Metcalfe DD. Analysis of plasma histamine levels in patients with mast cell disorders. Am J Med. 1989;87(6):649–54.

74. Grattan CE, Dawn G, Gibbs S, Francis DM. Blood basophil numbers in chronic ordinary urticaria and healthy controls: diurnal variation, influence of loratadine and prednisolone and relationship to disease activity. Clin Exp Allergy. 2003;33(3):337–41.

75. Nakamura Y, Nakano N, Ishimaru K, Ando N, Katoh R, Suzuki-Inoue K, et al. Inhibition of IgE-mediated allergic reactions by pharmacologically targeting the circadian clock. J Allergy Clin Immunol. 2016;137(4):1226–35.

76. Ando N, Nakamura Y, Aoki R, Ishimaru K, Ogawa H, Okumura K, et al. Circadian gene clock regulates Psoriasis-like skin inflammation in mice. J Investig Dermatol. 2015;135(12):3001–8.

19

Tiotropium in asthma: back to the future of anticholinergic treatment

Matteo Bonini[1]*⏺ and Nicola Scichilone[2]

Abstract

Asthma is among the most common chronic diseases worldwide; however, despite progresses in the understanding of the patho-physiological mechanisms and advances in the development of new therapeutic options and strategies, the disease remains uncontrolled in a not trivial proportion of subjects. Thus, the need of new molecules to treat the underlying biological and functional abnormalities and to control symptoms is strongly advocated by clinicians. In this scenario, the most recent GINA guidelines have included the use of tiotropium bromide in the most severe and uncontrolled forms of the disease, in addition to treatment with inhaled corticosteroid plus long acting beta adrenergic agents. Indeed, a large body of evidence has accumulated to support the use of tiotropium bromide in asthma. The current review paper provides a state of the art systematic revision of findings on the efficacy and safety of tiotropium in the adult and paediatric asthma population. To this aim, electronic searches were undertaken in the most common scientific databases from the date of inception to March 2017. Robust and high quality evidence showed that tiotropium is effective and safe in both adults and children/adolescents. Predictive markers of response have been also suggested, as well as cost–benefit analyses reported. The tiotropium bronchodilator effect seems to be not solely related to the reduction of the smooth muscle tone. However, the observations on anti-inflammatory properties or reduction in mucus production, despite highly interesting, have been only demonstrated in in vitro studies and animal models, therefore advocating for further specifically designed investigations.

Keywords: Anticholinergic, Antimuscarinic, Asthma, Bronchodilation, Control, Endotype, Exacerbation, Phenotype, Tiotropium

Background

Asthma is a major health concern worldwide, with a global prevalence of approximately 300 million, and an estimation of increasing figures up to 400 million people worldwide by 2025 [1]. Asthma is characterized by airway inflammation, reversible airway obstruction, and airway hyperresponsiveness which lead to respiratory symptoms that vary in terms of frequency and severity. Despite treatment per management guidelines [2], a vast proportion of patients experiences uncontrolled forms of the disease [3], thus representing a relevant unmet medical need. Indeed, uncontrolled asthma is responsible for impaired quality of life, increased number of visits to the emergency room and hospitalizations and disproportionate use of healthcare resources [4].

The observed variability in clinical response to currently available therapies has been related to distinctive asthma phenotypes and endotypes [5–8]. However, the evidence of poor control of symptoms despite novel and more targeted treatments [9] has led to explore novel treatment strategies. In this respect, anticholinergic drugs are being considered an alternative bronchodilator therapeutic option to beta-2 agonists for asthma. Beta-2 adrenergic drugs are the mainstay of asthma management and are the most commonly adopted treatment for preventing and reversing bronchial obstruction [10], however high heterogeneity in individual responses, occurrence of tolerance and side-effects have been reported with their use [11–13]. It is known that ancient Ayurvedic medicine already used *Datura stramonium* (a plant with anticholinergic effects) for asthma treatment.

*Correspondence: m.bonini@imperial.ac.uk
[1] Airways Division, Airways Disease Section, National Heart and Lung Institute (NHLI), Royal Brompton Hospital & Imperial College, Dovehouse Street, London SW3 6LY, UK
Full list of author information is available at the end of the article

Subsequently, the discovery of atropine, a potent competitive inhibitor of acetylcholine at postganglionic muscarinic receptors, and more importantly the demonstration of the importance of the parasympathetic nervous system in bronchoconstriction, renewed interest on the potential value of antimuscarinic agents in asthma [10]. Vagal innervation is in fact currently considered the major determinant of airway tone and represents the reversible component of airflow obstruction [14]. An up-regulated release of acetylcholine (ACh) causes an increased bronchial tone, bronchial hyperresponsiveness and reflex bronchoconstriction, thus leading to the narrowing of the airways. Bronchoconstriction is primarily regulated by five muscarinic receptors (M_R); M_1, M_2 and M_3 are expressed in the lung and in the bronchial tree. M_{1R} are mainly distributed in the peripheral lung tissue and in the alveolar walls within parasympathetic ganglia and regulate cholinergic transmission. M_{2R} are found in post-ganglionic nerves where they serve as auto-receptors, on smooth muscle cells (SM) and on fibroblasts. M_{3R} are predominantly expressed in SM cells and mediate SM ACh-induced contraction. In central airways, SM contraction is mediated by vagal innervation, whereas in the peripheral airways the function of M_{3R} is mediated by ACh released in response to inflammatory stimuli. M_{3R} can also be found in sub-mucosal glands where they are responsible for mucus secretion. Among the short-acting anti-cholinergic molecules, ipratropium bromide and oxitropium bromide have long been adopted as asthma relievers. Furthermore, a large body of evidence has accumulated in recent years to support the use of the long-acting anti-muscarinic tiotropium bromide in asthma [15, 16], and its use is now recommended by international guidelines (GINA 2016) for chronic treatment of adult patients with most severe and frequently exacerbated asthma [2], in addition to inhaled corticosteroids (ICS) in combination with long-acting beta-2 agonists (LABA). It has been also suggested that tiotropium exerts its beneficial effects through mechanisms other than the reduction on the cholinergic tone of the airways, some of which still need to be confirmed in humans [17].

The current paper aims at providing a state of the art systematic review of efficacy and safety of tiotropium in asthma. To this scope, the main findings on the role of tiotropium in pediatric and adult asthmatic populations were selected in a rigorous and unbiased manner, and reported in light of the current pharmacological treatment recommendations for asthma.

Methods

Electronic searches were undertaken in MEDLINE, Web of Science, the Cochrane Library and Scopus databases. The registers were searched using the keywords "asthma" AND "tiotropium" from the date of inception to March 2017. Following the removal of duplicates, the authors independently selected papers of potential interest on the basis of titles and abstracts for a full-text assessment and reached an agreement in cases of lack of consensus. Original studies of any design (except for single case reports due to low quality), published in English, performed in humans and primarily addressing the efficacy and/or safety of tiotropium in asthma were considered eligible for being included in the present review. In addition, reference lists of included manuscripts, recent reviews and textbooks were hand-searched for further relevant citations.

Results

The search strategy yielded 1864 articles (MEDLINE 211, Web of Science 420, the Cochrane Library 229 and Scopus 1004). Among these, 30 studies met the criteria for being included in the review and are reported below according to their primary aim (i.e. efficacy or safety). In regards to efficacy further distinctions have been also made depending on the target study population (i.e. adults or children/adolescents), the type of the effects investigated (bronchodilator or non-bronchodilator) and the findings on predictive markers of response and cost–benefit (Fig. 1).

Bronchodilator effects in adults

A proof of concept double blind, randomised, placebo-controlled, crossover study aiming to evaluate the effects of halving ICS dosage adding salmeterol, or salmeterol plus tiotropium was conducted in 2007 [18]. Eighteen non-smoking severe asthmatics were run-in for 4 weeks on HFA-fluticasone propionate 1000 mcg daily, and were then randomised to 4 weeks of either (a) HFA-fluticasone propionate 500 mcg twice a day + salmeterol 100 mcg twice a day + HFA-tiotropium bromide 18 mcg once a day; or (b) fluticasone propionate 500 mcg twice a day + salmeterol 100 mcg twice a day + matched placebo. Spirometry and body plethysmography were performed. Adding salmeterol to half the dose of fluticasone led to a significant improvement vs. baseline in the morning peak expiratory flow (PEF) and airway resistance (RAW). The combination salmeterol/tiotropium produced similar improvements in PEF and RAW, but also significantly improved the forced expiratory volume in the first second (FEV1) by 0.17 l (CI 0.01–0.32 l), FVC 0.24 l (CI 0.05–0.43 l) and reduced fraction exhaled NO (FeNO) by 2.86 ppb (CI 0.12–5.6 ppb).

In order to assess if there was any difference among the protective effect of ipratropium, oxitropium and tiotropium against methacholine-induced bronchoconstriction, 44 patients with intermittent asthma and a PD20

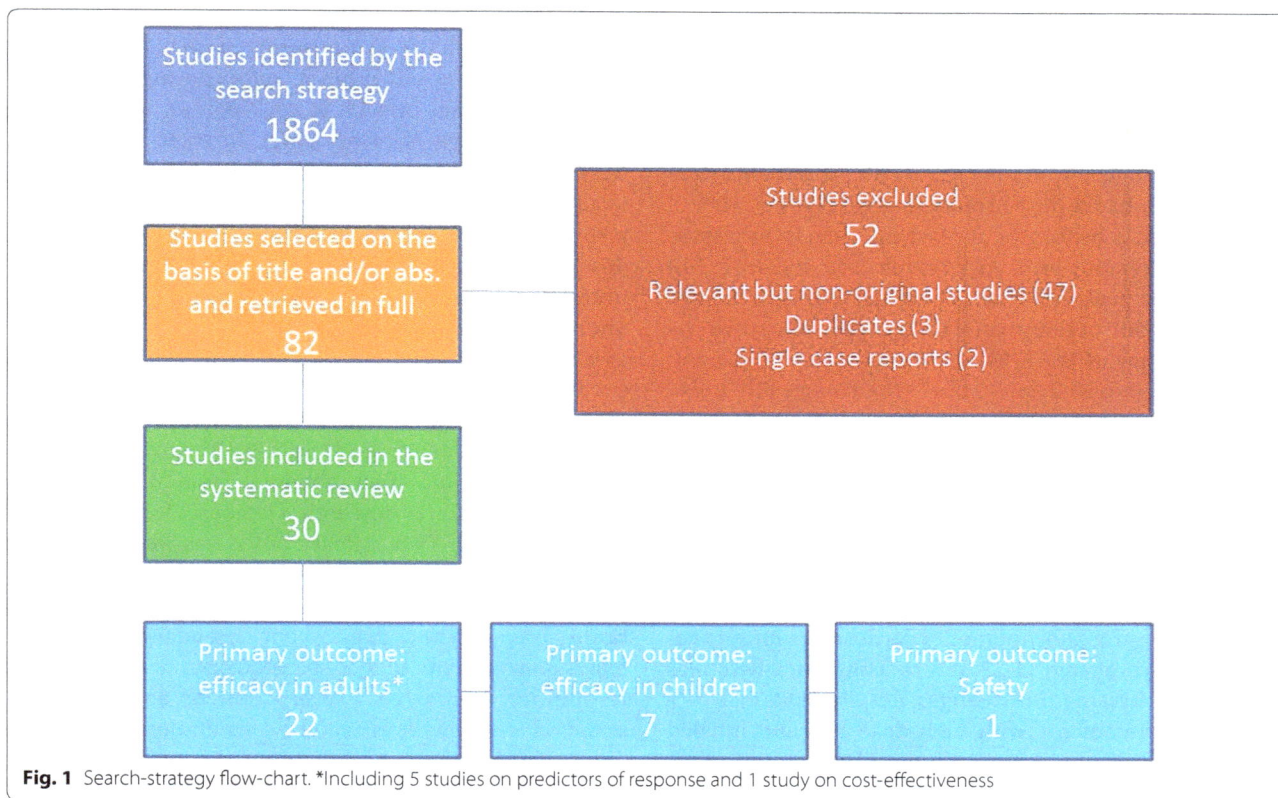

Fig. 1 Search-strategy flow-chart. *Including 5 studies on predictors of response and 1 study on cost-effectiveness

FEV1 < 200 mcg were selected [19]. At baseline, they had a mean FEV1% predicted of 98.8 ± 8.5 and mean PD15 FEV1 of 111.8 ± 61.0 mcg. After 72 h, all patients underwent a second methacholine challenge being given ipratropium (40 μg by MDI; n = 14), oxitropium (200 μg by MDI; n = 14) or tiotropium (18 μg by Handihaler; n = 16) 60 min before the test. The FEV1% increase was significantly higher in the oxitropium (6.7 ± 4.8%) and tiotropium groups (6.1 ± 2.5%) compared to the ipratropium group (3.8 ± 1.9%). Furthermore, after oxitropium and tiotropium, the PD15 (1628 ± 955.7 and 1595.5 ± 990 μg, respectively) was significantly higher in comparison to that following ipratropium (532.2 ± 434.8 μg).

In a three-way, double-blind, triple-dummy crossover trial involving 210 patients with inadequately controlled asthma, the addition of tiotropium to ICS, as compared with a doubling of the dose of the ICS (primary superiority comparison) or the addition of the LABA salmeterol (secondary non-inferiority comparison) was evaluated [20]. The use of tiotropium resulted superior in the primary outcome, when compared with a doubling of the dose of ICS, as assessed by measuring PEF, with a mean difference of 25.8 l/min (p < 0.001) and in most secondary outcomes (i.e. evening PEF, the proportion of asthma control days, FEV1 before bronchodilation and daily symptom scores). The addition of tiotropium was also non-inferior to the addition of salmeterol for all assessed outcomes and increased the pre-bronchodilator FEV1 more than what did salmeterol, with a difference of 0.11 l (p = 0.003).

Kerstjens et al. sought to compare through a randomized, double-blind, crossover study with three 8-week treatment periods, the efficacy and safety of 2 doses of tiotropium (5 and 10 mcg daily) administered through the Respimat inhaler compared with placebo as add-on therapy in patients with uncontrolled severe asthma, despite maintenance treatment with at least a high-dose ICS plus a LABA [21]. The primary endpoint was the peak FEV1 at the end of each treatment period. In the 107 adult patients enrolled, the peak FEV1 was significantly higher with 5 mcg (difference: 139 ml; 95% CI 96–181 ml) and 10 mcg (difference: 170 ml; 95% CI 128–213 ml) of tiotropium than with placebo (both p < 0.0001). No significant difference was observed between the active doses. Trough FEV1 and daily home PEF measurements at the end of the dosing interval were also higher with tiotropium at both doses. Adverse events (AE) were balanced across groups except for dry mouth, which was more common on tiotropium 10 mcg.

In two replicate, randomized, controlled trials involving 912 patients with asthma who were receiving ICS and LABA, authors compared the effect on lung function and exacerbations of adding tiotropium (a total dose of 5 µg) or placebo, both delivered by a soft-mist inhaler once daily for 48 weeks [22]. All the patients were symptomatic, had a post-bronchodilator FEV1 ≤ 80% of predicted and a history of at least one severe exacerbation in the previous year. At 24 weeks, the mean (± SE) change in the peak FEV1 from baseline was significantly greater with tiotropium than with placebo in the two trials: a difference of 86 ± 34 ml in trial 1 (p = 0.01) and 154 ± 32 ml in trial 2 (p < 0.001). The trough FEV1 also significantly improved in both trials with tiotropium, as compared with placebo. Furthermore, the addition of tiotropium increased the time to the first severe exacerbation (282 days vs. 226 days), with an overall reduction of 21% in the risk of a severe exacerbation (hazard ratio, 0.79; p = 0.03). AE were similar in the two groups and no deaths occurred.

The effects of a tiotropium single-dose on lung function were investigated in 18 severe asthmatics with and without emphysematous changes despite maximal recommended treatments with high-dose ICS and inhaled LABA through a double-blind, placebo-controlled, crossover study [23]. The primary efficacy outcome was the relative change in FEV1 from baseline to 60 min. Subsequently, the patients were treated with tiotropium inhaled once daily for 12 weeks in an open label manner, and lung function and symptoms were evaluated. At baseline, patients with emphysema had a mean FEV1% predicted of 55.9% before tiotropium and 56.8% before placebo, while in those without emphysema this was 77.4 and 77.6% respectively. In the first group, the increase from baseline FEV1 was 12.6% higher after tiotropium than placebo, while in the second the improvement was 5.4% higher after tiotropium than placebo. Chronic tiotropium administration also resulted in improved lung function and symptoms, particularly in asthmatics with emphysema.

To further investigate the efficacy and safety of three different doses of tiotropium Respimat as add-on to ICS in symptomatic patients with moderate persistent asthma, a randomised, double-blind, placebo-controlled, four-way crossover study, was conducted [24]. Patients were randomised to tiotropium Respimat 5, 2.5, 1.25 µg or placebo, once daily in the evening. Each treatment was administered for 4 weeks, without washout between treatment periods. Eligibility criteria included FEV1 60–90% of predicted and a seven-question Asthma Control Questionnaire (ACQ-7) score ≥ 1.5. Patients were required to continue maintenance treatment with stable medium-dose ICS for at least 4 weeks prior to and during the treatment period. LABA were not permitted during the treatment phase. The primary efficacy endpoint was peak FEV1 measured within 3 h after dosing (peak FEV1 0–3 h) at the end of each 4-week period, analysed as a response (change from baseline). In total, 149 patients were randomised and 141 completed the study. Statistically significant improvements in peak FEV1 0–3 h response were observed with each tiotropium Respimat dose versus placebo (all p < 0.0001) being the largest with tiotropium 5 µg (188 ml). Trough FEV1 and FEV1 area under the curve (AUC) responses were also significantly greater with each tiotropium dose than with placebo (all p < 0.0001). Occurrence of AE was comparable between placebo and all tiotropium Respimat groups.

Medical records of adults with asthma who were prescribed tiotropium were obtained from the UK Optimum Patient Care Research Database for the period 2001–2013 [25]. Two primary outcomes were compared in the year before (baseline) and the year after (outcome) addition of tiotropium: exacerbations (i.e. asthma-related hospital emergency department attendance, inpatient admission, or acute oral corticosteroid course) and acute respiratory events (i.e. exacerbation or antibiotic prescription with lower respiratory consultation). Secondary outcomes included lung function tests and short-acting β2 agonist (SABA) usage. Comparing baseline and outcome years of the 2042 study patients, the percentage of patients having at least one exacerbation decreased from 37 to 27% (p = 0.001) and the percentage of those having at least one acute respiratory event decreased from 58 to 47% (p = 0.001).

To investigate whether the dosing regimen of tiotropium, delivered via the Respimat SoftMist inhaler, affected 24 h bronchodilator efficacy and safety in asthmatic patients who were symptomatic despite medium-dose ICS, a randomised, double-blind, placebo-controlled, crossover study with 4-week treatment periods of tiotropium 5 mcg (once-daily) and 2.5 mcg (twice-daily) was performed [26]. The primary efficacy endpoint was FEV1 AUC from 0 to 24 h (0–24 h) at the end of each treatment period. Secondary endpoints included peak FEV1 0–24 h, trough FEV1, morning and evening PEF and pharmacokinetic assessments. Ninety-four patients were randomised and 89 (94.7%) completed the study. Significant and comparable bronchodilation was achieved over a 24-h period with both tiotropium dosing regimens. FEV1 AUC 0–24 h response (mean ± SE) was significantly greater with both tiotropium dosing regimens (once-daily 5 mcg: 158 ± 24 ml; twice-daily 2.5 mcg; 149 ± 24 ml; both p < 0.01) when compared with placebo. Improvements in peak FEV1 0–24 h, trough FEV1 and pre-dose a.m./p.m. PEF with both dosing regimens versus placebo were also statistically significant, with no difference between the tiotropium treatment regimens. Total systemic exposure and tolerability were comparable between study arms.

The study of Rajanandh and coworkers aimed to compare the 6 month efficacy and safety of formoterol (12 mcg), montelukast (10 mg), doxofylline (400 mg), or tiotropium (18 mcg) in combination with a low-dose budesonide (400 mcg) in patients with mild to moderate persistent asthma [27]. Outcomes included FEV1, Saint George Respiratory Questionnaire (SGRQ) scores, asthma symptom scores (daytime and night time), assessment of tolerability and rescue medication use. A total of 297 patients completed the study. In all 4 groups, significant improvements were observed in all the outcome measures, with formoterol treatment having greater and earlier improvements than the other 3 add-on medications. No patients discontinued the treatment because of AE.

Two 24-week, replicate, randomised, double-blind, placebo-controlled, parallel-group, active comparator trials were performed at 233 sites in 14 countries [28]. Eligible patients were aged 18–75 years with symptomatic asthma and a pre-bronchodilator FEV1 of 60–90% of predicted despite use of medium-dose ICS and had never smoked or were ex-smokers for $\geq$ 1 year with $\leq$ 10 pack-years. Patients were randomly assigned (1:1:1:1), with computer-generated pseudorandom numbers, to receive once-daily tiotropium 2.5 or 5 µg, twice-daily salmeterol 50 µg, or placebo, while maintaining ICS. Pre-specified co-primary endpoints, assessed at week 24, were peak FEV1 response, measured within the first 3 h after evening dosing; trough FEV1 response; and responder rate assessed according to the ACQ-7. Among the 2103 patients enrolled, 519 were randomly assigned to tiotropium 5 µg, 520 to tiotropium 2.5 µg group, 541 to salmeterol and 523 to placebo. A total of 1972 patients (94%) completed the study. Peak and trough FEV1 responses were significantly greater with tiotropium and salmeterol than with placebo and were similar in both studies. With pooled data, difference versus placebo in peak FEV1 was 185 ml (95% CI 146–223) in the tiotropium 5 µg group, 223 ml (95% CI 185–262) in the tiotropium 2.5 µg group, and 196 ml (95% CI 158–234) in the salmeterol group (all p < 0.0001); difference in trough FEV1 was 146 ml (95% CI 105–188), 180 ml (95% CI 138–221), and 114 ml (95% CI 73–155) respectively (all p < 0.0001). There were more ACQ-7 responders in the tiotropium 5 µg (OR 1.32, 95% CI 1.02–1.71; p = 0.035) and 2.5 µg (1.33, 1.03–1.72; p = 0.031) groups, and the salmeterol group (1.46, 1.13–1.89; p = 0.0039), than in the placebo group. Forty-eight patients had serious AE with no difference among the four arms (tiotropium 5 µg n = 11, tiotropium 2.5 µg n = 12, salmeterol n = 11, placebo n = 14).

The primary objective of the study performed by Paggiaro et al. was to evaluate the efficacy of once-daily tiotropium Respimat, compared to placebo, as add-on therapy to low- to medium-dose ICS in adults with symptomatic asthma [29]. A phase III, double-blind, placebo-controlled trial was conducted. Adults with symptomatic asthma (n = 464) receiving 200–400 mcg of budesonide or equivalent doses and a with pre-bronchodilator FEV1 of 60–90% of predicted normal values were randomized to 12 weeks of treatment with once-daily tiotropium Respimat 5, 2.5 mcg, or placebo, as add-on therapy. The primary endpoint was peak FEV1 (0–3 h) response. After 12 weeks, both tiotropium doses were superior to placebo (adjusted mean difference from placebo: 5 mcg = 128 ml; 2.5 mcg = 159 ml (both p < 0.001). Both doses of tiotropium were also superior to placebo with regard to the secondary endpoints (i.e. trough FEV1, FEV1 area under the curve, morning and evening PEF). At last, AE were comparable across the treatment groups.

A Phase II, randomized, double-blind, two-way crossover study comparing two daily dosing regimens of tiotropium for 4 weeks, once-daily 5 mcg (evening dosing) or twice-daily 2.5 mcg (morning and evening dosing), as add-on to maintenance therapy with ICS (400–800 mcg budesonide or equivalent) as controller medication, was conducted to confirm the 24-h bronchodilator efficacy and pharmacokinetic profile of tiotropium Respimat in adults with symptomatic asthma [30]. There was no washout between treatment periods. An increase in the area under the curve of the 24-h FEV1 profile from baseline was observed following once-daily tiotropium 5 mcg (217 ml) and twice-daily 2.5 mcg (219 ml), with no difference between the two regimens. In a subset of the study population, total tiotropium exposure, expressed as area under the plasma concentration versus time curve over 24 h, was comparable between dosing regimens. Unexpected tiotropium plasma levels were observed in two patients, possibly because of contamination.

The aim of the retrospective analysis performed by Abadoglu and Berkto was to assess the effectiveness of tiotropium as an add-on therapy to the standard treatment with high-dose ICS/LABA on asthma control and lung function in patients with severe asthma poorly controlled [31]. Of the 633 asthmatics, 64 (10.1%) patients who were tiotropium add-on treated at least for 3 months were evaluated. Number of exacerbations, emergency department visits, hospitalizations and lung functions of patients belonging to 12 months before starting add-on treatment were compared with those of 12 months after starting add-on treatment. The mean duration of add-on tiotropium treatment was 8.3 ± 0.5 months. Tiotropium improved asthma control in 42.2% of patients and decreased the number of emergency department visits and hospitalizations in 46.9 and 50.0% of them, respectively. While at baseline mean FEV1 and forced vital capacity (FVC) were 57.5 ± 1.9 and 74.3 ± 15.6% respectively, after 12 months of add-on tiotropium these rates increased to 65.5 ± 1.9 and 82.5 ± 15.1%.

A recent study aimed at assessing the effect of tiotropium on airway geometry and inflammation in patients with asthma who were symptomatic despite treatment with ICS/LABA [32]. A total of 53 patients with symptomatic asthma, who received ICS-LABA and who had a pre-bronchodilator FEV1 of 60–90% of the predicted value were randomized to the addition of tiotropium 5 mcg once daily (n = 25) or no add-on (n = 28) to maintenance therapy for 48 weeks. Quantitative computed tomography, FeNO and pulmonary function were measured. Compared to maintenance therapy, the addition of tiotropium significantly decreased airway wall area (WA) and wall thickness (T) corrected for the body surface area (BSA), and improved airflow obstruction. Changes in WA/BSA and T/BSA were significantly correlated with the change in predicted FEV1 (r = − 0.87, p < 0.001, and r = − 0.82, p < 0.001, respectively). No significant difference in the change of FeNO was instead observed between the two treatment groups.

At last, the effects of an inhaled single dose of tiotropium on lung function were investigated through a double-blind, placebo-controlled, crossover study in 9 smoking asthmatics and in 9 who have never smoked, all being treated with ICS and other asthma controllers [33]. Lung function was measured at baseline and at 1, 3, and 24 h after inhalation of 18 mcg of tiotropium or placebo. The primary outcome was a change in FEV1 from baseline. Tiotropium resulted in improved lung function and symptoms both in current smoker and non-smoker asthmatics.

Bronchodilator effects in children and adolescents

In a case series of 71 paediatric patients, tiotropium was shown to be beneficial in 3 distinct subgroups: as add-on therapy to asthmatics on maximal maintenance medication, as an alternative to high-dose ICS in patients experiencing significant side effects, and in subjects with chronic productive cough as predominant symptom [34]. Interestingly, almost half of the patients who started tiotropium were able to decrease the dose of ICS or stop the use of LABA.

The efficacy and safety of three doses of tiotropium (5, 2.5 and 1.25 μg), administered once-daily via Respimat SoftMist inhaler, were investigated compared to placebo in 139 asthmatic adolescents, symptomatic despite ICS treatment [35]. The change in peak FEV1 within 3 h post-dose from baseline (peak FEV1 0–3 h) was chosen as primary efficacy endpoint and resulted significantly improved in subjects who were administered tiotropium 5 μg. Overall incidence of AE, for the majority mild to moderate, was balanced across treatment groups, with no dose dependent observations.

In a similar Phase II, double-blind, placebo-controlled, incomplete-crossover, dose-ranging study, children aged 6–11 years with symptomatic asthma were randomised to receive once-daily tiotropium Respimat 5, 2.5, 1.25 μg or placebo, add-on to medium-dose ICS with or without a leukotriene modifier, during a 12-week treatment period [36]. For the primary end point (peak FEV1 0–3 h), the adjusted mean responses with tiotropium Respimat 5 μg (272 ml), 2.5 μg (290 ml) and 1.25 μg (261 ml) were all significantly greater than with placebo (185 ml; p = 0.0002, p < 0.0001 and p = 0.0011, respectively). Furthermore, the safety and tolerability of all doses of tiotropium were comparable with those of placebo, with no serious side effects and no events leading to discontinuation.

Eighty children with newly diagnosed moderate persistent asthma were randomly assigned to fluticasone propionate aerosol or fluticasone propionate aerosol plus tiotropium for 12 weeks [37]. Lung function was significantly improved in both groups at 4, 8, and 12 weeks compared with baseline (p < 0.01) and the control group (p < 0.05). There was no significant difference in the incidence of severe asthma between the two groups (36.3 and 26.8%, respectively). Compared with the control group, the number of days and frequency of SABA use, as well as the awakenings at night were significantly reduced in the tiotropium group. There were no severe AE in either of the study groups.

Hamelmann and coauthors sought to assess the efficacy and safety of once-daily tiotropium Respimat in a phase III trial in adolescent patients with moderate symptomatic asthma [38]. In this 48-week, double-blind, placebo-controlled, parallel-group study, 398 patients aged 12–17 years were randomized to receive 5 or 2.5 mcg of once-daily tiotropium or placebo, administered through the Respimat device every evening, as add-on treatment to ICS background therapy with or without a leukotriene receptor antagonist; LABA therapy was not permitted during the trial. Improvement in peak FEV1 0–3 h at 24 weeks (primary end point) was statistically significant with both tiotropium doses compared with placebo: 5 mcg of tiotropium, 174 ml (95% CI 76–272 ml); 2.5 mcg of tiotropium, 134 ml (95% CI 34–234 ml). Significant improvements in trough FEV1 at week 24 (secondary end point) were also observed with the 5 mcg dose only. Trends for improvement in asthma control and health-related quality of life over the 48-week treatment period were observed. The overall incidence of AE, most mild or moderate in intensity, was comparable across the 3 treatment groups.

The same authors enrolled 392 adolescents, aged 12–17 years, with severe symptomatic asthma in a phase III double-blind parallel-group trial, to receive once-daily tiotropium 5, 2.5 μg, or placebo, as an add-on to ICS plus other controller therapies over 12 weeks [39]. The primary and key secondary end-points were change from baseline (response) in peak FEV1 0–3 h and trough FEV1 after 12 weeks of treatment. Tiotropium 5 and 2.5 μg provided numerical improvements in peak FEV1 0–3 h (90 ml, p = 0.104; 111 ml, p = 0.046, respectively) and trough FEV1 response, as well as in asthma control were observed with both tiotropium doses, compared with placebo. The safety and tolerability of tiotropium were similar with those of placebo.

A 12-week, phase III, double-blind, placebo-controlled, parallel-group trial sought to assess the efficacy and safety of tiotropium Respimat as add-on to background therapy in children with severe symptomatic asthma. Participants aged 6–11 years (n = 401) were randomized to receive once-daily tiotropium Respimat 5 mcg (2 puffs of 2.5 mcg) or 2.5 mcg (2 puffs of 1.25 mcg), or placebo [40]. Compared with placebo, tiotropium 5 mcg, but not 2.5 mcg, significantly improved the primary endpoint (peak FEV1 0–3 h) and the key secondary endpoint (trough FEV1). The safety and tolerability of tiotropium were comparable with those of placebo.

Predictors of response

A total of 138 severe asthmatics with reduced lung function despite guideline recommended treatment were randomly assigned to additional tiotropium 18 mcg once a day and lung function parameters were measured every 4 weeks [41]. Responders were defined as those with an improvement of $\geq$ 15% or 200 ml in FEV1 that was maintained for at least 8 successive weeks. Single nucleotide polymorphisms (SNPs) in CHRM1–3 (coding muscarinic receptors M_1–M_3), as well as in the beta-2 adrenergic receptor (ADRB2) were recorded in 80 of the 138 asthmatics. Forty-six of the 138 asthmatics (33.3%) responded to tiotropium treatment. Logistic regression analyses (adjusted for age, gender, and smoking status) showed that ADRB2 Arg16Gly was significantly associated with a positive response to tiotropium.

The efficacy and safety of tiotropium compared to salmeterol and placebo in ADRB2 Arg16Arg adult patients with asthma not controlled by ICS alone was assessed in a double-blind, double-dummy, placebo-controlled trial [42]. After a 4-week run-in period with 50 mcg of twice-daily salmeterol, 388 asthmatic patients were randomized 1:1:1 to 16 weeks of treatment with 5 mcg of tiotropium Respimat administered once daily, 50 mcg of salmeterol administered twice daily through a metered-dose inhaler, or placebo. ICS regimens were maintained throughout

the trial. Changes in weekly PEF from the last week of the run-in period to the last week of treatment (primary endpoint) were $-$ 3.9 $\pm$ 4.87 l/min (n = 128) for tiotropium and $-$ 3.2 $\pm$ 4.64 l/min (n = 134) for salmeterol, both significantly superior to placebo ($-$ 24.6 $\pm$ 4.84 l/min, n = 125). Tiotropium was also non-inferior to salmeterol. AE were comparable across treatments.

More recently, a multisite, open-label, parallel-group, randomized clinical trial aimed to compare the effectiveness and safety of tiotropium vs LABA, when used with ICS in black adults with asthma and to determine whether allelic variation at the Arg16Gly locus of the ADRB2 gene was associated with treatment response [43]. It was in fact been reported that black populations may be disproportionately affected by LABA risks [44]. Patients eligible for, or receiving, step 3–4 combination therapy per National Heart Lung and Blood Institute (NHLBI) guidelines, were administered ICS plus either once-daily tiotropium (n = 532) or twice-daily LABA (n = 538) and were followed up for up to 18 months. Patients underwent genotyping at baseline and then attended study visits at 1, 6, 12 and 18 months, also completing monthly questionnaires. The primary outcome was time to asthma exacerbation. Secondary outcomes included patient-reported outcomes (Asthma Quality of Life Questionnaire, ACQ, Asthma Symptom Utility Index, and Asthma Symptom-Free Days questionnaire), FEV1, rescue medication use, asthma deteriorations, and AE. There was no difference between LABA + ICS vs tiotropium + ICS in time to first exacerbation, change in FEV1 at 12 and 18 months, ACQ score and other patient-reported outcomes at 18 months. Arg16Gly ADRB2 alleles were not associated with differences in the effects of tiotropium + ICS vs. LABA + ICS.

With the aim to describe individual and differential responses of asthmatic patients to salmeterol and tiotropium when added to ICS, as well as predictors of a positive clinical response, data from the double-blind, 3-way, crossover "NHLBI Asthma Clinical Research Network's Tiotropium Bromide as an Alternative to Increased Inhaled Glucocorticoid in Patients Inadequately Controlled on a Lower Dose of Inhaled Corticosteroid trial" were analysed [45]. Although approximately equal numbers of patients showed a differential response to salmeterol and tiotropium in terms of morning PEF (n = 90 and n = 78, respectively) and asthma control days (n = 49 and n = 53, respectively), more showed a differential response to tiotropium for FEV1 (n = 104) than salmeterol (n = 62). An acute response to SABA (i.e. albuterol) significantly predicted a positive clinical response to tiotropium for FEV1 and morning PEF, as did a decreased FEV1/FVC. Higher cholinergic tone was also a predictor, whereas ethnicity, sex, atopy, IgE level, sputum eosinophil count, fraction exhaled nitric oxide, asthma duration, and body mass index were not.

Additionally, to determine whether the efficacy of tiotropium add-on therapy is dependent on patients' baseline characteristics two randomized, double-blind, parallel-group, twin trials of once-daily tiotropium Respimat 5 mcg add-on to ICS plus LABA were performed in parallel in patients with severe symptomatic asthma [46]. Exploratory subgroup analyses were performed to determine whether results were influenced by baseline characteristics. Patients were randomized to receive tiotropium (n = 456) or placebo (n = 456). Tiotropium improved lung function, reduced the risk of asthma exacerbations and asthma worsening, and improved asthma symptom control, compared with placebo, independently from baseline characteristics including gender, age, body mass index, disease duration, age at asthma onset, FEV1% predicted and reversibility.

Non-bronchodilator effects

Although the use of tiotropium in asthma has been long advocated to exert its activity on airway tone, alternative mechanisms have been demonstrated in in vitro studies and in animal models to explain the efficacy of LAMA. Indeed, since the different cells involved in the inflammatory cascade express muscarinic receptors, it is plausible to hypothesize that tiotropium can act by interfering (or modulating) the function of these cells. These ancillary effects of tiotropium could corroborate the bronchodilator effect of the drug. Given the potential relevance of these findings for asthmatic patients, in addition to the evidence retrieved through the search strategy, the principal data on non-bronchodilator effects of tiotropium are summarized below.

The influx of eosinophils and neutrophils in the airways of asthmatics is in part modulated by M_{3R} activation [47]. Tiotropium has been found to cause a reduction in the eosinophil deposition in the airways [48], by acting directly on M_{3R} present on eosinophils or through the blocking of non-neuronal ACh release from macrophages and epithelial cells. Bühling and coauthors showed in vitro a suppressive activity of tiotropium on the ACh-mediated production of macrophages-derived chemotactic mediators [49]. Eosinophilic recruitment was shown to be affected also by a concomitant administration of tiotropium and budesonide or ciclesonide in animal models [50, 51]. In conjunction with olodaterol, tiotropium showed a synergistic protective effect against allergen-induced hyper-responsiveness in guinea pig models of asthma, inhibiting both the early and late asthmatic phases [52].

Even more important, M_{3R} seem to mediate airway smooth muscle thickening and extracellular matrix deposition. Profita et al. demonstrated an increased expression of M_{1R} and M_{3R} in fibroblasts from COPD and smoker subjects compared with those from healthy subjects [53]. After exposure to ACh, the proliferation of fibroblasts increased, and this phenomenon was downregulated by tiotropium and mediated by M_R, extracellular signal-regulated kinase (ERK) 1/2 and nuclear factor (NF) kappaB. The ACh-induced proliferation of fibroblasts was shown to be inhibited by tiotropium in a dose–response fashion [54]. The anti-remodelling effect of tiotropium was also confirmed by studies in animal models. In mice chronic asthma models tiotropium significantly decreased smooth muscle thickening and peribronchial collagen deposition, with a parallel reduction of Th2-mediated cytokines such as IL5 and IL13 [55].

An additional mechanism through which an anticholinergic drug may exert its beneficial effects in chronic airway diseases is by modulating mucus production. MUC5AC is recognized as the most common mucin gene whose expression is markedly increased in asthma and is mediated by M_{3R} in goblet cells [56]. MUC5AC production from goblet cells in mice was found to be inhibited by selective M_{3R} with tiotropium [57]. The effect of tiotropium on mucus production is not accompanied by modification of the rheological properties of mucus.

Finally, since cough is an important symptoms of asthma, and a cough-variant asthma has been described in clinical practice, the effect of LAMAs on cough reflex have been explored. Birrell and colleagues showed that tiotropium, but not glycopyrronium, was able to modulate the cough reflex through the transient-potential vanilloid receptor type-1 (TRPV1) with mechanisms that have not been fully understood, and perhaps not related to the intrinsic anticholinergic activity [58]. In this respect, Mutolo and coworkers recently demonstrated that the beneficial effect of tiotropium on cough involves acid-sensing ion channels and mechanoreceptors [59].

Cost effectiveness

The cost effectiveness of tiotropium therapy as add-on to usual care in asthma patients that are uncontrolled despite treatment with ICS/LABA combination was assessed from the perspective of the UK National Health Service (NHS). A Markov modelled analysis of two clinical trials, developed to determine levels of asthma control and exacerbations, found that add-on tiotropium provided an incremental 0.19 QALYs and £5389 costs over a lifetime horizon, resulting in an incremental cost-effectiveness ratio of £28,383 per QALY gained [60, 61].

Safety

Patients with symptomatic asthma (n = 285), despite treatment with ICS-LABA, were randomised to once-daily tiotropium (5 and 2.5 µg) Respimat for 1 year in a double-blind, placebo-controlled, parallel-group study to evaluate its long-term safety profile [62]. Secondary endpoints included trough FEV1, PEF response and ACQ-7 score. At week 52, AE rates with tiotropium 5, 2.5 µg and placebo were 88.6, 86.8 and 89.5%, respectively. Most commonly reported AE were pharyngitis, nasopharyngitis, asthma, bronchitis and gastroenteritis. In the tiotropium 5, 2.5 µg and placebo groups, 8.8, 5.3 and 5.3% of patients reported drug-related AE; 3.5, 3.5 and 15.8% reported serious AE. At week 52, adjusted mean trough FEV1 and PEF responses were significantly higher with tiotropium 5 µg (but not 2.5 µg) versus placebo. ACQ-7 responder rates were higher with tiotropium 5 and 2.5 µg versus placebo at week 24. Authors concluded that the long-term tiotropium Respimat safety profile was comparable with that of placebo, and associated mainly with mild to moderate AE in patients with symptomatic asthma despite ICS-LABA therapy.

Discussion

Collected findings strongly support a significant beneficial effect of tiotropium on several lung function parameters in both the adult and paediatric asthma populations. Retrieved evidence is of high quality being supported by studies with a robust design (i.e. randomized, double blind clinical trials), performed in large samples and published in top-ranked scientific journals. Most of the data addressed the role of tiotropium delivered by the Respimat soft-mist inhaler, showing best results for the once daily 5 mcg dose. Despite only one trial has been designed and powered for safety as primary outcome (prompting further ad-hoc investigations), the drug has been consistently shown a harmless profile when compared to placebo or other active treatments. Tiotropim has been proven to be effective irrespective of demographic patient characteristics (i.e. gender, age, body mass index, disease duration, age at asthma onset). The studies reporting scores from the Asthma Quality of Life Questionnaire (AQLQ) substantially failed in showing a significant and clinical relevant benefit of tiotropium over LABA/ICS alone despite the effect estimate favoured add-on tiotropium [63]. Conflicting data exist regarding a possible role of ADRB2 single nucleotide polymorphisms in predicting a positive drug response. This aspect might be of high clinical relevance and should deserve further assessment. The efficacy and safety of inhaled LABA in asthmatic patients with the ADRB2 Arg16Arg genotype has been in fact questioned, and the use of antimuscarinic agents may be proposed as an alternative treatment strategy in patients whose symptoms are not controlled by ICS.

In conclusion, the recent positioning of tiotropium as an additional treatment in some forms of asthma is the result of a growing evidence of its efficacy. The anticholinergic effect provides a rationale for the appropriate management of increased bronchomotor tone, which is paramount in chronic airway diseases. The renewing attention to the role of LAMA in asthma has led to the exploration of new pathways. It is plausible to hypothesize that the potent effect of tiotropium is to be attributed to mechanisms other than simply reducing the smooth muscle tone. The observations of anti-inflammatory properties or reduction in mucus production are interesting but at present demonstrated in in vitro studies and in animal models, and advocate for further, specifically designed investigations. Whether the efficacy of tiotropium is a class effect or, as suggested by several studies, a peculiar aspect of the drug is yet to be determined. The research developed and the ongoing/future studies on the demonstration of efficacy and safety of tiotropium in asthma represent an extremely valuable contribution for its optimal management.

Authors' contributions

Both authors equally contributed to the literature search, data collection and drafting of the article. Both authors read and approved the final manuscript.

Author details

[1] Airways Division, Airways Disease Section, National Heart and Lung Institute (NHLI), Royal Brompton Hospital & Imperial College, Dovehouse Street, London SW3 6LY, UK. [2] Department of Biomedicine and Internal and Specialistic Medicine (DIBIMIS), University of Palermo, Palermo, Italy.

References

1. Masoli M, Fabian D, Holt S, Beasley R, Global Initiative for Asthma (GINA) Program. The global burden of asthma: executive summary of the GINA Dissemination Committee report. Allergy. 2004;59(5):469–78.
2. Global INitiative on Asthma. http://ginasthma.org/. Accessed May 2017.
3. Bateman ED, Reddel HK, Eriksson G, Peterson S, Ostlund O, Sears MR, Jenkins C, Humbert M, Buhl R, Harrison TW, Quirce S, O'Byrne PM. Overall asthma control: the relationship between current control and future risk. J Allergy Clin Immunol. 2010;125(3):600–8.
4. Sullivan PW, Ghushchyan VH, Campbell JD, Globe G, Bender B, Magid DJ. Measuring the cost of poor asthma control and exacerbations. J Asthma. 2017;54(1):24–31.
5. Wenzel SE. Asthma: defining of the persistent adult phenotypes. Lancet. 2006;368(9537):804–13.
6. Kupczyk M, Ten Brinke A, Sterk PJ, Bel EH, Papi A, Chanez P, Nizankowska-Mogilnicka E, Gjomarkaj M, Gaga M, Brusselle G, Dahlén B, Dahlén SE, BIOAIR investigators. Frequent exacerbators–a distinct phenotype of severe asthma. Clin Exp Allergy. 2014;44(2):212–21.
7. Lefaudeux D, De Meulder B, Loza MJ, Peffer N, Rowe A, Baribaud F, Bansal AT, Lutter R, Sousa AR, Corfield J, Pandis I, Bakke PS, Caruso M, Chanez P, Dahlén SE, Fleming LJ, Fowler SJ, Horvath I, Krug N, Montuschi P, Sanak M, Sandstrom T, Shaw DE, Singer F, Sterk PJ, Roberts G, Adcock IM, Djukanovic R, Auffray C, Chung KF, U-BIOPRED Study Group. U-BIOPRED clinical adult asthma clusters linked to a subset of sputum omics. J Allergy Clin Immunol. 2016;139(6):1797–807.
8. Anderson GP. Endotyping asthma: new insights into key pathogenic mechanisms in a complex, heterogeneous disease. Lancet. 2008;372:1107.
9. Tan HT, Sugita K, Akdis CA. Novel biologicals for the treatment of allergic diseases and asthma. Curr Allergy Asthma Rep. 2016;16(10):70.

10. Bonini M, Usmani OS. Drugs for airway disease. Medicine. 2016;44(5):271–80.

11. Boulet LP, et al. Comparative efficacy of salbutamol, ipratropium, and cromoglycate in the prevention of bronchospasm induced by exercise and hyperosmolar challenges. J Allergy Clin Immunol. 1989;83:882.

12. Bonini M, Permaul P, Kulkarni T, Kazani S, Segal A, Sorkness CA, Wechsler ME, Israel E. Loss of salmeterol bronchoprotection against exercise in relation to ADRB2 Arg16Gly polymorphism and exhaled nitric oxide. Am J Respir Crit Care Med. 2013;188(12):1407–12.

13. Salpeter SR, Wall AJ, Buckley NS. Long-acting beta-agonists with and without inhaled corticosteroids and catastrophic asthma events. Am J Med. 2010;123(4):322–8.

14. Gelb AF, Nadel JA. Affirmation of the adoration of the vagi and role of tiotropium in asthmatic patients. J Allergy Clin Immunol. 2016;138(4):1011–3.

15. D'Amato M, Vitale C, Molino A, Lanza M, D'Amato G. Anticholinergic drugs in asthma therapy. Curr Opin Pulm Med. 2017;23(1):103–8.

16. Rodrigo GJ, Castro-Rodríguez JA. What is the role of tiotropium in asthma?: a systematic review with meta-analysis. Chest. 2015;147(2):388–96.

17. Bateman ED, Rennard S, Barnes PJ, Dicpinigaitis PV, Gosens R, Gross NJ, Nadel JA, Pfeifer M, Racké K, Rabe KF, Rubin BK, Welte T, Wessler I. Alternative mechanisms for tiotropium. Pulm Pharmacol Ther. 2009;22(6):533–42.

18. Fardon T, Haggart K, Lee DK, Lipworth BJ. A proof of concept study to evaluate stepping down the dose of fluticasone in combination with salmeterol and tiotropium in severe persistent asthma. Respir Med. 2007;101(6):1218–28.

19. Sposato B, Barzan R, Calabrese A, Franco C. Comparison of the protective effect amongst anticholinergic drugs on methacholine-induced bronchoconstriction in asthma. J Asthma. 2008;45(5):397–401.

20. Peters SP, Kunselman SJ, Icitovic N, Moore WC, Pascual R, Ameredes BT, Boushey HA, Calhoun WJ, Castro M, Cherniack RM, Craig T, Denlinger L, Engle LL, DiMango EA, Fahy JV, Israel E, Jarjour N, Kazani SD, Kraft M, Lazarus SC, Lemanske RF Jr, Lugogo N, Martin RJ, Meyers DA, Ramsdell J, Sorkness CA, Sutherland ER, Szefler SJ, Wasserman SI, Walter MJ, Wechsler ME, Chinchilli VM, Bleecker ER, National Heart, Lung, and Blood Institute Asthma Clinical Research Network. Tiotropium bromide step-up therapy for adults with uncontrolled asthma. N Engl J Med. 2010;363(18):1715–26.

21. Kerstjens HA, Disse B, Schröder-Babo W, Bantje TA, Gahlemann M, Sigmund R, Engel M, van Noord JA. Tiotropium improves lung function in patients with severe uncontrolled asthma: a randomized controlled trial. J Allergy Clin Immunol. 2011;128(2):308–14.

22. Kerstjens HA, Engel M, Dahl R, Paggiaro P, Beck E, Vandewalker M, Sigmund R, Seibold W, Moroni-Zentgraf P, Bateman ED. Tiotropium in asthma poorly controlled with standard combination therapy. N Engl J Med. 2012;367(13):1198–207.

23. Yoshida M, Nakano T, Fukuyama S, Matsumoto T, Eguchi M, Moriwaki A, Takata S, Machida K, Kanaya A, Matsumoto K, Nakanishi Y, Inoue H. Effects of tiotropium on lung function in severe asthmatics with or without emphysematous changes. Pulm Pharmacol Ther. 2013;26(2):159–66.

24. Beeh KM, Moroni-Zentgraf P, Ablinger O, Hollaenderova Z, Unseld A, Engel M, Korn S. Tiotropium Respimat® in asthma: a double-blind, randomised, dose-ranging study in adult patients with moderate asthma. Respir Res. 2014;15:61.

25. Price D, Kaplan A, Jones R, Freeman D, Burden A, Gould S, von Ziegenweidt J, Ali M, King C, Thomas M. Long-acting muscarinic antagonist use in adults with asthma: real-life prescribing and outcomes of add-on therapy with tiotropium bromide. J Asthma Allergy. 2015;8:1–13.

26. Timmer W, Moroni-Zentgraf P, Cornelissen P, Unseld A, Pizzichini E, Buhl R. Once-daily tiotropium Respimat(®) 5 µg is an efficacious 24-h bronchodilator in adults with symptomatic asthma. Respir Med. 2015;109(3):329–38.

27. Rajanandh MG, Nageswari AD, Ilango K. Assessment of montelukast, doxofylline, and tiotropium with budesonide for the treatment of asthma: which is the best among the second-line treatment? A randomized trial. Clin Ther. 2015;37(2):418–26.

28. Kerstjens HA, Casale TB, Bleecker ER, Meltzer EO, Pizzichini E, Schmidt O, Engel M, Bour L, Verkleij CB, Moroni-Zentgraf P, Bateman ED. Tiotropium or salmeterol as add-on therapy to inhaled corticosteroids for patients with moderate symptomatic asthma: two replicate, double-blind, placebo-controlled, parallel-group, active-comparator, randomised trials. Lancet Respir Med. 2015;3(5):367–76.

29. Paggiaro P, Halpin DM, Buhl R, Engel M, Zubek VB, Blahova Z, Moroni-Zentgraf P, Pizzichini E. The effect of tiotropium in symptomatic asthma despite low- to medium-dose inhaled corticosteroids: a randomized controlled trial. J Allergy Clin Immunol Pract. 2016;4(1):104–13.

30. Beeh KM, Kirsten AM, Dusser D, Sharma A, Cornelissen P, Sigmund R, Moroni-Zentgraf P, Dahl R. Pharmacodynamics and pharmacokinetics following once-daily and twice-daily dosing of tiotropium Respimat® in asthma using standardized Sample-contamination avoidance. J Aerosol Med Pulm Drug Deliv. 2016;29(5):406–15.

31. Abadoglu O, Berk S. Tiotropium may improve asthma symptoms and lung function in asthmatic patients with irreversible airway obstruction: the real-life data. Clin Respir J. 2016;10(4):421–7.

32. Hoshino M, Ohtawa J, Akitsu K. Effects of the addition of tiotropium on airway dimensions in symptomatic asthma. Allergy Asthma Proc. 2016;37(6):147–53.

33. Yoshida M, Kaneko Y, Ishimatsu A, Komori M, Iwanaga T, Inoue H. Effects of tiotropium on lung function in current smokers and never smokers with bronchial asthma. Pulm Pharmacol Ther. 2017;42:7–12.

34. Cook AL, Kinane TB, Nelson BA. Tiotropium use in pediatric patients with asthma or chronic cough: a case series. Clin Pediatr (Phila). 2014;53(14):1393–5.

35. Vogelberg C, Engel M, Moroni-Zentgraf P, Leonaviciute-Klimantaviciene M, Sigmund R, Downie J, Nething K, Vevere V, Vandewalker M. Tiotropium in asthmatic adolescents symptomatic despite inhaled corticosteroids: a randomised dose-ranging study. Respir Med. 2014;108(8):1268–76.

36. Vogelberg C, Moroni-Zentgraf P, LeonaviciuteKlimantaviciene M, Sigmund R, Hamelmann E, Engel M, Szefler S. A randomised dose-ranging study of tiotropium Respimat® in children with symptomatic asthma despite inhaled corticosteroids. Respir Res. 2015;16:20.

37. Huang J, Chen Y, Long Z, Zhou X, Shu J. Clinical efficacy of tiotropium in children with asthma. Pak J Med Sci. 2016;32(2):462–5.

38. Hamelmann E, Bateman ED, Vogelberg C, Szefler SJ, Vandewalker M, Moroni-Zentgraf P, Avis M, Unseld A, Engel M, Boner AL. Tiotropium add-on therapy in adolescents with moderate asthma: a 1-year randomized controlled trial. J Allergy Clin Immunol. 2016;138(2):441–50.

39. Hamelmann E, Bernstein JA, Vandewalker M, Moroni-Zentgraf P, Verri D, Unseld A, Engel M, Boner AL. A randomised controlled trial of tiotropium in adolescents with severe symptomatic asthma. Eur Respir J. 2017;49(1). doi:10.1183/13993003.01100-2016.

40. Szefler SJ, Murphy K, Harper T 3rd, Boner A, Laki I, Engel M, El Azzi G, Moroni-Zentgraf P, Finnigan H, Hamelmann E. A phase III randomized controlled trial of tiotropium add-on therapy in children with severe symptomatic asthma. J Allergy Clin Immunol. 2017. 10.1016/j.jaci.2017.01.014.

41. Park HW, Yang MS, Park CS, Kim TB, Moon HB, Min KU, Kim YY, Cho SH. Additive role of tiotropium in severe asthmatics and Arg16Gly in ADRB2 as a potential marker to predict response. Allergy. 2009;64(5):778–83.

42. Bateman ED, Kornmann O, Schmidt P, Pivovarova A, Engel M, Fabbri LM. Tiotropium is noninferior to salmeterol in maintaining improved lung function in B16-Arg/Arg patients with asthma. J Allergy Clin Immunol. 2011;128(2):315–22.

43. Wechsler ME, Yawn BP, Fuhlbrigge AL, Pace WD, Pencina MJ, Doros G, Kazani S, Raby BA, Lanzillotti J, Madison S, Israel E, BELT Investigators. Anticholinergic vs long-acting β-agonist in combination with inhaled corticosteroids in black adults with asthma: the BELT randomized clinical trial. JAMA. 2015;314(16):1720–30.

44. Nelson HS, Weiss ST, Bleecker ER, Yancey SW, Dorinsky PM, SMART Study Group. The salmeterol multicenter asthma research trial: a comparison of usual pharmacotherapy for asthma or usual pharmacotherapy plus salmeterol. Chest. 2006;129(1):15–26.

45. Peters SP, Bleecker ER, Kunselman SJ, Icitovic N, Moore WC, Pascual R, Ameredes BT, Boushey HA, Calhoun WJ, Castro M, Cherniack RM, Craig T, Denlinger LC, Engle LL, Dimango EA, Israel E, Kraft M, Lazarus SC, Lemanske RF Jr, Lugogo N, Martin RJ, Meyers DA, Ramsdell J, Sorkness CA, Sutherland ER, Wasserman SI, Walter MJ, Wechsler ME, Chinchilli VM, Szefler SJ, National Heart, Lung, and Blood Institute's Asthma Clinical Research Network. Predictors of response to tiotropium versus salmeterol in asthmatic adults. J Allergy Clin Immunol. 2013;132(5):1068–74.

46. Kerstjens HA, Moroni-Zentgraf P, Tashkin DP, Dahl R, Paggiaro P, Vandewalker M, Schmidt H, Engel M, Bateman ED. Tiotropium improves lung function, exacerbation rate, and asthma control, independent of baseline

characteristics including age, degree of airway obstruction, and allergic status. Respir Med. 2016;117:198–206.

47. Gosens R, Rieks D, Meurs H, Ninaber DK, Rabe KF, Nanninga J, Kolahian S, Halayko AJ, Hiemstra PS, Zuyderduyn S. Muscarinic M3 receptor stimulation increases cigarette smoke-induced IL-8 secretion by human airway smooth muscle cells. Eur Respir J. 2009;34(6):1436–43.

48. Buels KS, Jacoby DB, Fryer AD. Non-bronchodilating mechanisms of tiotropium prevent airway hyperreactivity in a guinea-pig model of allergic asthma. Br J Pharmacol. 2012;165(5):1501–14.

49. Bühling F, Lieder N, Kühlmann UC, Waldburg N, Welte T. Tiotropium suppresses acetylcholine-induced release of chemotactic mediators in vitro. Respir Med. 2007;101(11):2386–94.

50. Bos IS, Gosens R, Zuidhof AB, Schaafsma D, Halayko AJ, Meurs H, Zaagsma J. Inhibition of allergen-induced airway remodelling by tiotropium and budesonide: a comparison. Eur Respir J. 2007;30(4):653–61.

51. Kistemaker LE, Bos IS, Menzen MH, Maarsingh H, Meurs H, Gosens R. Combination therapy of tiotropium and ciclesonide attenuates airway inflammation and remodeling in a guinea pig model of chronic asthma. Respir Res. 2016;17:13.

52. Smit M, Zuidhof AB, Bos SI, Maarsingh H, Gosens R, Zaagsma J, Meurs H. Bronchoprotection by olodaterol is synergistically enhanced by tiotropium in a guinea pig model of allergic asthma. J Pharmacol Exp Ther. 2014;348(2):303–10.

53. Profita M, Bonanno A, Siena L, Bruno A, Ferraro M, Montalbano AM, Albano GD, Riccobono L, Casarosa P, Pieper MP, Gjomarkaj M. Smoke, choline acetyltransferase, muscarinic receptors, and fibroblast proliferation in chronic obstructive pulmonary disease. J Pharmacol Exp Ther. 2009;329(2):753–63.

54. Pieper MP, Chaudhary NI, Park JE. Acetylcholine-induced proliferation of fibroblasts and myofibroblasts in vitro is inhibited by tiotropium bromide. Life Sci. 2007;80(24–25):2270–3.

55. Kang JY, Rhee CK, Kim JS, Park CK, Kim SJ, Lee SH, Yoon HK, Kwon SS, Kim YK, Lee SY. Effect of tiotropium bromide on airway remodeling in a chronic asthma model. Ann Allergy Asthma Immunol. 2012;109(1):29–35.

56. Rogers DF. Motor control of airway goblet cells and glands. Respir Physiol. 2001;125(12):129–44.

57. Arai N, Kondo M, Izumo T, Tamaoki J, Nagai A. Inhibition of neutrophil elastase-induced goblet cell metaplasia by tiotropium in mice. Eur Respir J. 2010;35(5):1164–71.

58. Birrell MA, Bonvini SJ, Dubuis E, Maher SA, Wortley MA, Grace MS, Raemdonck K, Adcock JJ, Belvisi MG. Tiotropium modulates transient receptor potential V1 (TRPV1) in airway sensory nerves: a beneficial off-target effect? J Allergy Clin Immunol. 2014;133(3):679–87.

59. Mutolo D, Cinelli E, Iovino L, Pantaleo T, Bongianni F. Downregulation of the cough reflex by aclidinium and tiotropium in awake and anesthetized rabbits. Pulm Pharmacol Ther. 2016;38:1–9.

60. Willson J, Bateman ED, Pavord I, Lloyd A, Krivasi T, Esser D. Cost effectiveness of tiotropium in patients with asthma poorly controlled on inhaled glucocorticosteroids and long-acting β-agonists. Appl Health Econ Health Policy. 2014;12(4):447–59.

61. Willson J, Bateman ED, Pavord I, Lloyd A, Krivasi T, Esser D. Erratum to: cost effectiveness of tiotropium in patients with asthma poorly controlled on inhaled glucocorticosteroids and long-acting β-agonists. Appl Health Econ Health Policy. 2016;14(1):119–25.

62. Ohta K, Ichinose M, Tohda Y, Engel M, Moroni-Zentgraf P, Kunimitsu S, Sakamoto W, Adachi M. Long-term once-daily tiotropium Respimat® is well tolerated and maintains efficacy over 52 weeks in patients with symptomatic asthma in Japan: a randomised, placebo-controlled study. PLoS ONE. 2015;10(4):e0124109.

63. Kew KM, Dahri K. Long-acting muscarinic antagonists (LAMA) added to combination long-acting beta2-agonists and inhaled corticosteroids (LABA/ICS) versus LABA/ICS for adults with asthma. Cochrane Database Syst Rev. 2016;1:CD011721.

20

Immunosenescence in aging: between immune cells depletion and cytokines up-regulation

Maria Teresa Ventura[1], Marco Casciaro[2*], Sebastiano Gangemi[2] and Rosalba Buquicchio[3]

Abstract

Background: The immunosenescence is a relatively recent chapter, correlated with the linear extension of the average life began in the nineteenth century and still in progress. The most important feature of immunosenescence is the accumulation in the "immunological space" of memory and effector cells as a result of the stimulation caused by repeated clinical and subclinical infections and by continuous exposure to antigens (inhalant allergens, food, etc.). This state of chronic inflammation that characterizes senescence has a significant impact on survival and fragility. In fact, the condition of frail elderly occurs less frequently in situations characterized by poor contact with viral infections and parasitic diseases. Furthermore the immunosenescence is characterized by a particular "remodelling" of the immune system, induced by oxidative stress. Apoptosis plays a central role in old age, a period in which the ability of apoptosis can change. The remodelling of apoptosis, together with the Inflammaging and the up-regulation of the immune response with the consequent secretion of pro-inflammatory lymphokines represents the major determinant of the rate of aging and longevity, as well as of the most common diseases related with age and with tumors. Other changes occur in the innate immunity, the first line of defence providing rapid, but unspecific and incomplete protection, consisting mostly of monocytes, natural killer cells and dendritic cells, acting up to the establishment of a adaptive immune response, which is slower, but highly specific, which cellular substrate consists of T and B lymphocytes. The markers of "Inflammaging" in adaptive immunity in centenarians are characterized by a decrease in T cells "naive." The reduction of CD8 virgins may be related to the risk of morbidity and death, as well as the combination of the increase of CD8+ cells and reduction of CD4+ T cells and the reduction of CD19+ B cells. The immune function of the elderly is weakened to due to the exhaustion of T cell-virgin (CD95−), which are replaced with the clonal expansion of CD28- T cells.

Conclusions: The increase of pro-inflammatory cytokines is associated with dementia, Parkinson's disease, atherosclerosis, diabetes type 2, sarcopenia and a high risk of morbidity and mortality. A correct modulation of immune responses and apoptotic phenomena can be useful to reduce age-related degenerative diseases, as well as inflammatory and neoplastic diseases.

Background

Recent researches stigmatize that the steady increase in life expectancy in Europe, USA, Canada, Japan and England will allow many of the children born in 2000 to reach 100 years of life [1]. In this perspective, the main objective of the geriatrician is to analyze risk factors for diseases and conditions that can lead to functional limitations for the elderly, in order to avoid people to reach a disability state. In summary, the increase in life expectancy must coincide with an expectation of health, good health and self-sufficiency for the last part of life [2]. Old age is a situation in which a number of factors (molecular, cellular, physiological, immunological and psycho-social events) help to set up a scenario of "exhaustion of reserves"; this consist of a inability to functional adaptations and an

*Correspondence: mcasciaro@unime.it
[2] School and Operative Unit of Allergy and Clinical Immunology, Department of Clinical and Experimental Medicine, University of Messina, Messina, Italy
Full list of author information is available at the end of the article

accumulation of deficits of many organs [3]. This situation undergoes a dynamic process that oscillates between a "successful" and pathological aging, which establishes a situation of vulnerability that is identified with the fragility state. Undoubtedly, to the fragility state contribute the same factors that have contributed to the increased life expectancy, which is attested at the moment at 80 years of age [4]. Many factors have allowed this "stretching", i.e. the decrease of infant mortality, antibiotic therapy and prevention of cardiovascular and metabolic diseases, but also, especially in industrialized countries, the improvement of hygienic and nutrition conditions [5]. However, if aging is not accompanied by a healthy condition, the costs related to disabilities or frailty age-related could lead to the overgrowth of the public health expense with a negative impact on social welfare.

Immunosenescence

"The aging phenotype", including the immunosenescence is the result of an imbalance between inflammatory and anti-inflammatory mechanisms with the consequence of a state defined by some authors as "inflammaging" [6–8]. The "Inflammaging" is due to chronic antigen stimulation that occurs in the course of life and to the oxidative stress that involves the production of oxygen free radicals and toxic products. Both these factors are able to modify the potential of apoptotic lymphocytes. In fact, the phenomenon of "remodelling" and the "up-regulation" of pro-inflammatory cytokines (including IL-6) are the components most heavily implicated in the processes of longevity and diseases related to senescence [9–12]. As pro-inflammatory and anti-inflammatory chemokines and other signalling molecules, might propagate from already activated cells to adjacent ones and systemically by circulating products and microvesicles, recent studies claimed the possibility of understanding molecular basis of inflammaging by novel omic approaches [13].

In this sense, the state of good health in the elderly is the result not only of low pro inflammatory mechanisms, but also of an efficient network capable of neutralizing anti inflammatory antigenic insults received in the course of life. For this reason, the inflammaging would not only be important for the mechanisms of immunosenescence but also for the problem of longevity. It is reported that fragility is the result of an inflammatory state associated with the overproduction of certain lymphokines, including IL-6, called cytokine of geriatricians [14]. This factor, together with hormonal changes, nutritional deficiencies and physical inactivity would lead to one of the most important component of fragility that is sarcopenia [15, 16], as well as the reduction of bone mass. In this context, immunity appears to play an important role, both in the regulation of the mechanisms of aging as well as in the onset of the diseases typical of aging (i.e. infectious diseases, autoimmunity, cancer, metabolic diseases and neurodegenerative diseases).

Oxidative damage

Another factor influencing the Immune System, in addition to the antigenic stimulus, is the intervention of metabolites of oxygen (ROS), a consequence of the activation of the respiratory burst; as they can cause significant damage, is plausible to assume that aging is also due to an accumulation of free radicals [17]. The increase in oxygen metabolites and their accumulation causes damage to important cellular components (lipid membranes, the structural and enzymatic proteins and nucleic acids), which are contrasted by enzymatic and non-enzymatic defence systems, reparative enzymes, DNA damage and apoptotic processes damage-induced [18, 19]. These protective mechanisms become less effective as a result of continued exposure to oxidative stress and the accumulation of senescent and mutated cells, leading to an increased risk of cancer. The p53 protein counteracts the development of a neoplasm flaunting how cells respond to injury (DNA repair, or, if it fails, apoptosis). p53 plays an important role in senescence: if it increases, the incidence of neoplasia is reduced, but on the other hand it increases the speed of aging [20]. The result is a delicate balance between reduced p53 that leads to death by cancer and increased p53 leading to death for acceleration of senescence. Furthermore, an over expression of p53 generates reactive oxygen intermediates [21].

An important source of oxygen intermediates are the mitochondria. Although the main mitochondrial function is the production of energy, the isolated mitochondria generate oxygen radicals during oxidative phosphorylation. The mitochondrial electron transport chain is imperfect because it generates a superoxide radical by a process of reduction of O_2. The enzymatic dismutation of the superoxide radical produces H_2O_2, another important biological oxidant. Another factor contributing to the senescence is apoptosis, especially the one induced by acid metabolites arising from the paths of lipoxygenase and cyclooxygenase; however it is not clear whether these products induce the production of reactive intermediates or if they act independently as oxidants to induce apoptosis. Another intermediate product of oxygen metabolism is nitric oxide, a free radical known as an important regulator of mitochondrial function, capable of increasing the apoptotic phenomena, but also, at physiological levels, of preventing apoptosis and of interfering with the cascade of capsaicin [22]. In conclusion, high levels of oxidants can change the potential of oxido-reduction, by reducing the levels of ATP and increasing the porosity of the membranes leading to a progressive aging phenomenon of the cells, included the Immune System ones [23].

The "Remodelling" of the immune system

As a result of ROS accumulation, cells become resistant to apoptosis -induced damage and the number of senescent cells increases, while chronic antigenic stimulation induces increase of activated immune cells and overproduction of pro-inflammatory lymphokines that contribute to the remodelling of the immune system and of the 'inflammaging'. Senescence is a highly dynamic phenomenon characterised by continuous body adaptation to deteriorative changes [24].

ROS are closely linked to senescence and age-related diseases, in fact, genomic instability, caused by oxidative damage is the primary cause of aging. A caloric restriction can increase the average life-attenuating oxidative stress caused by normal metabolism [25].

As result of both inflammaging and of ROS increase, the modulation of apoptosis mechanisms becomes particularly delicate during senescence. The reduced sensitivity to the damage-induced apoptosis, typical of senescent cells, contributes to the accumulation of dysfunctional cells, clones of CD8+ and memory cells with a reduction of immunological space and an increased risk of infections and neoplastic diseases or degenerative disorders. The increase of the activation-induced apoptosis in response to inflammatory cytokines contributes to: the depletion of cells "naive", the reduction of the capacity of clonal expansion, the reduction of T cell responses with decreased ability to mount strong immune responses to antigenic stimuli and reduction of the immune repertoire.

The shortening of the telomeric DNA is age specific, and, regardless of the genetic influence, it is the result of the immunological history of each individual, with a close association between telomere length and mortality of individuals older than 65 years [26]. The input of virgin T cells gradually decreases, and, recently, the marker of the lymphocytes of the new generation are the T REC which represent markers of replication of T cells, with a progressive reduction of each subsequent division. Of course, the T REC decay dramatically with age in peripheral T lymphocytes.

Apoptosis

Apoptosis, a complex mechanism of programmed cell death, allows the maintenance of a physiological homeostasis mechanisms between survival and removal of damaged cells, allowing also the prevention of many diseases including neoplastic ones. Apoptosis is a strategic mechanism for the manifestation of the clonotypic diversity during lymphocyte selection, permitting to control the clonal expansion after antigenic stimulation. Apoptosis can be induced after a cellular damage (damage-induced cell death), or can be "activated" by a series of signals and anchor ligands to programmed-death receptors

(activation-induced cell death). Apoptosis is part of many changes typical of the immunosenescence, such as thymic involution, the alteration of the "repertoire" of T cells and the accumulation of effector memory cells, all events at the basis of autoimmunity. Studies about apoptosis in aging are controversial. In fact, during senescence both the two apoptotic process can be modulated differently, resulting in a variable impact in the process of senescence. A proper modulation of this important function can extend the lifespan and reduce the degenerative processes and inflammatory and neoplastic diseases that are very common during senescence [6, 27].

Hematopoietic bone and thymus

The immune system cells are constantly renewed from hematopoietic stem cells (HSC), but this ability declines during senescence and the total amount of hematopoietic tissue decreases. This event also seems to correlate with telomere shortening [28]. The changes affect also the myeloid and erythroid progenitors as B cells, with the consequence of a reduction in mature B cells. The precursors of T cells seem to suffer less; the changes that occur with age to the thymus gland, also lead to changes in the T cell compartment. The thymus undergoes a process of physiological involution, with volume reduction and replacement with adipose tissue in the functional part of both cortex and medulla, contraction of soluble factors and hormonal cytokines production. This process begins early in life and is almost complete at the age of 40–50 years [29].

Moreover, the immune system has the important function to protect the body from any form of damaging agent (chemical, traumatic or infectious). There are two kind of immunity working together in a cooperative manner: the natural immunity (innate) immunity and adaptive (acquired). The natural immunity is the first line of defence because it provides a fast protection, but unspecific and incomplete, consisting mostly of monocytes, natural killer cells and dendritic cells, which acts until the adaptive immune response is established; this immune response is slower, but highly specific and permanent, with a cellular substrate consisting of T and B lymphocytes.

T cells

The T cells are generated through a Thymic selection and they can be distinguished in CD4+ and CD8+, by their co-receptor molecules. These two cellular subtypes show during the aging process of the organism some changes in their percentages: the CD8+ cells increase their number during senescence. The CD4+ and the CD8+ cells express mutually exclusive the phenotype CD45RA and CD45RO. The first phenotype makes let to recognize naïve T cells, instead the second one to individuate memory/activated T cells [30]. The reduction of naïve lymphocytes may be a consequence of both thymic involution and chronic antigenic stimulation [31]. This event helps to explain the reduced ability of the elderly to resist to new infections [32].

Furthermore in the elderly naïve T-cells show multiple alterations, including the shortening of telomeres, the reduced production of IL-2 and the diminished ability to differentiate themselves into effector-cells. The loss in the number and function of the naïve T-cells is compensated in about 30% of the elderly, with the expansion of T CD8+, CD45RO+, CD25+ clones, capable of producing IL-2, and with a protective humoral capacity towards vaccinations with the expansion of effector "memory" cells [33]. In particular, in the elderly the vaccinations induce the accumulation of CD8+ effector cells with phenotypic changes, such as the loss of costimulatory CD8 molecules [32].

CD28-cells are responsible for the production of proinflammatory cytokines and are resistant to apoptosis. The origin of the CD28-cells has not yet been fully elucidated, but it is assumed that they represent cells undergoing a replicative senescence, due to the shortening of telomeres and to a reduction of the proliferative capacity [34]. The inversion of the CD4+/CD8+ cell number ratio, the increased number of the memory-effector cells and the seropositivity for the Citomegalvirus (CMV), identify an immune risk phenotype (IRP) in elderly patients [35]. At the same time in elderly patients it has been shown an increased production of IL-1, IL-4, IL-6 and IFN-gamma. These cytokines control B Cells differentiation through the isotype switch and the Ig production.

Further alterations concern a compromised response to the oxidative stress, that causes an increased susceptibility to damage-induced cell death [36], and calcium flow kinetics [37]. Recently it has been associated with the senescence a reduction of Mir 181 (MicroRNA precursor), that in T cell causes an impairment in the antigen recognition [38].

Regulatory T cells (Tregs) are a subset characterized by a high expression of CD25 and FOXP3, a transcriptional factor for the function and differentiation of Treg cells. The number of CD4+ FOXP3+ lymphocytes increases in the senile age. The accumulation of these cells in the elderly plays an important role in reactivating chronic infections and the change in the T17/Treg ratio can cause alterations in immune response with the appearance of inflammatory or autoimmune diseases [39].

B cells

Also the reservoir of B cells is influenced by age. In fact, humoral immunity undergoes both quantitative and qualitative alterations [40].

The reduced function of B cells was thought being due to a lack of helper T function in T-dependent responses. On the other hand, there are functions of B cells which are T-independent; one example is the response to the polysaccharide, which is crucial for antibacterial protection and that seems to be inefficient too [41].

In addition, some data suggest that B cells are important antigen-presenting cells themselves and that can be regulatory with key function for the development of T cells. Therefore, it is conceivable that some of the lack in the T cell functions may be due to an insufficient help from B cells. At the same time, changes are described in the number of B cells. In the elderly, there are also reported reduced levels of IgM and IgD (M and D type immunoglobulins) certainly connected to the transition from naive cells to memory B cells area [42]. On the contrary, during the senescence it occurs an increase of the IgG (G type immunoglobulins) level, especially of IgG1, IgG2 and IgG3; the level of IgA is also increased [43]. In particular, IgAs undergo significant changes, with a marked increase of monomeric IgA1, both in serum and saliva and a reduction of polymeric IgA2, especially in the sputum [44]. This imbalance could be charged to the reduction of the Peyer's patches at the level of the gastrointestinal mucosa as regards as IgA2, while the increase of IgA1 may be secondary to a deficiency of the activity of T "suppressor" subset and consequent hyperfunction of B lymphocytes [45]. The deficits taking place in this area are largely due to infectious events in the elderly, particularly in the gastrointestinal and respiratory system. The reduced number of plasma cells in the elderly bone marrow [46] causes a lack of antibody production, a reduced ability to respond to viruses and bacteria [47] and an altered response to vaccines against B hepatitis virus [48].

The innate immunity system

Alterations in innate immunity have a crucial role and the amount of related studies have identified a trend in the chapter of immunogerontology starting with the reduction of barriers in the epithelial layer of the skin and gastrointestinal and respiratory mucosa [49] with a consequent changes in local immunoglobulin ratio. Moreover, even some physiological events, such as the reduction of the thymic mass, seems to support the hypothesis that the immune system plays an important role in the phenomenon of aging, thus justifying a theory to explain some of the immunological diseases typical of this age such as autoimmune diseases, malignancies and infections. The high incidence of infectious events in old age can, however, be secondary to alterations in the phagocyte system [50].

With regard to the skin, immunosenescence is characterized by an impairment of all the structures with loss of the "barrier" function, reduction of the number and the volume of hairs, reduction of the number of sebaceous glands, loss of skin elasticity, impairment of the immunological defence of the skin [51].

Dendritic cells, responsible for the very first recognition of pathogens in the skin, show mitochondrial dysfunctions that interfere with their protective role [52].

In particular there is an impairment of the antigen uptake and of the apoptotic function [53].

Comparing the elderly plasmocytoid dendritic cell (PCD) capacity of antigen uptake with the one of the PCD of the young it is possible to observe a reduced ability of the elderly PCD to induce proliferation and stimulate secretion of INF gamma in CD4+ and CD8+ cells [54].

Macrophages

Macrophages, able to produce pro-inflammatory cytokines (TNF-alpha, IL-1, IL-6 e IL-8), have the function of processing and presenting antigens to T cells. During senescence, a decrease of macrophages precursors has been described, instead the number of monocytes appears unchanged [55]. The shortening of telomeres occurring in the senile age results in a reduction in the production of GS-CSF but also of Cytokines such as TNF-alpha and IL-6 [56]. In older animals it occurs a reduction of the production of superoxide anion after incubation with INF-gamma [57].

The phagocytic function appears to be reduced, while chemotaxis seems to be conserved, especially in the presence of certain factors such as stimulants of the complement fragment C5a. The production of lymphocyte derived chemotactic factors (LDCF) is reduced, as well as chemotaxis in the presence of this stimulator factor. In this case the inhibitory mechanism appears to be related to prostaglandins that are produced in high quantities, during senescence, and which exert an inhibitory action [58]. The reduced production of LDCF could be related to a low percentage of lymphocytes involved in the synthesis of the cytokine.

Neutrophils

Their number is preserved in the elderly, while the expression of CD16 Fc gamma receptor is reduced, with the consequence that, both the generation of superoxide mediated by the Fc receptor and the phagocytosis are impaired in the elderly; this suggests that the decline of the effector response of Fc receptors is particularly important for neutrophil dysfunction of the elderly [59].

In elderly people, the reduced response of these cells to Streptococcus Aureus is of fundamental clinical importance, because this event increases susceptibility to lung infections. At the same time in the aged mice the

migration of neutrophils into the lungs is reduced and this increases the risk of pulmonary infections and recurrences [60].

In addition, very recently, an alteration of the pathogen-mediated destruction of neutrophil extracellular Traps (NETs) has been described, confirming the reasons of the increase of infections in the elderly [61].

NK cells

The high incidence of immunoproliferative diseases in the elderly suggests that in this age a deficiency of an important mechanism of immune surveillance such as NK activity can be occur. In 1986, through the use of a "slow" target such as a cell line derived from an hepatocellular carcinoma, allowing an optimal evaluation of NK function, it was conceivable to demonstrate that in the elderly it was a significant reduction of the spontaneous cytotoxic capacity [62]. Recent studies pointed out that a high NK cytotoxicity is associated with longevity and good health, while a low NK function is associated with an increase in morbidity and mortality, and consequently, infections, mechanisms of atherosclerotic and neurodegenerative diseases. Furthermore, NK cells by producing cell lysis could cause the release of perforin and granzymes, which, in turn, activate caspases and provoke apoptosis of target cells. During senescence it occurs the reduction of an important lymphokine for the lymphocyte activation processes like the IL-2 and also for the killing of the NK-resistant cell lines in response to IL-2. This contributes to the deficit of the function, even in the presence of a normal number of NK cells [63].

Particularly during senescence there is a redistribution of NK cells with decreasing CD56 cells, characterized by a high density of surface CD56 antigen. In contrast, there is an increase in CD56–CD16 Nk cells [64]. This results in a reduction in IFN secretion for the elderly compared with the secreted quantity in young subjects [65]. In addition, during the senescence there is a decrease in the expression of the receptor activation expression, especially linked to the receptor NKp30 and NKp46 [66].

Of course, it's easy to imagine the consequences that may follow an alteration to the function of this population during senescence; in fact, NK cells intervene both in the elimination of tumor or viral-infected cells and also in the innate and adaptive immunological regulation, through the production of cytokines and chemokines [67].

Phenotype of immunological RISK (IRP) during senescence

According to recent studies, the IRP is predictive of the development of cognitive deficits and, as outlined by some authors, [35] is a prelude for a mortality rate over the next 4 years in 58% of cases. The IRP is defined, in the studies of this group of Swedish researchers carried out on elderly octogenarians and nonagenarians, by identifying some characteristic "markers" of this phenotype, including the inversion of the CD4/CD8 ratio, the increase in CD8 * CD28-memory/effector cells, the increase of proinflammatory cytokines such as IL-6, the reduction of B lymphocytes and a marked seropositivity for cytomegalovirus [68].

The pro-inflammatory profile resulting from an interaction between the genotype and environmental factors, becomes strategic trough the years; the increase of cytokine secretion also correlated with the impact of cytomegalovirus infection is responsible for an unsuccessful aging [69]. CMV-specific cells, both CD4+ and CD8+ cells have short telomeres and this leads to chromosomal instability and DNA damage repair processes in growth arrest and/or apoptosis. The consequence is that not all T memory cells differ in the same way and that can happen an expansion of this cell pool, whose clinical consequences consist in an increase in infectious diseases and neoplasms [70].

Conclusion

A shown above, immunosenescence is an unavoidable process typical of life being. Many immune system cells undergoes this process; however, the senescence process differ from one subject to the other. The development of a pro-inflammatory cytokines phenotype together with the counterbalance of an anti-inflammatory profile could let people reach an old age without disability. A correct modulation of immune responses and of apoptotic phenomena, in fact, can be useful to reduce age-related degenerative diseases, as well as inflammatory and neoplastic diseases in order to reach a successful aging.

Authors' contributions
VMT, BR and SG designed the study, made studies analysis and interpretation, and revised the manuscript. MC, SG carried out the bibliographic search, contributed to the draft of the manuscript. VMT and BR wrote and coordinated the draft of the manuscript. All authors read and approved the final manuscript.

Author details
[1] Department of Interdisciplinary Medicine, University of Bari, Policlinico, Piazza G. Cesare no 11, 70124 Bari, Italy. [2] School and Operative Unit of Allergy and Clinical Immunology, Department of Clinical and Experimental Medicine, University of Messina, Messina, Italy. [3] Dermatological Clinic, Department of Biomedical Science and Human Oncology, University of Bari Medical School, Policlinico, Italy.

References
1. Manton KG, Vaupel JW. Survival after the age of 80 in the United States, Sweden, France, England, and Japan. N Engl J Med. 1995;333:1232–5.
2. Christensen K, Doblhammer G, Rau R, Vaupel JW. Ageing populations: the challenges ahead. Lancet. 2009;374:1196–208.
3. Kirkwood TB. Understanding the odd science of aging. Cell. 2005;120:437–47.
4. Troen BR. The biology of aging. Mt Sinai J Med. 2003;70:3–22.
5. Jeune B, Brønnum-Hansen H. Trends in health expectancy at age 65 for various health indicators, 1987–2005, Denmark. Eur J Ageing. 2008;5:279.
6. Franceschi C, Capri M, Monti D, Giunta S, Olivieri F, Sevini F, Panourgia MP, Invidia L, Celani L, Scurti M, Cevenini E, Castellani GC, Salvioli S. Inflammaging and anti-inflammaging: a systemic perspective on aging and longevity emerged from studies in humans. Mech Ageing Dev. 2007;128:92–105.
7. Cevenini E, Monti D, Franceschi C. Inflamm-ageing. Curr Opin Clin Nutr Metab Care. 2013;16:14–20.
8. Minciullo PL, Catalano A, Mandraffino G, Casciaro M, Crucitti A, Maltese G, Morabito N, Lasco A, Gangemi S, Basile G. Inflammaging and anti-inflammaging: the role of cytokines in extreme longevity. Arch Immunol Ther Exp. 2016;64:111–26.
9. Ershler WB, Keller ET. Age-associated increased interleukin-6 gene expression, late-life diseases, and frailty. Annu Rev Med. 2000;51:245–70.
10. Gangemi S, Basile G, Monti D, Merendino RA, Di Pasquale G, Bisignano U, Nicita-Mauro V, Franceschi C. Age-related modifications in circulating IL-15 levels in humans. Mediat Inflamm. 2005;2005:245–7.
11. Gangemi S, Parisi P, Ricciardi L, Saitta S, Minciullo PL, Cristani MT, Nicita-Mauro V, Saija A, Basile G. Is interleukin-22 a possible indicator of chronic heart failure's progression? Arch Gerontol Geriatr. 2010;50:311–4.
12. Basile G, Paffumi I, D'Angelo AG, Figliomeni P, Cucinotta MD, Pace E, Ferraro M, Saitta S, Lasco A, Gangemi S. Healthy centenarians show high levels of circulating interleukin-22 (IL-22). Arch Gerontol Geriatr. 2012;54:459–61.
13. Monti D, Ostan R, Borelli V, Castellani G, Franceschi C. Inflammaging and human longevity in the omics era. Mech Ageing Dev. 2017;165(Part B):129–138.
14. Di Bona D, Vasto S, Capurso C, Christiansen L, Deiana L, Franceschi C, Hurme M, Mocchegiani E, Rea M, Lio D, Candore G, Caruso C. Effect of interleukin-6 polymorphisms on human longevity: a systematic review and meta-analysis. Ageing Res Rev. 2009;8:36–42.
15. Pel-Littel RE, Schuurmans MJ, Emmelot-Vonk MH, Verhaar HJ. Frailty: defining and measuring of a concept. J Nutr Health Aging. 2009;13:390–4.
16. Evans WJ, Paolisso G, Abbatecola AM, Corsonello A, Bustacchini S, Strollo F, Lattanzio F. Frailty and muscle metabolism dysregulation in the elderly. Biogerontology. 2010;11:527–36.
17. Liochev SI. Reactive oxygen species and the free radical theory of aging. Free Radic Biol Med. 2013;60:1–4.
18. Ginaldi L, De Martinis M, Monti D, Franceschi C. The immune system in the elderly: activation-induced and damage-induced apoptosis. Immunol Res. 2004;30:81–94.
19. De Martinis M, Franceschi C, Monti D, Ginaldi L. Apoptosis remodeling in immunosenescence: implications for strategies to delay ageing. Curr Med Chem. 2007;14:1389–97.
20. Minciullo PL, Inferrera A, Navarra M, Calapai G, Magno C, Gangemi S. Oxidative stress in benign prostatic hyperplasia: a systematic review. Urol Int. 2015;94:249–54.
21. Jackson JG, Pant V, Li Q, Chang LL, Quintas-Cardama A, Garza D, Tavana O, Yang P, Manshouri T, Li Y, El-Naggar AK, Lozano G. p53-mediated senescence impairs the apoptotic response to chemotherapy and clinical outcome in breast cancer. Cancer Cell. 2012;21:793–806.
22. Cristani M, Speciale A, Saija A, Gangemi S, Minciullo PL, Cimino F. Circulating advanced oxidation protein products as oxidative stress biomarkers and progression mediators in pathological conditions related to inflammation and immune dysregulation. Curr Med Chem. 2016;23:3862–82.

23. Dorn GW 2nd. Molecular mechanisms that differentiate apoptosis from programmed necrosis. Toxicol Pathol. 2013;41:227–34.

24. Ostan R, Bucci L, Capri M, Salvioli S, Scurti M, Pini E, Monti D, Franceschi C. Immunosenescence and immunogenetics of human longevity. Neuroimmunomodulation. 2008;15:224–40.

25. Ford DW, Jensen GL, Hartman TJ, Wray L, Smiciklas-Wright H. Association between dietary quality and mortality in older adults: a review of the epidemiological evidence. J Nutr Gerontol Geriatr. 2013;32:85–105.

26. Buchner N, Ale-Agha N, Jakob S, Sydlik U, Kunze K, Unfried K, Altschmied J, Haendeler J. Unhealthy diet and ultrafine carbon black particles induce senescence and disease associated phenotypic changes. Exp Gerontol. 2013;48:8–16.

27. Franceschi C, Bonafe M, Valensin S, Olivieri F, De Luca M, Ottaviani E, De Benedictis G. Inflamm-aging. An evolutionary perspective on immunosenescence. Ann N Y Acad Sci. 2000;908:244–54.

28. Maicher A, Kastner L, Dees M, Luke B. Deregulated telomere transcription causes replication-dependent telomere shortening and promotes cellular senescence. Nucleic Acids Res. 2012;40:6649–59.

29. George AJ, Ritter MA. Thymic involution with ageing: obsolescence or good housekeeping? Immunol Today. 1996;17:267–72.

30. Cossarizza A, Ortolani C, Paganelli R, Barbieri D, Monti D, Sansoni P, Fagiolo U, Castellani G, Bersani F, Londei M, Franceschi C. CD45 isoforms expression on CD4+ and CD8+ T cells throughout life, from newborns to centenarians: implications for T cell memory. Mech Ageing Dev. 1996;86:173–95.

31. Haynes L, Eaton SM, Burns EM, Randall TD, Swain SL. CD4 T cell memory derived from young naive cells functions well into old age, but memory generated from aged naive cells functions poorly. Proc Natl Acad Sci USA. 2003;100:15053–8.

32. Vallejo AN. CD28 extinction in human T cells: altered functions and the program of T-cell senescence. Immunol Rev. 2005;205:158–69.

33. Schwaiger S, Wolf AM, Robatscher P, Jenewein B, Grubeck-Loebenstein B. IL-4-producing CD8+ T cells with a CD62L ++(bright) phenotype accumulate in a subgroup of older adults and are associated with the maintenance of intact humoral immunity in old age. J Immunol. 2003;170:613–9.

34. Sansoni P, Vescovini R, Fagnoni F, Biasini C, Zanni F, Zanlari L, Telera A, Lucchini G, Passeri G, Monti D, Franceschi C, Passeri M. The immune system in extreme longevity. Exp Gerontol. 2008;43:61–5.

35. Wikby A, Ferguson F, Forsey R, Thompson J, Strindhall J, Lofgren S, Nilsson BO, Ernerudh J, Pawelec G, Johansson B. An immune risk phenotype, cognitive impairment, and survival in very late life: impact of allostatic load in Swedish octogenarian and nonagenarian humans. J Gerontol A Biol Sci Med Sci. 2005;60:556–65.

36. Sikora E. Activation-induced and damage-induced cell death in aging human T cells. Mech Ageing Dev. 2015;151:85–92.

37. Kollar S, Berta L, Vasarhelyi ZE, Balog A, Vasarhelyi B, Rigo J Jr, Toldi G. Impact of aging on calcium influx and potassium channel characteristics of T lymphocytes. Oncotarget. 2015;6:13750–6.

38. Li G, Yu M, Lee W-W, Tsang M, Krishnan E, Weyand CM, Goronzy JJ. Decline in miR-181a expression with age impairs T cell receptor sensitivity by increasing DUSP6 activity. Nat Med. 2012;18:1518–24.

39. Lages CS, Suffia I, Velilla PA, Huang B, Warshaw G, Hildeman DA, Belkaid Y, Chougnet C. Functional regulatory T cells accumulate in aged hosts and promote chronic infectious disease reactivation. J Immunol. 2008;181:1835–48.

40. Colonna-Romano G, Bulati M, Aquino A, Vitello S, Lio D, Candore G, Caruso C. B cell immunosenescence in the elderly and in centenarians. Rejuvenation Res. 2008;11:433–9.

41. Antonaci S, Jirillo E, Ventura MT, Garofalo AR, Bonomo L. Lipoprotein-induced inhibition of plaque-forming cell generation and natural killer cell frequency in aged donors. Ann Immunol. 1984;135:241–9.

42. Weksler ME, Szabo P. The effect of age on the B-cell repertoire. J Clin Immunol. 2000;20:240–9.

43. Paganelli R, Quinti I, Fagiolo U, Cossarizza A, Ortolani C, Guerra E, Sansoni P, Pucillo LP, Scala E, Cozzi E, et al. Changes in circulating B cells and immunoglobulin classes and subclasses in a healthy aged population. Clin Exp Immunol. 1992;90:351–4.

44. Ventura M. Determination of total IgA, IgA1 and IgA2 in the serum and saliva of an aged population. Recenti Prog Med. 1985;76:576–7.

45. Ventura MT. Evaluation of IgA1-IgA2 levels in serum and saliva of young and elderly people. Allergol Immunopathol. 1991;19:183–5.

46. Pritz T, Lair J, Ban M, Keller M, Weinberger B, Krismer M, Grubeck-Loebenstein B. Plasma cell numbers decrease in bone marrow of old patients. Eur J Immunol. 2015;45:738–46.

47. Buffa S, Pellicano M, Bulati M, Martorana A, Goldeck D, Caruso C, Pawelec G, Colonna-Romano G. A novel B cell population revealed by a CD38/CD24 gating strategy: CD38(−) CD24 (−) B cells in centenarian offspring and elderly people. Age. 2013;35:2009–24.

48. Rosenberg C, Bovin NV, Bram LV, Flyvbjerg E, Erlandsen M, Vorup-Jensen T, Petersen E. Age is an important determinant in humoral and T cell responses to immunization with hepatitis B surface antigen. Hum Vaccin Immunother. 2013;9:1466–76.

49. Nomellini V, Gomez CR, Kovacs EJ. Aging and impairment of innate immunity. Contrib Microbiol. 2008;15:188–205.

50. Antonaci S, Jirillo E, Ventura MT, Garofalo AR, Bonomo L. Non-specific immunity in aging: deficiency of monocyte and polymorphonuclear cell-mediated functions. Mech Ageing Dev. 1984;24:367–75.

51. De Martinis M, Sirufo MM, Ginaldi L. Allergy and Aging: an old/new emerging health issue. Aging Dis. 2017;8:162–75.

52. Simon AK, Hollander GA, McMichael A. Evolution of the immune system in humans from infancy to old age. Proc R Soc B Biol Sci. 2015;282:20143085.

53. Gupta S. Role of dendritic cells in innate and adaptive immune response in human aging. Exp Gerontol. 2014;54:47–52.

54. Prakash S, Agrawal S, Cao JN, Gupta S, Agrawal A. Impaired secretion of interferons by dendritic cells from aged subjects to influenza: role of histone modifications. Age. 2013;35:1785–97.

55. Della Bella S, Bierti L, Presicce P, Arienti R, Valenti M, Saresella M, Vergani C, Villa ML. Peripheral blood dendritic cells and monocytes are differently regulated in the elderly. Clin Immunol. 2007;122:220–8.

56. Davalos AR, Coppe JP, Campisi J, Desprez PY. Senescent cells as a source of inflammatory factors for tumor progression. Cancer Metastasis Rev. 2010;29:273–83.

57. Sebastian C, Herrero C, Serra M, Lloberas J, Blasco MA, Celada A. Telomere shortening and oxidative stress in aged macrophages results in impaired STAT5a phosphorylation. J Immunol. 2009;183:2356–64.

58. Ventura MT, Serlenga E, Tortorella C, Antonaci S. In vitro vitamin E and selenium supplementation improves neutrophil-mediated functions and monocyte chemoattractant protein-1 production in the elderly. Cytobios. 1994;77:225–32.

59. Butcher SK, Chahal H, Nayak L, Sinclair A, Henriquez NV, Sapey E, O'Mahony D, Lord JM. Senescence in innate immune responses: reduced neutrophil phagocytic capacity and CD16 expression in elderly humans. J Leukoc Biol. 2001;70:881–6.

60. Chen MM, Palmer JL, Plackett TP, Deburghgraeve CR, Kovacs EJ. Age-related differences in the neutrophil response to pulmonary pseudomonas infection. Exp Gerontol. 2014;54:42–6.

61. Brinkmann V, Zychlinsky A. Beneficial suicide: why neutrophils die to make NETs. Nat Rev Microbiol. 2007;5:577–82.

62. Ventura MT, Crollo R, Lasaracina E. In vitro zinc correction of natural killer (NK) activity in the elderly. Clin Exp Immunol. 1986;64:223–4.

63. Borrego F, Alonso MC, Galiani MD, Carracedo J, Ramirez R, Ostos B, Pena J, Solana R. NK phenotypic markers and IL2 response in NK cells from elderly people. Exp Gerontol. 1999;34:253–65.

64. Solana R, Campos C, Pera A, Tarazona R. Shaping of NK cell subsets by aging. Curr Opin Immunol. 2014;29:56–61.

65. Krishnaraj R. Senescence and cytokines modulate the NK cell expression. Mech Ageing Dev. 1997;96:89–101.

66. Almeida-Oliveira A, Smith-Carvalho M, Porto LC, Cardoso-Oliveira J, Ribeiro Ados S, Falcao RR, Abdelhay E, Bouzas LF, Thuler LC, Ornellas MH, Diamond HR. Age-related changes in natural killer cell receptors from childhood through old age. Hum Immunol. 2011;72:319–29.

67. Camous X, Pera A, Solana R, Larbi A. NK cells in healthy aging and age-associated diseases. J Biomed Biotechnol. 2012;2012:195956.

68. Wikby A, Nilsson BO, Forsey R, Thompson J, Strindhall J, Lofgren S, Ernerudh J, Pawelec G, Ferguson F, Johansson B. The immune risk phenotype is associated with IL-6 in the terminal decline stage: findings from the Swedish NONA immune longitudinal study of very late life functioning. Mech Ageing Dev. 2006;127:695–704.

21

A 13-year real-life study on efficacy, safety and biological effects of *Vespula* venom immunotherapy

Marcello Albanesi[1*], Andrea Nico[1], Alessandro Sinisi[1], Lucia Giliberti[1], Maria Pia Rossi[1], Margherita Rossini[2], Georgios Kourtis[1], Anna Simona Rucco[1], Filomena Loconte[1], Loredana Muolo[1], Marco Zurlo[1], Danilo Di Bona[1], Maria Filomena Caiaffa[3] and Luigi Macchia[1]

Abstract

Background: *Hymenoptera* venom immunotherapy (VIT) is a clinically effective treatment. However, little is known about its long-term clinical efficacy and biological effects. Several mechanisms have been proposed to account for VIT efficacy, including reduction of specific IgE and induction of allergen-specific IgG_4, but the overall picture remains elusive. We investigated *Vespula* VIT clinical efficacy up to 8 years after discontinuation and the kinetics of *Vespula*-specific IgE and IgG_4. Out of 686 consecutive patients we retrospectively selected and analysed a series of 23 patients with *Vespula* allergy that underwent a 5-year IT course, followed by a prolonged follow-up.

Methods: Clinical efficacy of VIT was assessed as number and severity of reactions to *Vespula* re-stinging events. The presence of *Vespula*-specific IgE and IgG_4 was also monitored over time.

Results: During the VIT treatment, patients were protected, reporting no reactions or mild reactions in occasion of re-stinging events. This protection was entirely maintained during the follow-up, up to 8 years. Skin reactivity (reflecting mast cell-bound *Vespula*-specific IgE) and circulating *Vespula*-specific IgE levels declined substantially during VIT. Notably, this reduction was maintained over time during the follow-up. Moreover, all the patients were analysed for IgG_4. A robust induction of *Vespula*-specific IgG_4 was observed during the VIT course, with a substantial decline during the follow-up.

Conclusions: We conclude that *Vespula* VIT is a clinically effective treatment, which induces long-term protection after discontinuation. The reduction of specific IgE, assessed by skin tests and RAST, closely matches the VIT- induced protection, while the IgG_4 induction seems not to be associated with VIT clinical efficacy in the long term.

Keywords: *Hymenoptera* venom allergy, Allergen immunotherapy, VIT, AIT, Long-term efficacy, Venom-specific IgE, Venom-specific IgG_4

Background

Insect sting allergy is responsible for severe and, sometimes, life-threatening reactions. Venom immunotherapy (VIT) was proven to be effective and safe in patients with venom allergy-induced anaphylaxis [1, 2]. The clinical efficacy of VIT is commonly defined by a reduction of the severity of the allergic reactions after *Hymenoptera* stings. In clinical practice, the reduction of both skin reactivity to insect venom and specific IgE levels in serum helps corroborate the assessment of the IT clinical efficacy [3]. Indeed, taken together, these two parameters define the global levels of allergen-specific IgE, as skin reactivity is quantitatively proportional to mast cell bound IgE. Of note, the vast majority of IgE are mast cell bound, whereas serum IgE reflect the minor pool of unbound/circulating IgE.

*Correspondence: marcello.albanesi@uniba.it
[1] School and Chair of Allergology and Clinical Immunology, Department of Emergency and Organ Transplantation, University of Bari-Aldo Moro, Piazza Giulio Cesare 13, Policlinico, 70124 Bari, Italy
Full list of author information is available at the end of the article

Only some reports exist on the long-term clinical efficacy of VIT and the kinetics of bound and unbound IgE after IT discontinuation (Additional file 1: Table S1) [4–10].

In the present study, we investigated, retrospectively, the real-life long-term efficacy of *Vespula* (*Vespula* spp.) VIT and its effects of specific IgE and IgG_4. Thus, 23 patients (18 men and 5 women), with a history of severe allergic reaction to *Vespula* sting, underwent *Vespula* VIT for 5 years, followed by an 8-year follow-up. During the study period, we monitored: (i) allergic reactions to *Vespula* stings; (ii) performed rigorously standardized quantitative skin testing; (iii) evaluated *Vespula*-specific IgE levels.

Several mechanisms have been proposed to account for VIT-induced clinical efficacy, including drop of the allergen specific IgE levels and induction of protective IgG_4 antibodies [11–14]. In fact, IgG_4 are considered protective antibodies for several reasons: (i) among all the IgG subtypes, they have a weak capacity to bind Fcγ Receptors and thereby a reduced ability to activate immune cells [15]; (ii) the Fc portion of IgG_4 molecule does not fix complement, due to the low affinity for complement factor C1q [16]; (iii) IgG_4 are functionally monovalent and unable to form immune complexes. Indeed, IgG_4 are dynamic molecules that exchange Fab arms by swapping heavy-light chain pairs with IgG_4 molecules of different specificities [17, 18]. This results in the production of bispecific antibodies with a substantially decreased capacity for antigen cross-linking [15, 17, 18].

Thus, we also investigated the kinetics of IgG_4 in the 23 patients during the 5-year VIT course and the follow-up.

Methods
Patients
Twenty-three patients (18 men, 5 women) with severe *Vespula* allergy that underwent VIT for 5 years were retrospectively analysed in this study. These patients were monitored for allergic reactions to *Vespula* stings during 8 additional years, after VIT discontinuation.

Inclusion criteria
We carefully analysed the clinical files of 686 patients that had access to our Hymenoptera Venom Allergy Service, from 1989 to 2010 and applied a stringent selection process based on the following criteria:

Diagnostic criteria
a. History of severe adverse reaction to *Vespula* stinging events: only the patients that had a grade III/IV [19] reaction to a *Vespula* stinging events were included in this study.

b. Clear recognition of the culprit insect in the entomological display case: only the patients that recognized clearly *Vespula* as the culprit insect were included in this study.

c. Sensitization to *Vespula* venom as revealed by both skin test and RAST: patient missing either of these two parameters were excluded from this study.

Therapeutic criteria
Requirement of 5-year *Vespula* VIT: patients that underwent either shorter/longer VIT courses or multiple ITs for different *Hymenoptera* (e.g. *Vespula* and *Polistes*) were excluded from this study.

Follow-up criteria
Requirement of at least one follow-up clinical assessment (at least 3 years after VIT discontinuation), with skin tests execution and serum collection for RAST determination (see below): if one of these determinations was missing the patient was excluded from the study.

Vespula venom IT
All patients had been treated with *Vespula* spp. VIT, subcutaneously (n = 13 were from ALK-Abellò VIT supplier, Milan, Italy; n = 10 were from Dome Hollister Stier Miles VIT supplier, Spokane, WA, USA). As for the ALK-Abellò VIT, the venom was purified, biologically standardized in Quality Units (SQ-U) and absorbed onto alum hydroxide gel. The maintenance dosage was 100.000 SQ-U. The amount of alum hydroxide contained in the maintenance dose was 1.35 mg. The DHS VIT was an aqueous solution of purified *Vespula* venom. The maintenance dosage was 100 µg, fully comparable with the ALK-Abellò maintenance dosage [20]. After 10–15 weeks of induction with increasing doses of *Vespula* venom, the maintenance dose was given every 6 weeks, for 5 years. Adverse reactions to the VIT injections were recorded on the clinical logbook of the patient. In particular, local reactions of less than 10 cm in diameter were considered mild local reactions. The IT protocols used are summarized in Additional file 2: Table S2 and Additional file 3: Table S3.

The insect-sting challenge test was not performed at the end of the VIT course, due to local ethical policies.

Stings events recording
Patients were asked to recognize the stinging insect using an entomological display case.

All the patients were interviewed for re-stings and possible related adverse reactions. During VIT course, the interview process was performed every 6 weeks, at every VIT administration. During the follow-up, patients were interviewed approximately 3 and 8 years, respectively, upon VIT discontinuation.

Vespula re-stinging events were also recorded in the clinical logbook of the patient (along with a few occasional stings by other *Hymenoptera*). The severity of adverse reaction to stinging events was classified according to Müller [19].

Quantitative skin testing

Skin tests were performed at baseline and 3 and 5 years after the beginning of VIT. Moreover, the tests were performed at year 3.5 ± 1.4 and 8.1 ± 3.8 after discontinuation. Skin testing was carried out in a strictly quantitative fashion by two distinct techniques: skin prick testing and intradermal testing, as described [21]. Both techniques were carried out in a single session, sequentially, in a three-step procedure. Thus, the patients were first subjected to skin prick testing, using a 100 µg/ml *Vespula* venom solution (see below) and, successively, to intradermal tests with the same allergen at two different tenfold concentrations (viz. 0.1 and 1 µg/ml, respectively).

Lyophilized *Vespula* allergen *(Vespula* spp.) was supplied by Dome–Hollister-Stier Miles, Spokane, WA, USA, and reconstituted in 1% albumin saline. Histamine hydrochloride 10 mg/ml in 50% glycerol solution (Stallergenes, Antony, France) was used as the positive control in skin prick testing. A 0.002 mg/ml aqueous solution of the same reagent was used as the positive control in intradermal testing. Saline with 1% albumin was used as the negative control in both skin prick testing and intradermal testing. Both skin prick tests and intradermal tests were performed on the volar side of the forearms.

As for skin reactivity quantitative assessment, the area of the wheals generated was calculated as described [21]. In order to achieve normalization for inter and intra-individual variations, results were expressed in terms of ratio between the *Vespula* wheal area and the homologous histamine area, referred to as Skin Index [22].

Serum antibody measurement

Allergen-specific *(Vespula* spp.) IgE levels were measured by RAST (ImmunoCAP Thermo Fischer, Milan, Italy) in serum samples collected at baseline, approx. 3 and 6 months, respectively, from starting and, then, yearly during the VIT course. During the follow-up, serum collection took place at the same time-points as for skin testing. The sera were not diluted before the IgE assessment. Results were expressed in mass units (assuming $1U = 2.4$ ng).

Vespula-specific IgG_4 levels were determined in the above sera using a *Vespula* IgG_4 ELISA kit (Dr. Fooke Laboratories, Neuss, Germany). Thus, *Vespula* pre-coated strips were used. The sera of the patients were diluted 1:101, in dilution buffer (supplied), and then added into the correspondent wells. After incubation

(1 h at 37 °C) and extensive washing, 100 µl of anti-human IgG_4-antibody conjugated with horseradish peroxidase were added, followed by 1 h incubation at 37 °C. Upon further washing, 100 µl of Substrate (also supplied by Dr. Fooke Laboratories) was added and incubated for 10 min, in the dark, at room temperature, revealing the presence of specific IgG_4. Upon addition of 50 µl of stop solution, optical density (O.D.) measurement was carried out using a microplate reader (Biorad, model 450, Milan, Italy), at λ 450 nm. Results were expressed in mass units.

Vespula-specific IgG_4 were also determined by an additional experimental approach, based on an in-house adaptation of two different commercially available antibody-revealing tools. Thus, anti-human IgG_4 pre-coated 96-well plates (Cayman Chemical Company, Ann Arbor, USA) were used. Upon blocking with 10% non-fat dried milk, overnight, the wells were incubated at 37 °C with 50 µl of ALLERgen Basic Kit incubation buffer (RADIM, Pomezia, Italy) and 50 µl of serum of the patients, for 1 h. Subsequently, after extensive washing, biotinylated *Vespula* allergen (100 µl; also from RADIM) was added, followed by 30 min incubation at 37 °C. Upon further washing and incubation with streptavidin-conjugated horseradish peroxidase (30 min at 37 °C; RADIM) addition of the substrate (15 min at room temperature) revealed the presence of specific IgG_4. O.D. measurement was carried out as above, at λ 450 nm.

Vespula-specific IgG_4 levels were also measured in 20 adult healthy controls (14 female, 6 male; average age 32.4 ± 8.1) by the commercial kit. Only five of them were studied with the in-house technique.

Statistical analysis

IgE and IgG_4 changes were analysed using one-way Anova with Bonferroni post-test (N.S.: > 0.01, *$p < 0.01$, **$p < 0.001$). Error bars in figures correspond to standard error means. Moreover, the IgG_4 results obtained in the patients were analysed against results in healthy controls, using the Student's t Test (N.S. $p > 0.05$, *$p < 0.05$). Average and standard deviation are used in the text.

Results
Clinical efficacy and safety of *Vespula* VIT

Twenty-three patients were analysed in this retrospective study: 18 men and 5 women (out of a cumulative series of 686 *Hymenoptera*-allergic patients). All these patients had been diagnosed with *Vespula* venom allergy and had a clinical history of severe allergic reactions to *Vespula* stings. Moreover, they had undergone a 5-year *Vespula* VIT course, with a subsequent prolonged follow-up of up to 8 years. The clinical features of the patients at the time of diagnosis are summarized in Table 1.

Table 1 Clinical features of the patients enrolled in the study

Patient	Gender	Severity of reaction Pre VIT (according to Müller)	Age (years)	VIT duration (months)	Follow-up duration (months)	Total VIT dose (SQ-U ×10⁶)	Total VIT dose (mg)	VIT supplier
N.G.	M	IV	60	61	53	4.51		Alk
T.G.	M	IV	33	58	182		5.9	DHS
P.G.	M	IV	49	59	122		4.7	DHS
C.G.	F	III	21	60	184		5.1	DHS
C.G.	M	III	45	59	36		5.7	DHS
C.G.	M	III	35	60	199		6.5	DHS
D.F.T.	M	IV	51	58	103	1.82		Alk
R.F.	M	IV	44	59	151	2.05		Alk
G.G.	F	III	39	73	41	4.41		Alk
C.M.	F	IV	37	61	38	2.18		Alk
D.M.S	M	III	54	61	36	4.44		Alk
I.N.	M	IV	54	63	36	2.36		Alk
A.A.	M	III	13	63	62	2.11		Alk
C.M.	M	IV	39	64	43	2.19		Alk
D.F.	M	IV	59	64	66		5.8	DHS
T.A.	M	IV	49	62	28		5.7	DHS
V.V.	M	IV	50	59	51		5.6	DHS
T.A.	M	III	46	60	44	2.57		Alk
S.S.	F	III	29	50	36	3.85		Alk
M.S.	M	III	52	64	56	1.71		Alk
M.A.	F	III	33	64	27	2.28		Alk
V.R.	M	IV	52	62	37		6.5	DHS
M.F.	M	IV	40	64	31		5.7	DHS
Mean			42.78	61.22	72.26	5.73	2.80	
SD			11.81	4.02	55.37	0.54	1.07	

DHS Dome Hollister Stier, *ALK* ALK-Abellò

At first, we evaluated clinical efficacy of *Vespula* VIT. The single stinging events were assessed and the symptoms associated with their severity. During the VIT course, patients were carefully interviewed every 6 weeks, at every VIT administration. Likewise, during the follow-up, patients were personally interviewed at two different time points after VIT discontinuation (approximatively 3 and 8 years). During the VIT course, 16 patients (69.6%) were stung by a *Vespula*, with a total of 44 stinging events, evenly distributed over time (on average, 8.8 stinging events/year ± 5.4). Particularly, during the first year of VIT there were 13 stinging events in 8 patients. All the stung patients were protected. In fact, none of these events led to a major systemic reaction (grade IV according to Müller) [19], 8 events (18.2%) were followed by a mild to moderate systemic reaction (grade II–III), whereas 36 events (81.8%) were either followed by a local reaction (grade I) or were completely asymptomatic (Fig. 1a).

During the follow-up, 14 patients (60.8%) were stung by *Vespula*, with a total of 46 stings. Importantly, the vast majority of these stinging events were either followed by a local reaction or asymptomatic (43 events, 93.5%), whereas only three stings (6.5%) were followed by a moderate systemic reaction (grade III; Fig. 1a). The severity of the adverse reaction towards re-stinging events decreased over time in the same allergic individuals undergoing *Vespula* IT and subjected to multiple stings and this protection was maintained long after VIT discontinuation (data not shown).

Furthermore, we assessed the safety of VIT. To this aim, we monitored the possible adverse reactions to the subcutaneous VIT injections. During the 5-year VIT course, 998 injections in total were given. Of these, 990 (99.2%) were followed by no adverse reaction of any kinds, whereas eight injections (0.8%) were followed by a local immediate reaction. None of the injections was followed by a systemic anaphylactic reaction (Fig. 1b).

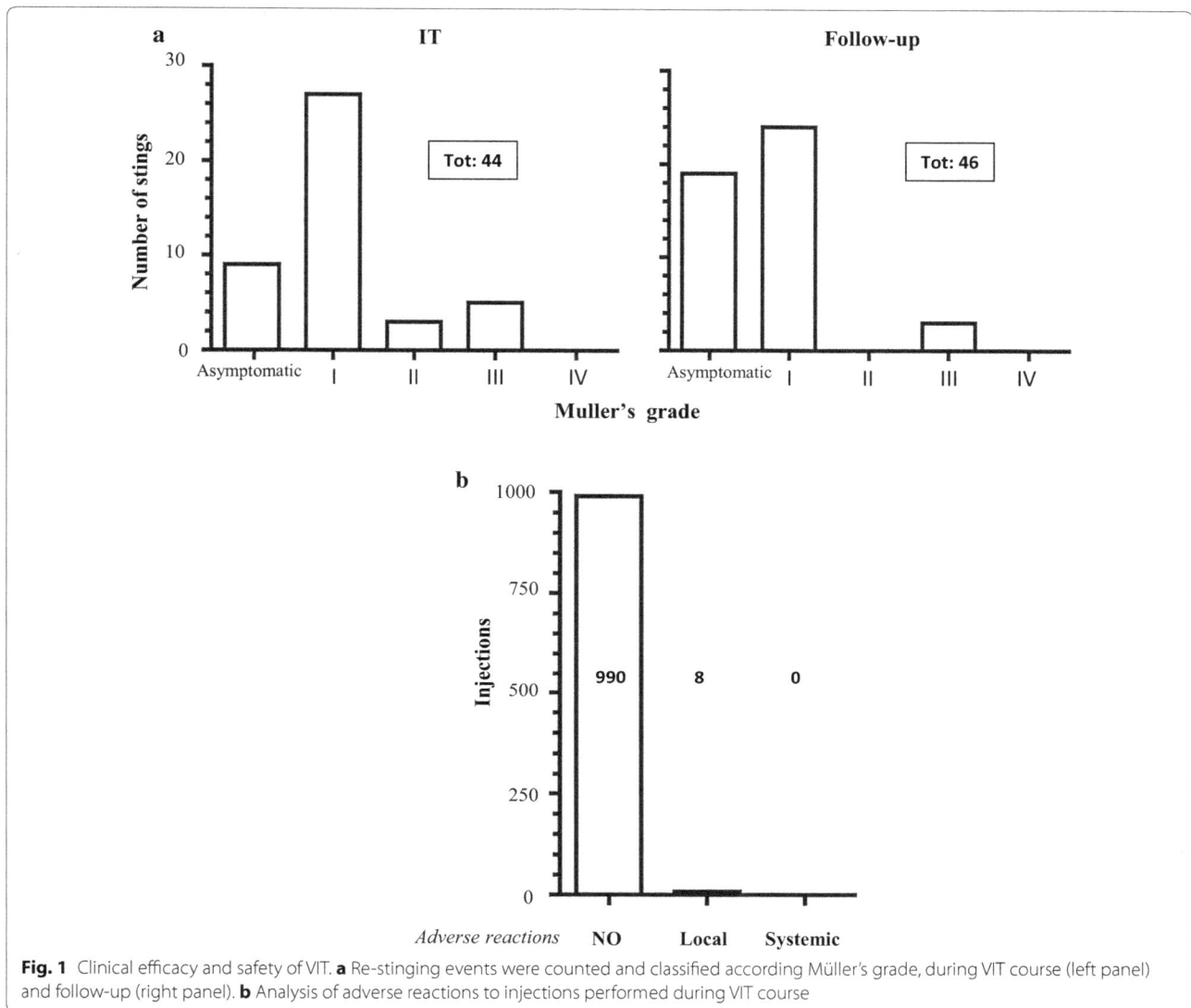

Fig. 1 Clinical efficacy and safety of VIT. **a** Re-stinging events were counted and classified according Müller's grade, during VIT course (left panel) and follow-up (right panel). **b** Analysis of adverse reactions to injections performed during VIT course

Kinetics of *Vespula*-specific IgE

IgE interact via the Fc portion with FcεRI, expressed on different cell types, in particular mast cells. FcεRI is a high affinity receptor that has a dissociation constant (K_d) of 10^{-9} [23]. As a consequence, the vast majority of IgE is linked to tissue resident mast cells (i.e. the bound pool). The remaining part of IgE (i.e. the much lesser unbound pool) circulates in plasma [24]. In allergic subjects, the amount of specific IgE bound on mast cell surface may be assessed through quantitative skin testing [21, 25]. The amount of unbound IgE may be evaluated by RAST [26]. Thus, using these techniques, we evaluated the kinetics of both bound and unbound *Vespula*-specific IgE, during the VIT course and the follow-up.

As shown in Fig. 2a, during the VIT course, the skin reactivity (reflecting the bound pool of *Vespula*-specific IgE) steadily declined over time, with a 62.5% reduction after 5 years (Skin Index from 0.8 ± 0.6 to 0.3 ± 0.3). This reduction was essentially maintained throughout the follow-up.

In contrast, soon after the beginning, VIT induced a significant increase in *Vespula*-specific circulating IgE (from $20.8 \times 10^3 \pm 27.0 \times 10^3$ ng/ml to $42.1 \times 10^3 \pm 44.8 \times 10^3$ ng/ml; $p < 0.001$), peaking approximately 3 months after VIT initiation. After this initial transient increase, circulating IgE levels steadily declined over time, reaching an average value of $17.1 \times 10^3 \pm 20.2 \times 10^3$ ng/ml, at the end of the treatment, as expected [27]. During the follow-up

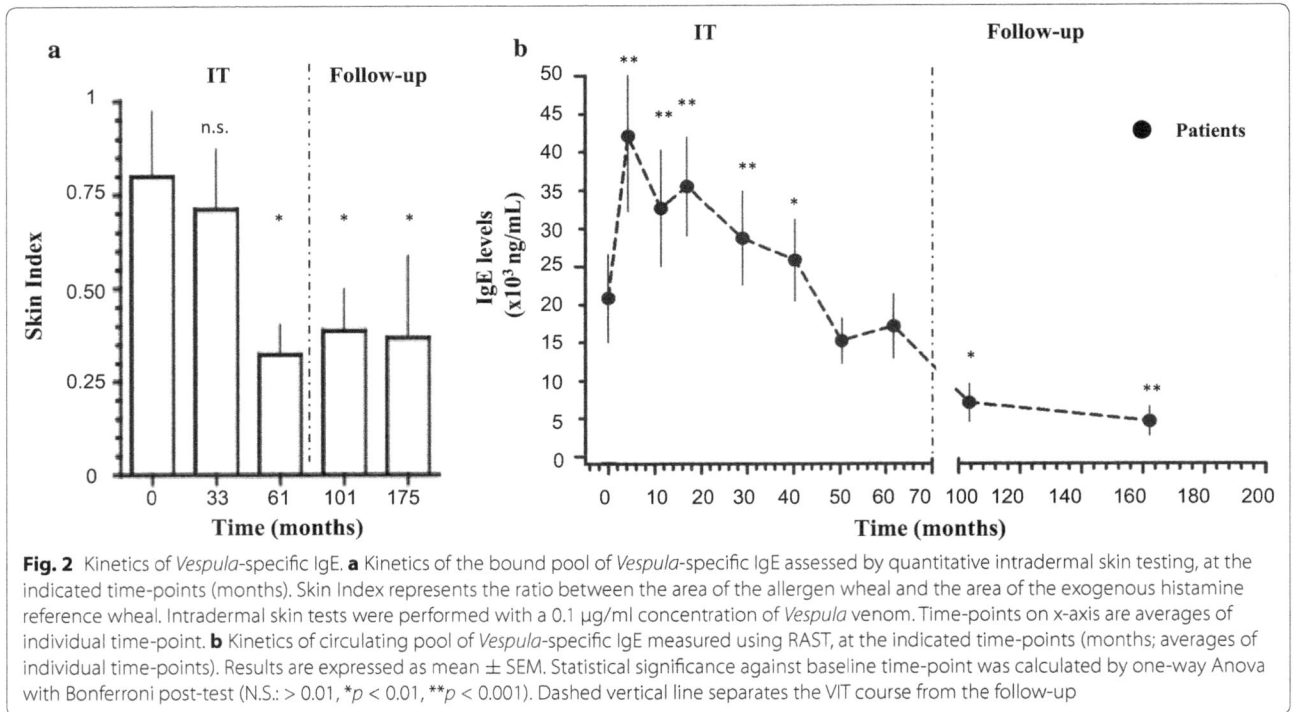

Fig. 2 Kinetics of *Vespula*-specific IgE. **a** Kinetics of the bound pool of *Vespula*-specific IgE assessed by quantitative intradermal skin testing, at the indicated time-points (months). Skin Index represents the ratio between the area of the allergen wheal and the area of the exogenous histamine reference wheal. Intradermal skin tests were performed with a 0.1 µg/ml concentration of *Vespula* venom. Time-points on x-axis are averages of individual time-point. **b** Kinetics of circulating pool of *Vespula*-specific IgE measured using RAST, at the indicated time-points (months; averages of individual time-points). Results are expressed as mean ± SEM. Statistical significance against baseline time-point was calculated by one-way Anova with Bonferroni post-test (N.S.: > 0.01, *p < 0.01, **p < 0.001). Dashed vertical line separates the VIT course from the follow-up

we observed a further drop of the circulating *Vespula*-specific IgE levels, down to $4.5 \times 10^3 \pm 6.1 \times 10^3$ ng/ml (71.1% reduction; Fig. 2b). No differences in the kinetics of mast-cell bound and circulating IgE were observed when patients treated with ALK-Abellò and patients treated with DHS VIT were compared with each other (Additional file 4: Figure S1A).

Kinetics of *Vespula*-specific IgG₄

We assessed the *Vespula*-specific IgG_4 levels, at the same time-points as for circulating IgE. Interestingly, in all these patients an increase of *Vespula*-specific IgG_4 was detected during the VIT course (from 293.2 ± 292.8 ng/ml at baseline to 718.2 ± 527.2 ng/ml at 29 months, during the VIT course, to 630.5 ± 475.5 ng/ml at the end of the IT course). The induction of IgG_4 was not maintained over time, during the follow-up. Indeed, a drop in the IgG_4 levels after VIT discontinuation was observed, down to 328.3 ± 260.1 ng/ml and 323.9 ± 259.2 ng/ml at 103 and 162 months, respectively (Fig. 3a).

No differences in the kinetics *Vespula*-specific IgG_4 were observed when patients treated with ALK-Abellò and patients treated with DHS VIT were compared with each other (Additional file 4: Figure S1B).

In order to validate the technical approach used to assess the IgG_4 levels, we developed an in-house IgG_4 assay, based on the adaptation of two different commercially available antibody-revealing tools. Thus, in 6 out of

the 23, patients we evaluated the IgG_4 levels using two different assays.

The set of results obtained were comparable with each other (Fig. 3b).

It is also worth noticing that *Vespula*-specific IgG_4 levels in healthy controls at the baseline were significantly lower compared with the 23 patients.

Discussion

It is widely accepted that *Vespula* VIT induces protection from stings in allergic patients during VIT and after discontinuation. In 2004, Golden and Colleagues monitored children with allergy to insect stings that had undergone VIT [8]. Importantly, they demonstrated that VIT in children leads to a significantly lower risk of systemic reactions to stings, up to 20 years after the treatment is stopped, suggesting that clinical efficacy is long lasting [8]. In 2008, Hafner et al. performed a long-term survey in adult patients who had previously discontinued VIT. The majority of the patients reported that the symptoms experienced with stinging events after VIT discontinuation were milder than symptoms before VIT, suggesting again long-term efficacy [9]. Moreover, Pravettoni and co-workers, analysing a series of 232 patients, found that 35.2% of the patients who could be monitored (159) reported at least one field sting up to 10 years after VIT discontinuation. None of them suffered from any systemic reactions [28].

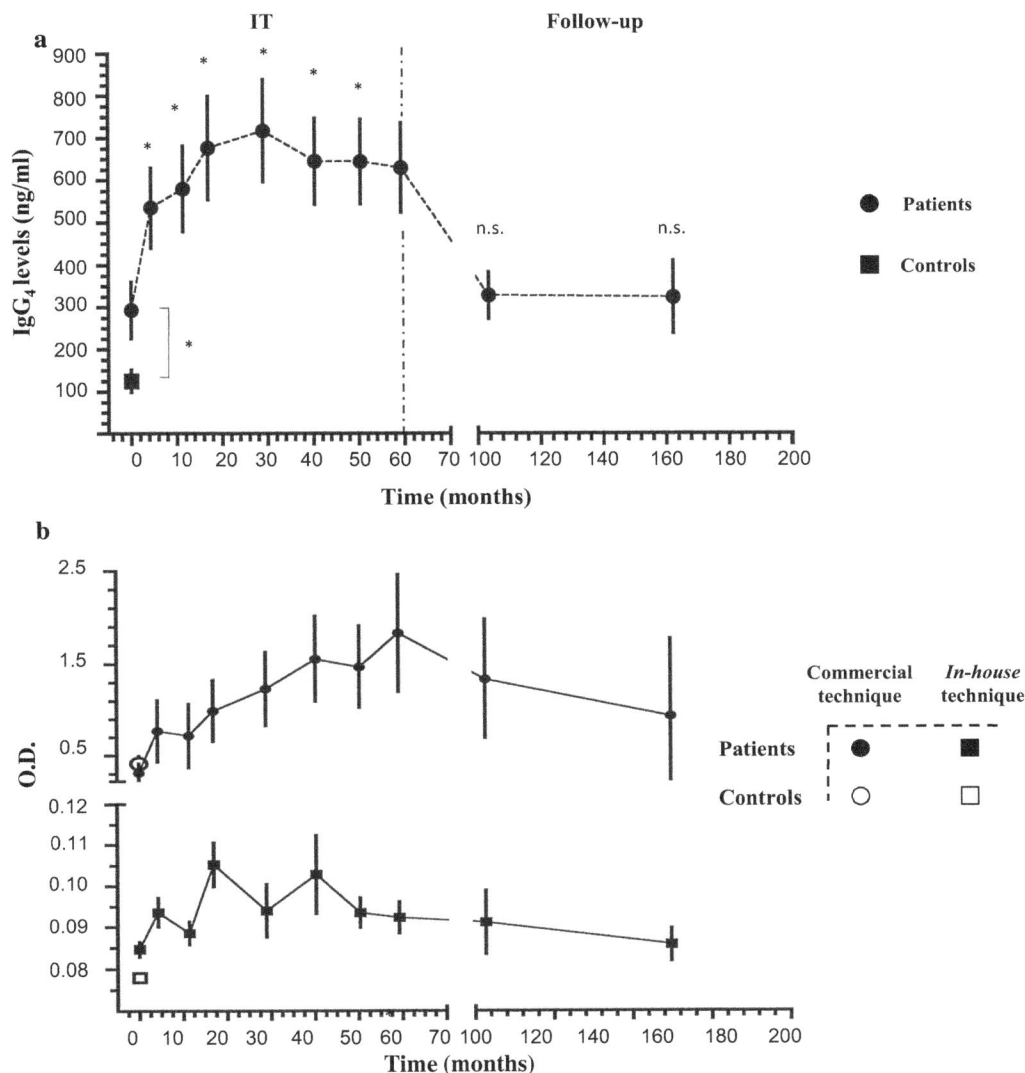

Fig. 3 Kinetics of Vespula-specific IgG$_4$. **a** Kinetics of serum Vespula-specific IgG$_4$ measured using commercial ELISA kit at the indicated time-points, in months (averages of individual time-points). N = 23 patients and 20 healthy controls. Statistical significance against baseline time-point was calculated by one-way Anova with Bonferroni post-test (N.S.: > 0.01, *p < 0.01, **p < 0.001). Dashed vertical line separates the VIT course from the follow-up. **b** Comparison of measurement (O.D.) obtained with the IgG$_4$ commercial kit versus the in-house technique at the indicated time-points, in months (averages of individual time-points). N = 6 patients and five healthy controls. Results are expressed as mean ± SEM

However, few reports exists on VIT clinical efficacy long after discontinuation in adult patients (Additional file 1: Table S1) and most of them rely on data obtained through mail questionnaires sent to the patients after VIT discontinuation or telephone interviews.

Moreover, near-all these studies present some points of relative weakness, mostly because of considerable heterogeneity at different levels (Additional file 1: Table S1): (i) age of the patients, (ii) duration of the IT, (iii) type(s) of venom(s) administered during VIT (e.g. honeybee, Vespula) and (iv) VIT supplier used.

As for the age of patients, the outcome of the immune response is age-related [29]. Therefore, the final outcome of VIT and its long-term efficacy may vary accordingly. Moreover for duration of VIT, some of the studies on long-term efficacy included patients that underwent variable periods of VIT (from 3 to 5 years). Nonetheless, such difference might influence the outcome of the long-term immunological memory and therefore the extent of the long-term protection. Moreover, Hymenoptera venoms are, to some extent, cross-reactive and this could introduce biases in the assessment of VIT outcomes, when two therapies are given together. As an example, *Vespula* antigen 5 (Ves v 5), one of the major *Vespula* allergen, contains 204 amino acids residues and shares 60% of sequence identity with *Polistes dominulus* antigen 5 (Pol d 5) [30]. Therefore, patients undergoing VIT for these two different venoms could possibly develop a longer and more robust protection compared to patients receiving VIT for a single venom.

Finally, in near-all the reports present in the literature the VIT supplier is not declared. This latter point appears to be particularly relevant as *Hymenoptera* venoms comprise a complex mixture of different proteins that might all contribute to sensitization. Indeed, in vespid venom three main allergens have been described: Phospholipase A1, Hyaluronidase and Antigen 5 [31]. Importantly, the purification process of the venom extracts may vary between manufacturers [32, 33] and, therefore, the final quality and composition of the venom extracts might not be fully comparable. Thus, a different outcome in the final immune response might be obtained using different venom preparations.

In our work, we analysed a homogenous group of adult patients (mean age of 42.8 years ± 11.8) that underwent *Vespula* VIT only, for almost exactly 5 years (on average 61.2 months ± 4.0). After VIT discontinuation, we monitored all the patients over a prolonged follow-up (Table 1). Moreover, in our study, 11 patients were treated with DHS and 12 with ALK-Abellò ITs. It has to be noticed that in all the patients nearly the same induction/maintenance protocol was used (Additional file 2: Table S2 and Additional file 3: Table S3) and the final dose of venom received was fully comparable, regardless of the suppliers [20]. Interestingly, no differences were observed in terms of clinical protection in the patient treated with VIT of either of the two suppliers (data not shown). Moreover, both DHS and ALK-Abellò ITs induced comparable effects on circulating *Vespula*-specific IgE and IgG$_4$ (Additional file 4: Figure S1A, B). This latter observation indirectly confirms that the immunogenicity of the VIT used was also similar.

We demonstrated that *Vespula* VIT confers a robust protection not only during the VIT course, but also long after its discontinuation. Indeed, during the follow-up, 60% of the patients were re-stung, of whom 93% were minimally symptomatic or asymptomatic and none of the patients needed to resume *Vespula* VIT, which suggests that a 5-year IT course is possibly protective and can be recommended, at least in *Vespula* allergic patients. In order to evaluate clinical efficacy of *Vespula* VIT the patients in our study were interviewed for stinging events at each single administration during VIT and at two time (at least) points during the follow-up. In the case of a sting, they were asked to recognize the culprit insect at

every interview, using an entomologic display case. It has to be noticed that *Vespula* appears to be correctly recognized in 72.3% of the cases from *Vespula* allergic patients [34]. This rather stringent approach represents a novelty.

Moreover, aside clinical efficacy, we also evaluated the biological effects of *Vespula* VIT. Indeed, as shown in Additional file 1: Table S1, few reports assessed the long-term biological effects of venom IT. Even though a drop of circulating specific IgE titres was sometimes observed in up to 70% of the patients undergoing VIT [35], only little information is present in the literature on the kinetics of venom-specific IgE long after treatment discontinuation.

As it is known, IgE molecules have a unique immunological behaviour. Indeed, at the steady state, the vast majority of IgE is bound on the surface of the mast cells via the interaction with FcεRI, a high affinity receptor, able to bind a single IgE molecule with K$_d$ of 10^{-9} [23]. The remaining smaller pool of IgE circulates in plasma in unbound form. Therefore, in our study, we monitored both bound and unbound pools of *Vespula*-specific IgE.

On the one hand, changes in the bound pool of IgE were assessed with skin testing, performed in a strictly quantitative fashion. Data of this kind are particularly scarce in the context of long-term studies. Indeed, skin test results might be influenced by several factors such as circadian rhythm and technical expertise of the operator performing skin testing, thus demanding methodological rigour. Moreover, in order to render our data comparable with each other, we put emphasis on achieving normalization of the results. To this aim, we expressed this parameter by a Skin Index, previously defined as the ratio between the area of the wheal generated by the *Vespula* allergen and the area of the wheal generated by exogenous histamine [21]. Remarkably, we observed a robust reduction of skin reactivity (62.5% reduction after 5 years of VIT) after VIT that was maintained throughout the follow-up (Fig. 2a). To our knowledge, few works have so far analysed skin reactivity/variation in mast cell-bound specific IgE in a strictly quantitative fashion at different time points. In particular, before VIT, during the VIT course and long after VIT discontinuation.

On the other hand, the unbound pool of *Vespula* specific IgE was assessed by RAST. In line with other reports [36, 37], we observed a transient increase of circulating *Vespula*-specific IgE early after VIT initiation, peaking at 3 months (Fig. 2b). This time-point corresponds to the end of the IT induction phase, during which the allergen is administered weekly, at increasing doses. Thus, the increase in *Vespula*-specific IgE titres might be explained by the presence in allergic subjects of memory IgE B cells. These cells are able to differentiate into

IgE-producing plasma cells upon allergen encounter [38, 39]. Interestingly, during this initial phase of VIT, the patients are already protected towards re-stinging events. Indeed, during the first year of VIT course, we observed 13 re-stinging events (in 8 patients) that were either asymptomatic or followed by a reaction of grade I of the Müller scale. This observation suggests that the clinical protection is already present early during the VIT course, despite the high *Vespula*-specific IgE levels. This initial increase was followed by a progressive and steady decline during the maintenance period. Surprisingly, we observed a persistent and further reduction of circulating IgE levels long after VIT discontinuation. This latter data suggest the induction of immunological changes, possibly inducing tolerance, resulting in the decline of specific IgE levels (Even though mast-cell bound *Vespula*-specific IgE levels seemed not to decline further during the follow-up) (Fig. 2a, b).

The cross-comparison between the clinical data, the quantitative skin test analysis and the data on circulating *Vespula*-specific IgE seems to suggest that the drop of *Vespula*-specific IgE levels might be mechanistically related to the long-term efficacy of VIT. As a consequence, based on our data, one can propose to use the venom-specific IgE levels (assessed after discontinuation) as a biomarker for long-term VIT clinical efficacy, at least in *Vespula* allergy.

However, the precise immunological mechanisms underlying VIT efficacy are probably more diverse and complex and still unclear [40–43]. Particularly, VIT has been shown to induce a rise in specific IgG$_4$ levels. It is well known that a regular and persistent exposure to an antigen is able to induce IgG$_4$ antibodies [44]. As mentioned above, IgG$_4$ should be considered anti-inflammatory antibodies. Indeed, IgG$_4$ are dynamic molecule that behave as monovalent antibodies and therefore cannot form immune complexes [17]. Moreover IgG$_4$, due to their poor binding capacity to both complement and FcγRs, activate only weakly Fc-dependent immune mechanisms, such as antibody dependent cytotoxicity or the complement cascade [15, 16]. However, even though IgG$_4$ have been previously proposed as a contributing factor to the clinical efficacy of VIT [45, 46], no reports have analysed the changes in the IgG$_4$ levels long-after VIT discontinuation, so far (Additional file 1: Table S1).

Thus, we evaluated changes in the levels of *Vespula*-specific IgG$_4$ throughout VIT and follow-up in the 23 patients studied. Remarkably, we found that *Vespula*-specific IgG$_4$ rose and then reached a plateau during the VIT course but declined substantially during the follow-up, since the IgG$_4$ titres at 3 and 8 years follow-up timepoints are comparable to the ones observed before VIT (Fig. 3a).

This latter result suggests that long-term protection induced by VIT could be IgG$_4$-independent. Interestingly, a previous report by Varga et al. [47] analysed the role of honeybee specific IgG$_4$ in a group of 10 children that had undergone honeybee VIT. In line with our results, the authors of this study after a 2-year follow-up found no correlation between honeybee specific IgG$_4$ levels and long-term efficacy of VIT.

In our study we evaluated, for the first time, *Vespula*-specific IgG$_4$ using two different technical approaches. In particular, the commercial kit for *Vespula*-specific IgG$_4$ was based on the use of *Vespula* allergen pre-coated strips. In this assay, after the incubation with the patient serum, the presence of IgG$_4$ is revealed using of anti-human IgG$_4$-antibody conjugated with horseradish peroxidase. Nonetheless, in this experimental setting, the total amount of IgG$_4$ revealed might be underestimated. Indeed, during the incubation, other *Vespula*-specific antibodies with different isotypes (e.g. IgG$_2$, IgE), present in the patient serum, will most likely compete with IgG$_4$ for the binding to the cognate antigen. In order to overcome this possible competition and to ascertain the results obtained with the commercial kit for *Vespula*-specific IgG$_4$, we developed an *in house*-technique that we applied to six patients and nine normal controls. This assay relies on the use of pre-coated anti-IgG$_4$ wells. After incubation with the patients' sera, *Vespula*-specific IgG$_4$ are revealed using biotinylated *Vespula* allergen. Remarkably, the results obtained with the two distinct technique were comparable, thus validating our findings on IgG$_4$ (Fig. 3b).

It has to be noticed that IgG$_4$ titres at the beginning of the VIT were already higher compared to the 20 healthy controls, suggesting that in *Hymenoptera* venom allergic subjects an IgG-driven immune response already occurs independently from VIT. To our knowledge, this is the only study in which pre-VIT values of IgG$_4$ in *Vespula* allergic patients are compared to those found in a group of normal adult individuals. Finally, we analysed the trend of the ratio between the *Vespula*-specific IgE and IgG$_4$ over all the study period. Interestingly, this ratio progressively declines (from 70.1 to 27.2, at the end of the VIT course). This decline appears to be even more pronounced at the end of the follow-up (14.2) (Additional file 4: Figure S1C). This latter result seems to corroborate the hypothesis that indeed *Vespula* venom VIT induces long-lasting immunological changes.

Conclusions

In conclusion, our results obtained in a relatively small but well-controlled cohort of patients (out of a series of 686 patients) show that *Vespula* VIT induces a robust and long-lasting protection towards re-stinging events. The results obtained on *Vespula*-specific IgE levels show that IgE levels

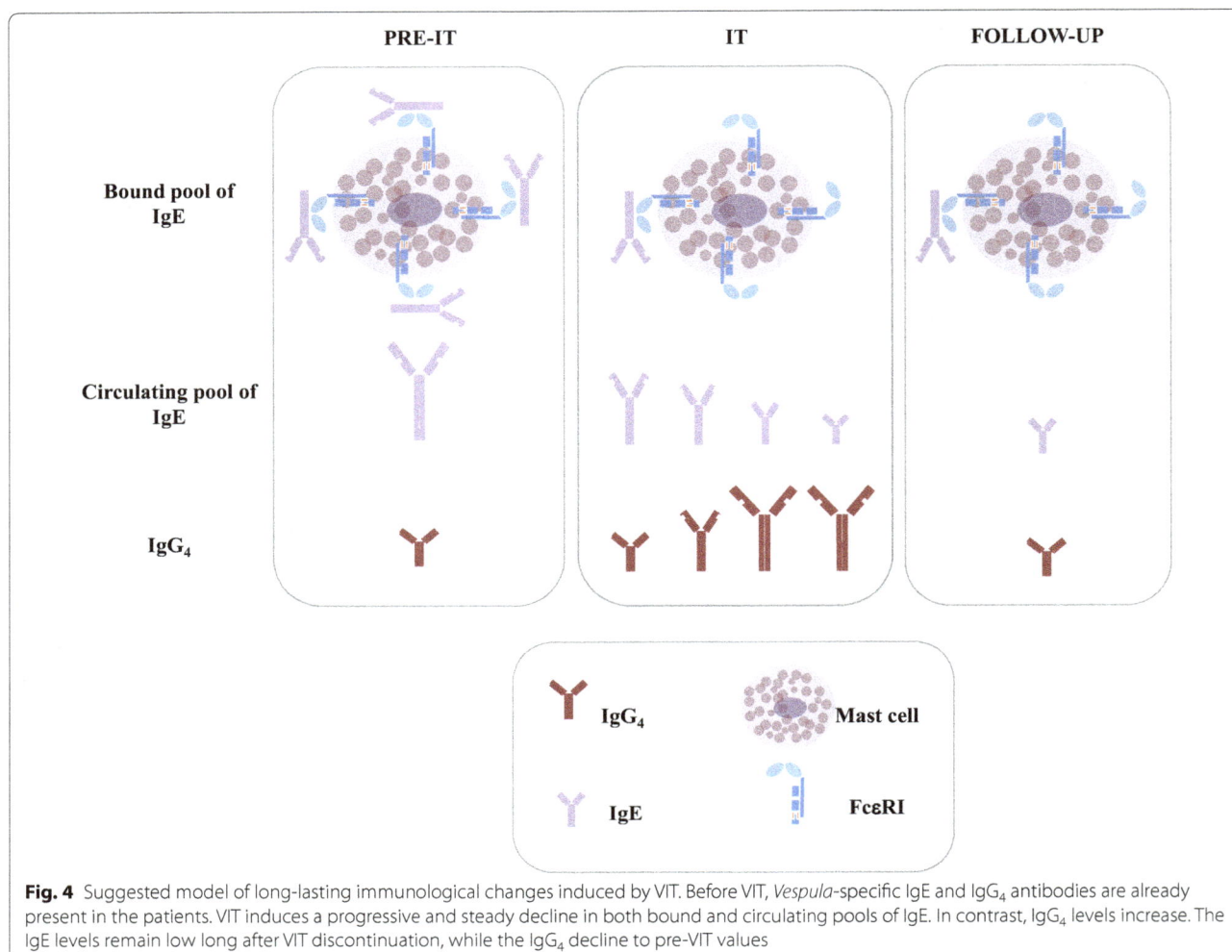

Fig. 4 Suggested model of long-lasting immunological changes induced by VIT. Before VIT, *Vespula*-specific IgE and IgG$_4$ antibodies are already present in the patients. VIT induces a progressive and steady decline in both bound and circulating pools of IgE. In contrast, IgG$_4$ levels increase. The IgE levels remain low long after VIT discontinuation, while the IgG$_4$ decline to pre-VIT values

(bound and unbound) closely match the VIT clinical efficacy. Particularly, IgE levels in the follow-up, are perhaps the best predictor of clinical efficacy of *Vespula* VIT. Furthermore, IgG$_4$ levels were sustained during VIT course but declined substantially after the end of VIT and, therefore, are less useful in assessing clinical efficacy of VIT in the long term. Rather, specific IgG$_4$ could be used as a signature of valid immune stimulation induced by VIT (Fig. 4).

helped with the analysis of the data and clinical assistance; LG performed the experiments with the help of MPR and MR, LM; AS, AR, GK and FL helped with the clinical assistance; MZ helped with analysis of the data; MFC discussed results, provided ideas, helped with the clinical and scientific work organization; DDB participated in the data analysis and provided critical reading of the manuscript; LM apart from clinical involvement, conceived and supervised the study, secured the financial support and revised the manuscript. All authors read and approved the final manuscript.

Abbreviations
VIT: venom immunotherapy; RAST: radioallergosorbentest; OD: optical density; DHS: Dome–Hollister Stier; SQ-U: Standard Quality Unit.

Author details
[1] School and Chair of Allergology and Clinical Immunology, Department of Emergency and Organ Transplantation, University of Bari-Aldo Moro, Piazza Giulio Cesare 13, Policlinico, 70124 Bari, Italy. [2] Unit of Clinical Pathology, Policlinico di Bari, Piazza Giulio Cesare 13, Policlinico, 70124 Bari, Italy. [3] School and Chair of Allergology and Clinical Immunology, Department of Medical and Surgical Sciences, University of Foggia, Via Luigi Pinto 1, 70100 Foggia, Italy.

Authors' contributions
MA analysed the data, wrote the manuscript, performed some of the IgG$_4$ work, helped with the project design and patient clinical assistance; AN

Acknowledgements

We are thankful to F. Frisenda and M. Di Giacomo from the University of Bari-Aldo Moro for the help with the experimental work and to F. Joensson from the Antibody in Therapy and Pathology Laboratory, Institute Pasteur, Paris for providing critical reading of the manuscript.

Funding

The authors declare that this study was carried out with institutional resources only.

References

1. Moffitt JE, et al. Stinging insect hypersensitivity: a practice parameter update. J Allergy Clin Immunol. 2004;114(4):869–86.
2. Bonifazi F, et al. Prevention and treatment of Hymenoptera venom allergy: guidelines for clinical practice. Allergy. 2005;60(12):1459–70.
3. Bilo BM, et al. Diagnosis of Hymenoptera venom allergy. Allergy. 2005;60(11):1339–49.
4. Keating MU, et al. Clinical and immunologic follow-up of patients who stop venom immunotherapy. J Allergy Clin Immunol. 1991;88(3):339–48.
5. Golden DB, et al. Discontinuing venom immunotherapy: outcome after five years. J Allergy Clin Immunol. 1996;97(2):579–87.
6. Golden DB, et al. Discontinuing venom immunotherapy: extended observations. J Allergy Clin Immunol. 1998;101(3):298–305.
7. Lerch E, Muller UR. Long-term protection after stopping venom immunotherapy: results of re-stings in 200 patients. J Allergy Clin Immunol. 1998;101(5):606–12.
8. Golden DB, et al. Outcomes of allergy to insect stings in children, with and without venom immunotherapy. N Engl J Med. 2004;351(7):668–74.
9. Hafner T, DuBuske L, Kosnik M. Long-term efficacy of venom immunotherapy. Ann Allergy Asthma Immunol. 2008;100(2):162–5.
10. Reisman RE. Duration of venom immunotherapy: relationship to the severity of symptoms of initial insect sting anaphylaxis. J Allergy Clin Immunol. 1993;92(6):831–6.
11. Oka T, et al. Rapid desensitization induces internalization of antigen-specific IgE on mouse mast cells. J Allergy Clin Immunol. 2013;132(4):922–932.e1–16.
12. Zhao D, et al. The functional IgE-blocking factor induced by allergen-specific immunotherapy correlates with IgG4 antibodies and a decrease of symptoms in house dust mite-allergic children. Int Arch Allergy Immunol. 2016;169(2):113–20.
13. Gawlik R, et al. Effects of venom immunotherapy on serum level of CCL5/RANTES in patients with Hymenoptera venom allergy. Immunopharmacol Immunotoxicol. 2015;37(4):375–9.
14. Cavkaytar O, Akdis CA, Akdis M. Modulation of immune responses by immunotherapy in allergic diseases. Curr Opin Pharmacol. 2014;17:30–7.
15. Bruhns P, et al. Specificity and affinity of human Fcgamma receptors and their polymorphic variants for human IgG subclasses. Blood. 2009;113(16):3716–25.
16. Vidarsson G, Dekkers G, Rispens T. IgG subclasses and allotypes: from structure to effector functions. Front Immunol. 2014;5:520.
17. van der Neut Kolfschoten M, et al. Anti-inflammatory activity of human IgG4 antibodies by dynamic Fab arm exchange. Science. 2007;317(5844):1554–7.
18. Aalberse RC, Schuurman J. IgG4 breaking the rules. Immunology. 2002;105(1):9–19.
19. Müller UR. Insect sting allergy: clinical picture, diagnosis, and treatment. Stuttgart: Gustav-Fischer Verlag; 1990.
20. Patriarca G et al. Sublingual desensitization in patients with wasp venom allergy: preliminary results. Int J Immunopathol Pharmacol. 2008;21:669–77.
21. Corallino M, et al. Skin testing technique and precision in stinging insect allergy. J Clin Nurs. 2007;16(7):1256–64.
22. Macchia L, et al. Changes in skin reactivity, specific IgE and IgG levels after one year of immunotherapy in olive pollinosis. Allergy. 1991;46(6):410–8.
23. Jonsson F, Daeron M. Mast cells and company. Front Immunol. 2012;3:16.
24. Diane F, Jelinek I, James T. Immunoglobulin structure and functions. In: Franklin Adkinson N, Bochner B, Wesley Burks A, Holgate ST, Lemanske RF, editors. Middleton's, allergy. Elsevier Saunders; 2014. 1: p. Chapter 3:30–45.
25. Carr TF, Saltoun CA. Chapter 2: Skin testing in allergy. In: Allergy Asthma Proceedings. 2012. 33;1:S6–8.
26. Golden DB. Insect sting anaphylaxis. Immunol Allergy Clin N Am. 2007;27(2):261–72.
27. Randolph CC, Reisman RE. Evaluation of decline in serum venom-specific IgE as a criterion for stopping venom immunotherapy. J Allergy Clin Immunol. 1986;77(6):823–7.
28. Pravettoni V, et al. Determinants of venom-specific IgE antibody concentration during long-term wasp venom immunotherapy. Clin Mol Allergy. 2015;13:29.
29. Ginaldi L, et al. The immune system in the elderly: II. Specific cellular immunity. Immunol Res. 1999;20(2):109–15.
30. King TP, et al. Yellow jacket venom allergens, hyaluronidase and phospholipase: sequence similarity and antigenic cross-reactivity with their hornet and wasp homologs and possible implications for clinical allergy. J Allergy Clin Immunol. 1996;98(3):588–600.
31. King TP, et al. Protein allergens of white-faced hornet, yellow hornet, and yellow jacket venoms. Biochemistry. 1978;17(24):5165–74.
32. Frick M, et al. Predominant Api m 10 sensitization as risk factor for treatment failure in honey bee venom immunotherapy. J Allergy Clin Immunol. 2016;138(6):1663–71.
33. Blank S, et al. Api m 10, a genuine *A. mellifera* venom allergen, is clinically relevant but underrepresented in therapeutic extracts. Allergy. 2011;66(10):1322–9.
34. Baker TW, et al. The HIT study: Hymenoptera Identification Test—how accurate are people at identifying stinging insects? Ann Allergy Asthma Immunol. 2014;113(3):267–70.
35. Golden DB, et al. Natural history of Hymenoptera venom sensitivity in adults. J Allergy Clin Immunol. 1997;100(6):760–6.
36. Durham SR, Till SJ. Immunologic changes associated with allergen immunotherapy. J Allergy Clin Immunol. 1998;102(2):157–64.
37. Wuthrich B, Arrendal H, Lanner A. Antibody response pattern (specific IgE and IgG) of insect sting allergic patients in immunotherapy with venom preparations. Schweiz Med Wochenschr. 1981;111(46):1756–65.
38. Zuidscherwoude M, van Spriel AB. The origin of IgE memory and plasma cells. Cell Mol Immunol. 2012;9(5):373–4.
39. Wong KJ, et al. IgE+ B cells are scarce, but allergen-specific B cells with a memory phenotype circulate in patients with allergic rhinitis. Allergy. 2015;70(4):420–8.
40. Pilette C, et al. Grass pollen immunotherapy induces an allergen-specific IgA2 antibody response associated with mucosal TGF-beta expression. J Immunol. 2007;178(7):4658–66.
41. Kerstan A, et al. Wasp venom immunotherapy induces activation and homing of CD4(+) CD25(+) forkhead box protein 3—positive regulatory T cells controlling T(H)1 responses. J Allergy Clin Immunol. 2011;127(2):495–501.
42. Nouri-Aria KT, et al. Grass pollen immunotherapy induces mucosal and peripheral IL-10 responses and blocking IgG activity. J Immunol. 2004;172(5):3252–9.
43. Ozdemir C, et al. Mechanisms of immunotherapy to wasp and bee venom. Clin Exp Allergy. 2011;41(9):1226–34.
44. Adjobimey T, Hoerauf A. Induction of immunoglobulin G4 in human filariasis: an indicator of immunoregulation. Ann Trop Med Parasitol. 2010;104(6):455–64.
45. Akdis CA, Akdis M. Mechanisms of allergen-specific immunotherapy and immune tolerance to allergens. World Allergy Organ J. 2015;8(1):17.
46. Akdis M, Akdis CA. Mechanisms of allergen-specific immunotherapy: multiple suppressor factors at work in immune tolerance to allergens. J Allergy Clin Immunol. 2014;133(3):621–31.
47. Varga EM, et al. Time course of serum inhibitory activity for facilitated allergen-IgE binding during bee venom immunotherapy in children. Clin Exp Allergy. 2009;39(9):1353–7.

High frequency of IgE sensitization towards kiwi seed storage proteins among peanut allergic individuals also reporting allergy to kiwi

Jenny van Odijk[1,2]* **iD**, Sigrid Sjölander[3], Peter Brostedt[3], Magnus P. Borres[3,4] and Hillevi Englund[3]

Abstract

Background: IgE sensitization to storage proteins from nuts and seed is often related to severe allergic symptoms. There is a risk of immunological IgE cross-reactivity between storage proteins from different species. The potential clinical implication of such cross-reactivity is that allergens other than the known sensitizer can cause allergic symptoms. Previous studies have suggested that kiwi seed storage proteins may constitute hidden food allergens causing cross-reactive IgE-binding with peanut and other tree nut homologs, thereby mediating a potential risk of causing allergy symptoms among peanut ant tree nut allergic individuals. The objective of this study was to investigate the degree of sensitization towards kiwi fruit seed storage proteins in a cohort of peanut allergic individuals.

Methods: A cohort of 59 adolescents and adults with peanut allergy was studied, and self reported allergies to a number of additional foods were collected. Quantitative IgE measurements to seed storage proteins from kiwi and peanut were performed.

Results: In the cohort, 23 out of the 59 individuals were reporting kiwi fruit allergy (39%). The frequency of IgE sensitization to kiwi fruit and to any kiwi seed storage protein was higher among peanut allergic individuals also reporting kiwi fruit allergy ($P = 0.0001$ and $P = 0.01$). A positive relationship was found between IgE levels to 11S globulin ($r = 0.65$) and 7S globulin ($r = 0.48$) allergens from kiwi and peanut, but IgE levels to 2S albumin homologs did not correlate. Patients reporting kiwi fruit allergy also reported allergy to hazelnut ($P = 0.015$), soy ($P < 0.0001$), pea ($P = 0.0002$) and almond ($P = 0.016$) to a higher extent than peanut allergic individuals without kiwi allergy.

Conclusions: Thirty-nine percent of the peanut allergic patients in this cohort also reported kiwi fruit allergy, they displayed a higher degree of sensitization to kiwi storage proteins from both kiwi and peanut, and they also reported a higher extent of allergy to other nuts and legumes. On the molecular level, there was a correlation between IgE levels to 11S and 7S storage proteins from kiwi and peanut. Taken together, reported symptoms and serological findings to kiwi in this cohort of patients with concurrent allergy to peanut and kiwi fruit, could be explained by a combination of cross-reactivity between the 11S and 7S globulins and co-sensitization to the 2S albumin Act d 13.

Keywords: 2S albumin, 7S globulin, 11S globulin, IgE, Seeds, Storage proteins, Kiwi, Peanut

*Correspondence: jenny.van.odijk@vgregion.se
[1] Dept of Respiratory Medicine and Allergology, Sahlgrenska Academy
at Göteborg University, Göteborg, Sweden
Full list of author information is available at the end of the article

Background

Fruits, tree nuts and legumes like peanuts commonly cause allergic reactions in both children and adults affected by food allergy [1]. When prescribing an elimination diet, foods containing homologous proteins able to cause IgE cross-reactive reactions also need to be considered. As extensive food eliminations can lead to impaired quality of life, pin-pointing and exclusion of the clinically relevant foods only is of outmost importance [2]. There are common IgE epitopes on allergens from peanut and other plant foods [3], but the clinical relevance is not always known and both cross-reactivity and co-sensitization to these allergens must be considered [4, 5].

IgE sensitization to storage proteins has been associated with severe allergic reactions to several plant foods, especially tree nuts, peanuts and other legumes [6]. In 2014, storage proteins were identified also in seeds from green kiwi fruit, Act d 12 from the 11S globulin family and Act d 13 from the 2S albumin family [7]. Kiwi fruit is a common food allergen with allergic symptoms ranging from mild oral allergy symptoms to anaphylaxis [7, 8]. Evidence of IgE cross-reactivity between kiwi fruit storage proteins and homologs from nuts and legumes was presented in an in vitro study where binding of kiwi fruit specific IgE was inhibited by hazelnut, peanut and walnut protein extracts [9]. Recently, in silico studies also identified similar IgE-binding epitopes on Act c 12 from golden kiwi fruit seeds and other 11S globulins [10]. Considering the reports of concurrent peanut allergy and kiwi fruit allergy, in combination with the severity of allergic reactions caused by storage proteins, the objective of this study was to investigate the degree of IgE sensitization towards kiwi fruit seed storage protein in a cohort of peanut allergic individuals.

Methods

In this study, a cohort of 59 peanut allergic adults living in the western area of Sweden (demographic data in Table 1) from a previously published study was studied. Detailed data about the group has been described previously [11]. In the original study, 74 patients were included, however limited by the amount of sera available the patient number was reduced to 59 in this study. Inclusion criteria were a known peanut sensitization (SPT positive and/or positive IgE to peanut and a convincing history of

Table 1 IgE sensitization to peanut and kiwi seed storage proteins, allergic symptoms after peanut ingestion and other allergies in a cohort of peanut allergic individuals (n = 59) whereof 39% also reported kiwi allergy

	All patients	Reporting kiwi allergy	Not reporting kiwi allergy	P
Demographic data				
N	59	23	36	
Median age (min–max)	23 (14–39)	23 (15–38)	23 (14–39)	
% female	69	74	67	
% sensitized (> 0.35 kU/l) in the group				
Any peanut storage protein	61	52	67	*0.04*
Any kiwi seed storage protein	41	52	33	*0.01*
Ara h 3 (11S globulin)	39	35	42	0.38
Act d 12 (11S globulin)	36	43	31	0.11
Ara h 1 (7S globulin)	49	39	56	*0.02*
Act d 7S (7S globulin)	36	43	31	0.11
Ara h 2 (2S albumin)	56	43	64	*0.005*
Act d 13 (2S albumin)	20	22	19	0.73
Ara h 8 (PR-10)	54	83	36	*< 0.0001*
Act d 8 (PR-10)	59	83	44	*< 0.0001*
Peanut	90	87	92	0.36
Kiwi fruit	36	52	25	*0.0001*
% with reported allergy to				
Hazelnut	54	65	47	*0.015*
Soy	22	39	11	*< 0.0001*
Lentil	14	17	11	0.31
Pea	32	48	22	*0.0002*
Almond	46	57	39	*0.016*

P values from Fisher's exact test between frequencies in "with kiwi allergy" and "without kiwi allergy" groups, italics means P < 0.05

suspected peanut allergy). The participants completed a questionnaire about food allergies and specific questions about whether they suffered from allergies like birch or timothy grass pollen, and several foods like legumes, tree nuts and fruits [11]. Commercial ImmunoCAP reagents (Thermo Fisher Scientific, Uppsala, Sweden) were used for quantitative IgE-analyses to allergen extracts from peanut (f13) and kiwi (f84) and to recombinant Ara h 1, Ara h 2, Ara h 3, Ara h 8 and Act d 8. Analyses to Ara h 9 (LTP), Bet v 2 (profilin) and CCD were also performed. Experimental ImmunoCAP with native Act d 7S globulin, Act d 13 and Act d 12 purified from kiwi seeds were developed in house (Thermo Fisher Scientific, Uppsala, Sweden) as described previously [12]. The cut-off for positive IgE-level was defined as > 0.35 kU$_A$/l. Group differences of IgE-levels were analyzed using Mann–Whitney test. Comparisons of frequency distributions between groups were analyzed by Fisher's exact test (two tailed). Spearman's rank correlation test was used to analyze the relationship between IgE concentrations. P values < 0.05 were considered significant.

Ethics approval
The study was approved by the Regional Ethical Review Board at Göteborg University and the collected personal data was treated according to the Swedish personal data act.

Results
Of the 59 individuals with peanut allergy (age 14–39 years, median 23 years, Table 1), 23 (39%) reported to suffer from allergy symptoms when eating kiwi. Of these 23, 12 (52%) displayed IgE sensitization to kiwi fruit and 12 (52%) to one or more of the kiwi seed storage proteins (Table 1). The frequency of IgE sensitization to kiwi fruit and to any kiwi storage protein were higher among patients reporting kiwi allergy than those who did not ($P = 0.0001$ and $P = 0.01$, Table 1).

The opposite was found for peanut storage proteins where the frequency of sensitization to one or more peanut storage protein was higher among the individuals not reporting kiwi fruit allergy (67% vs 52%, $P = 0.04$). For individual components, a higher degree of sensitization to Ara h 1 and Ara h 2 was noted among the non-kiwi fruit allergic ($P = 0.02$ and $P = 0.005$, Table 1).

IgE levels to kiwi fruit were higher among the patients reporting kiwi allergy than those who did not (mean level 3.0 vs 0.3 kU/l, $P = 0.009$), however IgE levels towards whole peanut, peanut storage proteins and kiwi seed storage proteins did not differ between groups (data not shown). IgE concentrations to homologous 11S globulins (Act d 12 and Ara h 3) and 7S globulins (Act d 7S globulin and Ara h 1) from peanut and kiwi displayed a positive correlation, but the 2S albumins (Act d 13 and Ara h 2) did not (Fig. 1). For individual patients with concurrent peanut and kiwi allergy, there was no clear pattern regarding primary sensitizing allergens. In seven patients a general pattern of higher IgE-levels to peanut storage proteins was observed, while in five patients the levels of IgE to kiwi storage proteins were higher (Table 2).

For the PR-10 proteins, Ara h 8 and Act d 8, a higher degree of sensitization towards these proteins ($P < 0.0001$ for both Act d 8 and Ara h 8, Table 1), was demonstrated in the group reporting kiwi allergy. Additionally, the IgE levels towards these proteins were higher in the group reporting kiwi allergy ($P = 0.004$ for Act d 8 and $P < 0.0001$ for Ara h 8). For all patients, a low degree of sensitization to Ara h 9 (LTP), Bet v 2 (profilin) and CCD was observed and levels did not differ significantly between groups (Table 2).

The group reporting kiwi fruit allergy also reported significantly higher frequencies of allergies to other foods including hazelnut ($P = 0.015$), soy ($P < 0.0001$), pea ($P = 0.0002$) and almond ($P = 0.016$), but not for lentils ($P = 0.31$) (Table 1).

Discussion
IgE sensitization to storage proteins have been associated with severe clinical reactions for several nuts, seeds, legumes and now recently also for fruit seeds [5–7, 9]. In this study of peanut allergic adolescents and adults, more than a third reported allergy symptoms when eating kiwi and more than half of them presented with IgE to one or more kiwi seed storage proteins, underlining the importance of also including seeds from fruits in the diagnostic work-up of peanut allergic individuals.

The frequency of concurrent kiwi and peanut allergy in this study, is in line with studies by Lucas et al. and Sirvent et al. [9, 13] studying peanut allergy among kiwi allergic subjects. In the study by Lucas et al., it was noted that more than half of the children with kiwi fruit allergy experiencing severe symptoms also reported peanut and tree nut allergies [13]. A number of these children reacted to their first known exposure of kiwi fruit indicating that they were primarily sensitized to a cross reacting allergen from another source like peanut and/or tree nuts [13]. This IgE cross-reactions was confirmed in vitro in a study by Sirvent et al., where peanut, almond, hazelnut and walnut inhibited the binding of IgE to both Act d 12 and Act d 13 [9] in sera from Spanish adults diagnosed with kiwi allergy, implying that the proteins share common epitopes. Existence of shared epitopes on homologous 11S globulin proteins was also noted in another in silico study by Barre et al. [10].

On the molecular level, there was some correlation between IgE-levels specific for the 11S and 7S globulins

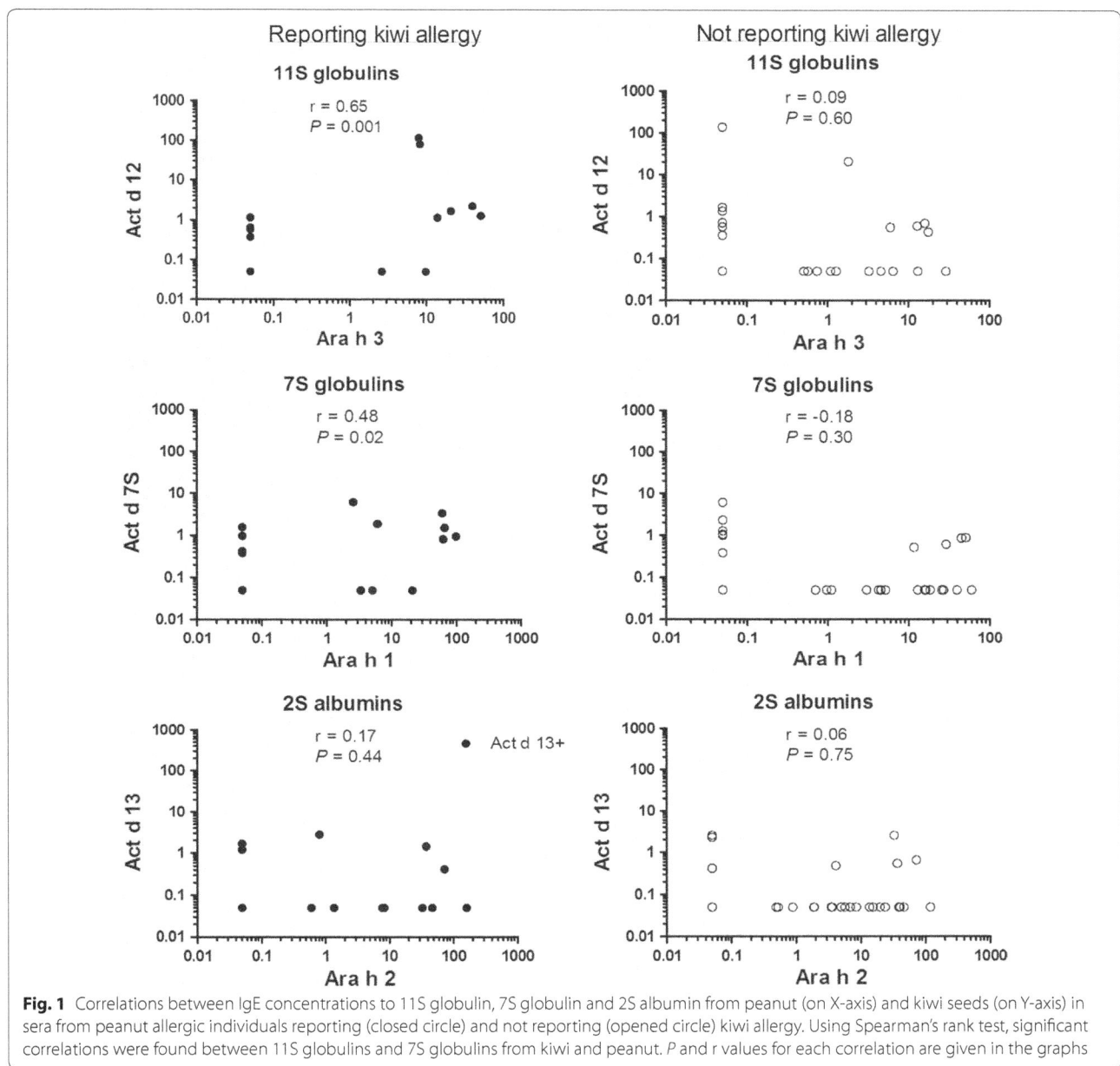

Fig. 1 Correlations between IgE concentrations to 11S globulin, 7S globulin and 2S albumin from peanut (on X-axis) and kiwi seeds (on Y-axis) in sera from peanut allergic individuals reporting (closed circle) and not reporting (opened circle) kiwi allergy. Using Spearman's rank test, significant correlations were found between 11S globulins and 7S globulins from kiwi and peanut. P and r values for each correlation are given in the graphs

from kiwi and peanut, but not for the 2S albumins. The results are supported by a study by Ballabio et al., where 11S globulins were demonstrated to be the protein which mediated the highest degree of IgE cross-reactivity between proteins from several legumes and peanut [4]. Similar to the results in this study, IgE antibodies towards 2S albumins from hazelnut (Cor a 14) was demonstrated to not cause cross-reactive allergic reactions to the homologous protein from peanut (Ara h 2), although peanut allergy was common among hazelnut allergic individuals [5].

The peanut allergic patient's reporting concurrent kiwi fruit allergy, to a higher extent also reported allergies to other storage protein containing foods than peanut allergic patients without kiwi allergy. This may indicate the presence of cross-reactive IgE antibodies to these other foods, but could also be explained by these individuals being more susceptible to develop new allergies in general. The presence of a general cross-reactive pattern is strengthened by the observation that the patients with concurrent allergy to kiwi fruit and peanut, additionally to displaying a higher frequency of cross-sensitization to

Table 2 Individual data of patients included in the study

Patient#	IgE analyses, kU/l													Age	Gender	Reported foods to cause allergy symptoms					
	Peanut	Kiwi	Ara h 1	Ara h 2	Ara h 3	Act d 12	Act d 7S	Act d 13	Ara h 8	Act d 8	Ara h 9	Bet v 2	CCD			Hazelnut	Soy	Lentils	Pea	Almond	Kiwi
1	1.8	2.5	0	0	0	0.4	0.4	0	59.3	12.7	0	0	0	19	F	X				X	X
2	173	9.5	99.0	73.5	51.2	1.3	0.9	0.4	12.7	3.9	0	0	0	25	F	X	X	X	X		X
3	27.7	13.3	2.6	0	7.9	115	6.2	0	47.5	35.9	0	0	0	15	M	X	X	X	X	X	X
4	2.3	0.8	1.4	0	0	0	0	0	7.7	0	0	0	0	23	F	X	X		X	X	X
5	17.5	18.8	6.0	0	8.3	78.9	1.9	1.7	20.4	2.1	0.6	0	0	15	F			X			X
6	0	0	0	0	0	0	0	0	0.6	0.4	0	0	0	15	M	X					X
7	0.5	0	0	0	0	0	0	0	2.7	2.4	0	0	0	26	F	X					X
8	169	5.4	61.0	33.3	39.6	2.2	3.4	0	0	1.1	0	0	0	19	M		X	X	X	X	X
9	0.9	0	0	0.6	0	0	0	0	2.8	0.4	0	0	0	28	F	X				X	X
10	0.6	0	0	0	0	0	0	0	2.4	2.3	0	0	0	35	F	X				X	X
11	9.9	3.6	0	0	0	0.6	1.0	0	64.7	63.0	0.4	0	0	17	F	X				X	X
12	64.4	1.4	21.0	47.2	9.8	0	0	0	6.7	3.1	0	0	0	37	F	X	X		X		X
13	16.8	0	3.4	7.7	0	0	0	0	2.9	5.1	0	0.8	0	19	F						X
14	169	0.4	66.3	160	20.8	1.7	1.5	0	5.8	1.5	0	0	0	15	F		X		X		X
15	22.5	0	5.1	8.4	2.6	0	0	0	0	0	0	0	0	25	F		X		X		X
16	112	0	63.1	37.7	13.9	1.1	0.8	1.4	1.4	1.9	0	0	0	24	F						X
17	0	0	0	0	0	0	0	0	0	0	0	0	0	20	M				X		X
18	4.7	0	0	0	0	0	0	0	35.7	58.2	0	0	0	18	M					X	X
19	0.5	2.1	0	0	0	0	0	0	5.9	5.5	0	0	0	33	F	X			X	X	X
20	0	0.5	0	0	0	0	0	1.2	3.4	3.3	0	0	0	24	F	X			X	X	X
21	1.9	10.0	0	0	0	0	0.4	0	42.6	33.7	0	0	0	26	F	X	X			X	X
22	0.8	0	0	0	0	0.6	1.5	2.8	0	0	0	0	0	38	M	X	X			X	X
23	0.7	0	0	0	0	1.1	0	0	5.4	0.8	0	0	0	23	F	X	X			X	X
% of patients > 0.35 kU/l / % reporting allergy symptoms	87	52	39	43	35	43	43	22	83	83	9	4	0	74		65	39	17	48	57	100
24	8.1	0	5.2	5.0	0	0	0	0	0	0	0	0	0	30	M						
25	7.2	0	0	1.9	0	0	0	0	0	0	0	0	0	15	M						
26	195	0	45.0	72.2	16.0	0.7	0.8	0.7	0	0	0	2.0	0	17	M	X				X	
27	3.0	0	3.0	0.5	0	0	0	0	1.0	0.9	0	0	0	18	F						
28	77.3	0	26.9	40.6	6.5	0	0	0	0	0	0	0	0	17	F						
29	5.3	0	1.0	1.9	0	0	0	0	0	0	0	0	0	19	F	X					
30	1.0	0	0.5	0.5	0	0	0	0	4.0	4.6	0	0	0	24	F	X					
31	70.9	0	39.5	15.3	13.1	0	0	0	0	0	0	0	0	18	F	X					

Table 2 continued

Patient#	IgE analyses, kU/l													Age	Gender	Reported foods to cause allergy symptoms					
	% of patients > 0.35 kU/l for each allergen															% reporting allergy symptoms					
	Peanut	Kiwi	Ara h 1	Ara h 2	Ara h 3	Act d 12	Act d 7S	Act d 13	Ara h 8	Act d 8	Ara h 9	Bet v 2	CCD			Hazelnut	Soy	Lentils	Pea	Almond	Kiwi
32	195	0	59.8	38.9	29.1	0	0	0	0	0	0	0	0	18	F						
33	2.2	1.4	0	0	0	1.6	2.3	0	0	0	0	0	1.3	27	F						
34	0.5	0	0	0	0	0	0	0	0	12.4	0	0	0	14	M	×				×	
35	1.1	0	0	0.9	0	0	0	0	0	0	0	0	0	16	M						
36	1.5	0.6	0	0	0	0.6	1.3	0	0	0	0	0	0.8	14	F						
37	9.4	0	4.5	4.1	0	0	0	0.5	0	0	0	0	0	15	M	×					
38	0	0	0	0	0	0.7	1.0	2.5	0	0	0	0	0	18	F	×				×	
39	4.3	0.6	0	0	1.8	20.4	1.0	2.3	2.1	3.5	0	0.9	0	22	F						
40	0.6	0.5	0	0	0	0	0	0	2.0	3.8	0.9	0	0	30	F	×					
41	19.5	0	15.7	5.7	0.6	0	0	0	0	0	0	0	0	25	M	×			×	×	
42	13.1	0	1.1	8.4	0.5	0	0	0	0	0	0	0	0	37	F						
43	115	1.0	50.8	36.7	12.9	0.6	0.9	0.5	5.1	4.1	11.3	1.0	1.0	16	M	×	×	×	×	×	
44	35.3	0	18.5	13.6	1.3	0	0	0	0	0	0	0	0	38	F	×	×	×	×	×	
45	89.7	0	25.7	19.9	0.7	0	0	0	0	0	0	0	0	19	M					×	
46	14.5	0	4.2	3.6	1.1	0	0	0	1.4	0.9	0	0	0	34	F				×		
47	72.2	0	16.3	46.5	3.2	0	0	0	0	0	0	0	0	34	M		×	×	×		
48	16.4	0	4.5	6.8	0	0	0	0	12.8	22.6	0	0	0	28	F						
49	0	1.6	0	0	0	0	0	0	4.4	8.7	0	0	0	29	F				×		
50	149	0.7	29.1	119	17.6	0.4	0.6	0	7.3	7.1	0	0	0	28	F			×	×		
51	0.8	0.6	0	0	0	0	0	0	3.0	2.0	0	0	0	27	M	×			×	×	
52	41.7	0	12.9	23.8	4.6	0	0	0	0	0	0	0	0	39	F	×					
53	19.5	1.3	0	0	0	135	6.1	0.4	14.2	1.0	1.2	0	0.8	22	F						
54	61.8	0	11.7	33.0	6.0	0.6	0.5	2.5	2.8	0.7	0	0	0	23	F	×				×	
55	0.9	0	0	0	0	1.3	1.0	0	0	0.5	0	0	0	22	M	×				×	
56	0.4	0	0	0	0	0	0	0	0	0	0	0	0	28	F					×	
57	0.5	0	0	0	0	0	0	0	1.6	0.5	1.2	0	0	29	F	×				×	
58	9.4	0	0.7	3.5	0	0	0	0	0	0	0	0	0	23	F						
59	0	0	0	0	0	0.4	0.4	0	0	1.6	0	0	0	25	F	×			×	×	0
	92	25	56	64	42	31	31	19	36	44	11	8	11	14	67	47	11	11	22	39	

11S and 7S globulins, also presented with a high degree of cross-reactivity to PR-10 proteins. The group of peanut allergic patients *not* reporting kiwi allergy in this study displayed a higher frequency of peanut storage protein sensitization, higher degree of sensitization to the peanut allergy marker Ara h 2, and less symptoms to other nuts and legumes.

Evidence of immunological cross-reactivity between homologous storage proteins in nuts, seeds and legumes is well-known. In addition, there are several reports also for allergy symptoms among peanut and tree nut allergic individuals caused by cross-reactions to storage proteins from fruit and plant seeds [14–20]. In this study, this nut and fruit seed cross-reactivity is further highlighted by the findings from patients reporting allergy to both peanut and kiwi. Storage proteins have stable IgE-binding epitopes that often are resistant to both heating and gastrointestinal processing [5, 14]. Seeds from fruits can be ingested both intentionally and accidentally, as seed storage proteins can leak during food processing leading to unintentional contamination of for example fruit juices [15]. From a safety perspective for the patient with a peanut or tree nut allergy, it is important to investigate also the risk of allergic reactions caused by cross-reactive IgE antibodies to fruit storage proteins, especially since fruit seeds can present as hidden allergens.

The major limitation of this study is the use of data from self-reported, and not food challenge proven, kiwi fruit allergy. The major kiwi fruit allergen—Act d 1—is abundant in kiwi pulp and in kiwi fruit protein extract, and sensitization to Act d 1 is a marker of severe kiwi allergy [8]. In addition, sensitization towards kiwi seed storage proteins has been reported as a marker of kiwi allergy [7]. Of the 23 individuals reporting allergy symptoms in this study, a vast majority (n = 15, 65%) were sensitized either to kiwi fruit extract or kiwi seed storage proteins, supporting the validity of their self-reported kiwi allergy symptoms.

Conclusions

The frequency of reported allergy to kiwi fruit was high in a cohort of Swedish adolescents and adults with peanut allergy. Further, in the group of patients that reported concurrent symptoms to kiwi fruit, a majority displayed IgE-reactivity to storage proteins from kiwi seeds and a correlation between IgE-levels to 11S and 7S globulins and PR-10 proteins from kiwi and peanut. These patients also reported a high frequency of symptoms to other nuts and legumes. In the group of peanut allergic patients not reporting kiwi allergy, the individuals displayed a higher frequency of peanut storage protein sensitization, especially to Ara h 2, and presented with fewer symptoms to other nuts and legumes. The results implicate

the presence of at least two phenotypes of peanut allergic individuals in this cohort. One group with a broader cross-sensitization profile and having co-existing symptoms to both kiwi and other plant foods as well as co-sensitization to kiwi Act d 13, and a second group with a strong peanut sensitization to the major allergen Ara h 2 and less symptoms to other plant foods. The clinical relevance and implication of these results remains to be elucidated.

Abbreviations

IgE: immunoglobulin E; kU/l: kilounits of allergen-specific IgE per liter.

Authors' contributions

JO has been responsible for this cohort from the beginning and has been participating in the planning, collection of the data. HE, SS and PB have carried out the majority of laboratory work and data analysis. All authors have written the manuscript together. All authors read and approved the final manuscript.

Author details

[1] Dept of Respiratory Medicine and Allergology, Sahlgrenska Academy at Göteborg University, Göteborg, Sweden. [2] Internal Medicine and Clinical Nutrition, Sahlgrenska Academy at Göteborg University, Göteborg, Sweden. [3] R&D, ImmunoDiagnostic Division, Thermo Fisher Scientific, Uppsala, Sweden. [4] Department of Women's and Children's Health, Uppsala University, Uppsala, Sweden.

Competing interests

Sigrid Sjölander, Peter Brostedt, Hillevi Englund and Magnus Borres are employed by Thermo Fisher Scientific, Uppsala, Sweden. Jenny van Odijk declares that she has no competing interests.

Funding

This study was supported by Association of Asthma and Allergy, Sweden and the analysis funded by Thermo Fisher Scientific, Uppsala,

References

1. Nwaru BI, Hickstein L, Panesar SS, Roberts G, Muraro A, Sheikh A. Prevalence of common food allergies in Europe: a systematic review and meta-analysis. Allergy. 2014;69(8):992–1007.
2. Le TM, Lindner TM, Pasmans SG, Guikers CL, van Hoffen E, Bruijnzeel-Koomen CA, et al. Reported food allergy to peanut, tree nuts and fruit: comparison of clinical manifestations, prescription of medication and impact on daily life. Allergy. 2008;63(7):910–6.
3. Barre A, Sordet C, Culerrier R, Rance F, Didier A, Rouge P. Vicilin allergens of peanut and tree nuts (walnut, hazelnut and cashew nut) share structurally related IgE-binding epitopes. Mol Immunol. 2008;45(5):1231–40.
4. Ballabio C, Magni C, Restani P, Mottini M, Fiocchi A, Tedeschi G, et al. IgE-mediated cross-reactivity among leguminous seed proteins in peanut allergic children. Plant Foods Hum Nutr. 2010;65(4):396–402.
5. Masthoff LJ, van Hoffen E, Mattsson L, Lidholm J, Andersson K, Zuidmeer-Jongejan L, et al. Peanut allergy is common among hazelnut-sensitized subjects but is not primarily the result of IgE cross-reactivity. Allergy. 2015;70(3):265–74.

6. Ebisawa M, Moverare R, Sato S, Maruyama N, Borres MP, Komata T. Measurement of Ara h 1-, 2-, and 3-specific IgE antibodies is useful in diagnosis of peanut allergy in Japanese children. Pediatr Allergy Immunol. 2012;23(6):573–81.

7. Sirvent S, Canto B, Cuesta-Herranz J, Gomez F, Blanca N, Canto G, et al. Act d 12 and Act d 13: two novel, masked, relevant allergens in kiwifruit seeds. J Allergy Clin Immunol. 2014;133(6):1765–7.

8. Le TM, Bublin M, Breiteneder H, Fernandez-Rivas M, Asero R, Ballmer-Weber B, et al. Kiwifruit allergy across Europe: clinical manifestation and IgE recognition patterns to kiwifruit allergens. J Allergy Clin Immunol. 2013;131(1):164–71.

9. Sirvent S, Canto B, Gomez F, Blanca N, Cuesta-Herranz J, Canto G, et al. Detailed characterization of Act d 12 and Act d 13 from kiwi seeds: implication in IgE cross-reactivity with peanut and tree nuts. Allergy. 2014;69(11):1481–8.

10. Barre AD, Simplicien M, Benoist H, Rougé P. Molecular basis of cross-reactivity between Act c 12 and other seed 11S-globulin allergens. Revue Française d'Allergologie. 2017;57(2):58–66.

11. Moverare R, Ahlstedt S, Bengtsson U, Borres MP, van Hage M, Poorafshar M, et al. Evaluation of IgE antibodies to recombinant peanut allergens in patients with reported reactions to peanut. Int Arch Allergy Immunol. 2011;156(3):282–90.

12. Nilsson C, Brostedt P, Hidman J, van Odijk J, Borres MP, Sjolander S, et al. Recognition pattern of kiwi seed storage proteins in kiwifruit allergic children. Pediatr Allergy Immunol. 2015;26(8):817–20.

13. Lucas JS, Grimshaw KE, Collins K, Warner JO, Hourihane JO. Kiwi fruit is a significant allergen and is associated with differing patterns of reactivity in children and adults. Clin Exp Allergy. 2004;34(7):1115–21.

14. O'Sullivan MD, Somerville C. Cosensitization to orange seed and cashew nut. Ann Allergy Asthma Immunol. 2011;107(3):282–3.

15. Turner PJ, Gray PE, Wong M, Varese N, Rolland JM, O'Hehir R, et al. Anaphylaxis to apple and orange seed. J Allergy Clin Immunol. 2011;128(6):1363–5.

16. Brandstrom J, Lilja G, Nilsson C, Ingemarsson N, Borres MP, Brostedt P, et al. IgE to novel citrus seed allergens among cashew-allergic children. Pediatr Allergy Immunol. 2016;27(5):550–3.

17. Glaspole IN, de Leon MP, Rolland JM, O'Hehir RE. Anaphylaxis to lemon soap: citrus seed and peanut allergen cross-reactivity. Ann Allergy Asthma Immunol. 2007;98(3):286–9.

18. Vocks E, Borga A, Szliska C, Seifert HU, Seifert B, Burow G, et al. Common allergenic structures in hazelnut, rye grain, sesame seeds, kiwi, and poppy seeds. Allergy. 1993;48(3):168–72.

19. Wensing M, Knulst AC, Piersma S, O'Kane F, Knol EF, Koppelman SJ. Patients with anaphylaxis to pea can have peanut allergy caused by cross-reactive IgE to vicilin (Ara h 1). J Allergy Clin Immunol. 2003;111(2):420–4.

20. Oppel T, Thomas P, Wollenberg A. Cross-sensitization between poppy seed and buckwheat in a food-allergic patient with poppy seed anaphylaxis. Int Arch Allergy Immunol. 2006;140(2):170–3.

The control of allergic rhinitis in real life

Federica Gani[1]* ⓘ, Carlo Lombardi[2], Laura Barrocu[1], Massimo Landi[3], Erminia Ridolo[4], Massimo Bugiani[5], Giovanni Rolla[6], Gianenrico Senna[7] and Giovanni Passalacqua[8]

Abstract

Background: Allergic Rhinitis (AR) is a high-prevalence disease. In Europe about 25% of the general population is affected, and in Italy the prevalence is estimated to be 19.8%. The Allergic Rhinitis and its Impact on Asthma (ARIA) international document underlined that the prevalence of severe or refractory or overlapping rhinitis is increasing and represents a non-negligible socio-economic burden. In general, despite the social healthcare costs, allergic rhinitis remains underestimated, not sufficiently controlled and often undertreated.

Aim of the study: In this multi-center Italian observational and prospective study we assessed the control of AR in patients (> 16 years) without previous asthma diagnosis, referred to Allergy Centers.

Methods: Patients of both sexes and older than 16 with rhinitis symptoms and without asthma were studied. A Visual Analogue Scale (VAS) and the CARAT (Control of Allergic Rhinitis and Asthma Test) were used as patient reported outcome. The possible causes of poor control of AR, as per protocol, were assessed accordingly.

Results: We observed 250 patients in a real-life setting: more than 60% of them had an uncontrolled AR, only about 50% used multiple medications, and only a minority were receiving allergen immunotherapy.

Conclusion: This survey, conducted in a real-life setting, confirmed that AR is overall poorly controlled. The VAS assessment well correlates with the structured CARAT questionnaire and with the relevant symptoms of AR.

Keywords: Allergic rhinitis, Control, Real-life

Background

Allergic Rhinitis (AR) is a high-prevalence disease. In Europe about 25% of the general population is affected and in Italy, the prevalence is estimated to be 19.8% [1]. The Allergic Rhinitis and its Impact on Asthma (ARIA) international document [2] underlined that severe or refractory or mixed forms of AR are increasing and represent a not negligible socio-economic burden [3]. In addition, it was observed that more than one half of patients use multiple medications, but many of them don't feel satisfied with the symptoms scores [4]. Finally, since AR is considered a trivial disease, many patients do not seek medical care or specific diagnosis and primarily refer to pharmacies for self medications [5], or refer

to alternative/complementary medicines [6], whereas allergen specific immunotherapy (AIT) is neglected [7]. Currently, topical/systemic antihistamines and intranasal corticosteroids are considered the first-line therapy, but many other treatments (such as decongestants, cromones or anti-muscarinic agents) are available over the counter.

Despite the social health costs [8], it emerges that generally AR is underestimated, often poorly controlled and undertreated. Thus, a more detailed education for healthcare workers and patients would be needed and a better awareness of the disease should be disseminated. It is true that, so far, there are no predictive biomarkers to appropriately address the therapeutic approach, or to predict the response, for instance, to AIT [9]. According to these considerations, in the last decade greater attention has been devoted to a more comprehensive approach to AR [10], looking specifically to the severity of symptoms, exacerbations, impact on the quality of

*Correspondence: fedgani@tin.it
[1] Allergy Service, Azienda Ospedaliera "San Luigi Orbassano", Turin, Italy
Full list of author information is available at the end of the article

life, course of disease, use of medications. The web-based instruments are a promising example of the possibility of day-by-day monitoring of patients [3].

Currently in real life the most feasible and practical instrument to evaluate the presence, severity and control of symptoms remains the Visual Analogue Scale (VAS), consisting in a single patient-reported outcome of the effect of the disease and of the treatment. Patients with a VAS > 5 are considered not controlled [11–13]. Accordingly, most patients agreed that VAS evaluation could be considered a good instrument [14, 15].

Other instruments to assess the impact of AR are available, for example the CARAT ("Control of Allergic Rhinitis and Asthma Test") questionnaire evaluates in few questions the perceived control of AR and concomitant asthma, also assessing the overall use of pharmacotherapy [16]. Other more detailed questionnaires are also available. It has been identified that the major reasons for an unsatisfactory control of rhinitis are incorrect diagnosis, intrinsic severity of the disease [17], incorrect use/misuse of the intranasal treatment [11].

The aim of this study was to assess through the use of VAS and CARAT instruments the level of control of AR in patients (> 16 years) without previous asthma diagnosis referred to Allergy Centers. The possible causes of poor control were also further investigated.

Methods

This was a multi-center observational cross-sectional study involving patients with AR, referred for the first time to Allergy centers of Northern Italy (Turin, Verona, Parma, Brescia) between May and December 2015. Only patients with ascertained symptoms of AR in the previous month and without a previous asthma diagnosis were included. The level of control was assessed by the VAS (0 = troublesome symptoms, 10 = no symptoms) and the CARAT instrument [16]. CARAT is a tool created and validated to measure disease control of both allergic rhinitis and asthma. It is a self-administered questionnaire that quantifies not only nasal, ocular, oropharyngeal, lower respiratory tract symptoms, sleep impairment, activities, psychosocial impediments, but also treatment and exacerbation. The more the patient is symptomatic and has a poor quality of life, the lower the CARAT score. In addition, the relevant demographic and clinical data (age, sex, duration of the disease, allergen sensitizations) were recorded for the analyses. The type of medications (e.g. antihistamines, nasal steroids, decongestants), their frequency of dosing and possible incremental use were assessed. The AR was better controlled when the VAS was lower and the CARAT scores were higher.

All statistical procedures were performed using the statistical package STATA version 14 for Windows [STATA®

(Stata Corp-LP-College Station-TX-USA)] [18]. All tests of significativity were carried out at a 0.05 level. For the analysis of symptom severity and symptomatic treatment changes, the ratings "present always, never, less than or more than 2/week" were used. Age was categorized in 10-year intervals. The time of symptoms' duration was classified as < 1, 1–4, 5–10, 11–20, > 20 years. All categorized variables were used in the analysis as ordinal variables when appropriate. The relationship between VAS and symptoms score was measured by means of quantile (median) regression with VAS-score as dependent and Symptom-score as predictive variables [19–21].

Statistical methods were used to investigate which factors could influence the VAS score and the relationship between VAS score (dependent variables) and symptoms, medication use and life quality.

Ordinal logistic regression with VAS score as dependent variable, measuring the increase in the log odds of being in a higher level of VAS-score for a class increase in each predictive variable (i.e., going from 0 to 4), given all the other variables in the model are held stable. The Parallel Regression Assumption was tested by Brant Test [20, 21]. The same analysis was repeated by means of binomial logistic regression categorizing VAS score as < 5 or ≥ 5. The predicted marginal probabilities of VAS ≥ 5 (in % scale) were computed and reported by age strata. To assess the influence of category of drug used on the probability of VAS > 5 we performed logistic model analysis. In all analysis bootstrap estimation of standard error was used.

Results

Symptoms and treatment

Within the considered period, 250 patients (54% female, age between 16 and 80 years, 2% over 65 years) were studied (Table 1). Overall 45% of patients had symptoms of AR for less than 5 years, and 12% of the patients reported a persistence of symptoms greater than 20 years. Most patients reported no comorbidity associated with rhinitis and among patients with comorbid conditions 20.8% had nasal polyposis and 2.6% had an acetylsalicylic acid-exacerbated disease. 79% were polysensitized, mainly to grass (68.4%), house dust mites (38%) and cat dander (31.6%). In 52% of the cases the most frequently reported symptom was nasal obstruction (daily or > 2/week). 29% of patients reported mild obstruction, whereas 18% had no obstruction during the previous 4 weeks. The second relevant symptom was rhinorrhea, frequent in 50%, mild in 33% and absent in 17%. Sneezing and itching were overall less frequent. According to the ARIA guidelines [1], 34% patients reported a relevant impact of AR on their daily activities. Nocturnal awakenings were reported by 52% of patients (Table 2).

Table 1 Demographic data of the population

Sex	
Male	115/250 (46%)
Female	135/250 (54%)
Age range (years)	
10–20	45/250 (18%)
20–45	143/250 (57%)
45–65	57/250 (23%)
> 65	5/250 (2%)
Onset of symptoms (years)	
1–5	113/250 (43%)
5–10	37/250 (15%)
10–20	70/250 (28%)
> 20	30/250 (12%)
Allergen sensitization	
Monosensitized	52/250 (21%)
Polysensitized	198/250 (79%)

Table 2 Symptoms frequency

Nasal obstruction	
Never	45/250 (18%)
1–2/week	73/250 (29%)
> 2/week	72/250 (29%)
Always	59/250 (23%)
Rhinorrhea	
Never	42/250 (17%)
1–2/week	82/250 (33%)
> 2/week	74/250 (29%)
Always	52/250 (21%)
Sneezing	
Never	34/250 (14%)
1–2/week	94/250 (38%)
> 2/week	66/250 (26%)
Always	56/250 (22%)
Itching	
Never	61/250 (24%)
1–2/week	89/250 (36%)
> 2/week	65/250 (26%)
Always	35/250 (14%)
Quality of life	
Never	77/250 (31%)
1–2/week	85/250 (34%)
> 2/week	70/250 (28%)
Always	18/250 (7%)
Awakenings	
Never	119/250 (48%)
1–2/week	68/250 (27%)
>2/week	53/250 (21%)
Always	10/250 (4%)

Within the population, 71% of patients (178/250) were assuming symptomatic drugs, such as antihistamines (68% as regular treatment and 32% on demand), nasal steroids (75% regular and 25% on demand), nasal lavages (14% on demand). 59% of the subjects taking any therapy did not report an increase in drug consumption for more than 1 week/month.

Risk factors of severe disease

More importantly, 62% of the patients scored a VAS ≥ 5, suggesting a non-optimal control of the disease in the previous last 4 weeks. By the median regression, a negative weak correlation (Spearman's rho $= -0.65$ p < 0.01) was seen between VAS and symptom scores (Fig. 1). The ordinal logistic regression analysis showed that, controlling for other symptoms, the probability of an higher VAS-score level increases significantly with stuffy nose and sneezing symptoms (OR 2.06–CI 95% 1.57–2.71), quality of life compromised (OR 1.64 CI 95% 1.17–2.28) and night awakenings (OR 1.44 CI 95% 1.03–2.00) (Table 3). In those patients with uncontrolled AR, nasal obstruction resulted to be the most relevant symptom.

The risk of uncontrolled disease is associated considering the probability of having VAS score > 5 (as lack of control of disease) the logistic regression analysis showed that itching and nocturnal awakenings have less influence on the control of AR (Table 4) than nasal obstruction and sneezing frequency. The frequency of nasal obstruction in linearly associated with VAS score > 5, (OR 1.78 for each nasal obstruction frequency grade, CI 95% 1.24–2.55) (Fig. 2). There was no significant association between control of the disease and demographic characteristics (age, sex, comorbidities, duration of the disease).

Treatment of rhinitis

In patients with uncontrolled disease (VAS > 5), oral antihistamines were the most used medications (p = 0.005), whereas nasal steroids (as suggested by ARIA guidelines) were less used (p = 0,604) and allergen immunotherapy was the least employed (p = 0.037) (Table 5). In patients who needed to increase therapy (23/178), the most used drugs were steroids, both topical and systemic, and the steroid/antihistamine topical combination.

Discussion and conclusions

It is well known that AR is considered as a "trivial" disorder in the general population. Nonetheless, it probably remains the most common immune-mediated disease, with prevalence continuously increasing, and being responsible for a not negligible economic burden in term of absenteism or presenteeism [22, 23]. It has recently become clear that, despite the easy diagnosis, AR remains often uncontrolled or inappropriately treated. This can

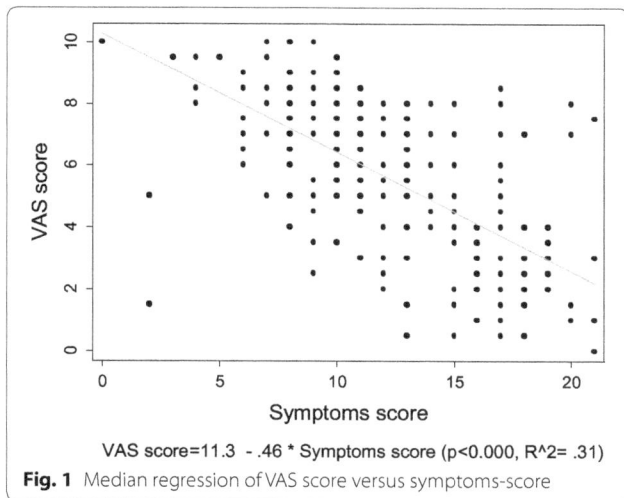

VAS score=11.3 - .46 * Symptoms score (p<0.000, R^2= .31)

Fig. 1 Median regression of VAS score versus symptoms-score

Table 3 Risk of higher VAS-symptoms score by QoL and CARAT items score adjusted each-other and for age by means of ordinal logistic regression)

VAS-score	Odds ratio	95% CI		p value
Age (media 34 years old)	0.98	0.97	1.00	0.020
Nasal obstruction (204/250)	2.06	1.57	2.71	0.000
QoL (169/250)	1.64	1.17	2.28	0.004
Awakenings (131/250)	1.44	1.03	2.00	0.031
Itching (189/250)	1.20	0.91	1.58	0.191
Drug consumption (178/250)	1.22	0.80	1.86	0.349

Table 4 Risk of VAS > 5—uncontrolled disease—by level of CARAT item (categorical) controlling each-other

	Odds ratio	95% Confidence interval	p value
Nasal obstruction			
Never	2.04	0.74–5.60	0.168
1–2/week	3.59	1.21–10.63	0.021
> 2/week	6.76	1.87–24.50	0.004
Linear trend	1.78	1.24–2.55	0.002
Sneezing			
Never	0.32	0.10–1.03	0.056
1–2/week	1.34	0.37–4.88	0.655
> 2/week	6.84	1.17–40.11	0.033
Linear trend	1.99	1.27–3.13	0.003
Itching			
Never	3.43	1.30–9.05	0.013
1–2/week	2.58	0.83–8.09	0.103
> 2/week	3.21	0.60–17.22	0.173
Linear trend	1.52	0.99–2.33	0.053
Awakenings			
Never	1.44	0.59–3.50	0.421
1–2/week	3.63	1.09–12.03	0.035
> 2/week	2.38	0.20–28.40	0.493
Linear trend	1.67	1.04–2.69	0.034

Result of logistic regression analysis using VS > 5 as dependent and CARAT Items as predictive variables

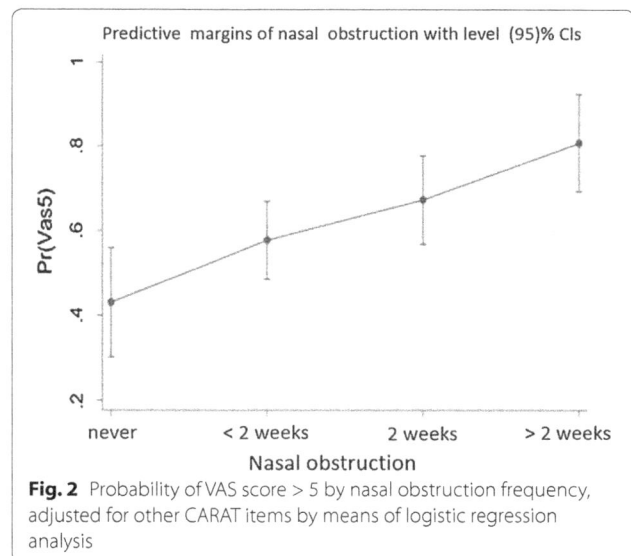

Fig. 2 Probability of VAS score > 5 by nasal obstruction frequency, adjusted for other CARAT items by means of logistic regression analysis

have a reflection on the natural history of the disease, as AR is the most relevant risk factor for the future development of allergic asthma [24–26]. In this multi-center cross-sectional study, conducted in Northern Italy, we aimed at evaluating the level of control of AR by means of a simple tool, the VAS, that can be easily filled by patients and reflects the presence of symptoms and their burden in the previous month. A VAS score > 5 suggests a not satisfactory control of symptoms. This parameter was correlated with CARAT, single symptoms, and the consumption of AR-related drugs. More than 60% of the patients analysed had an uncontrolled AR, providing evidence in line with the available literature data [4]. A European survey evidenced that a satisfactory control of AR symptoms can be achieved only in about 45% of the patients, independently of the drugs used [23]. It is also true that in our survey, including selected patients, only about one half was using multiple medications, and that only a minority was undergoing AIT. This survey confirmed that the VAS assessment is a reliable clinical tool, as it well correlates with the structured CARAT questionnaire and with the relevant symptoms of AR. In

our study, nasal obstruction, the quality of life and nocturnal awakenings significantly impacted on the VAS, but the best index of the failure to control was the presence of nasal obstruction. Even this observation conforms to what can be found in the literature, as nasal obstruction

Table 5 Risk of VAS > 5—uncontrolled disease—by therapeutic approaches used in patients

	Odds ratio	95% CI		p value > z
Antihistamines	2.33	1.30	4.20	0.005
AIT	0.37	0.15	0.94	0.037
Nasal steroids	0.82	0.38	1.76	0.604
Antihistamines plus nasal steroids	0.74	0.16	3.52	0.704
Nasal lavage	1.32	0.60	2.91	0.485
Systemic steroids	0.48	0.13	1.82	0.28

is the most difficult symptom to treat being it reported by most troublesome patients. This finding suggests to always evaluate this symptom as a predictive marker of poor control of the disease. We could not show any correlation between the lack of AR control and asthma, since our patients were selected without asthma and in a cross-sectional fashion [18, 19]. Finally, the most alarming fact that emerges is that the ARIA guidelines are still poorly followed. In fact, our AR patients, even if not controlled, mainly used antihistamines but not nasal steroids. Also, AIT is poorly used in our sample, although this observation could be biased by the fact that the most part of patients was at the first allergologic visit. Our series included patients who came after the evaluation of general practitioners, post-Emergency Room or specialists (ENT, paediatricians, pulmonologists). This suggests that not only general practitioners, but also other medical categories ignore or do not follow the ARIA guidelines, which must therefore have a greater circulation in order to obtain a better control of allergic rhinitis.

Authors' contributions
All the signing authors equally contributed in the clinical work, collected the data and drafted the manuscript. All authors read and approved the final manuscript.

Author details
[1] Allergy Service, Azienda Ospedaliera "San Luigi Orbassano", Turin, Italy. [2] Departmental Unit of Allergology & Respiratory Diseases, Fondazione Poliambulanza, Brescia, Italy. [3] Primary Care Pediatrician, National Healthcare System, Turin, Italy. [4] Experimental and Clinical Medicine, University of Parma, Parma, Italy. [5] Consultant Physician of Professional Diseases Observatory, Procura della Repubblica, Turin, Italy. [6] Allergology and Immunology, University of Turin, AO Mauriziano, Turin, Italy. [7] Asthma Center and Allergy Unit, Verona University and General Hospital, Verona, Italy. [8] Allergy and Respiratory Diseases, IRCCS San Martino-IST University of Genoa, Genoa, Italy.

Acknowledgements
None to disclose.

References
1. Bauchau V, Durham SR. Prevalence and rate of diagnosis of allergic rhinitis in Europe. Eur Respir J. 2004;24(5):758–64.
2. Bousquet J, Schünemann HJ, Zuberbier T, Bachert C, Baena-Cagnani CE, Bousquet PJ, Brozek J, Canonica GW, et al. Development and implementation of guidelines in allergic rhinitis—an ARIA-GA2LEN paper. Allergy. 2010;65(10):1212–21.
3. Bousquet J, Hellings PW, Agache I, Bedbrook A, Bachert C, Bergmann KC, Bewick M, Bindslev-Jensen C, et al. ARIA 2016: Care pathway implementing emerging technologies predictive medicine in rhinitis and asthma across the life cicle. Clin Transl Allergy. 2016;30(6):47.
4. WHO Collaborating Center for Asthma and Rhinitis, Bousquet J, Anto JM, Demoly P, Schünemann HJ, Togias A, Akdis M, et al. Severe chronic allergic (and related) diseases: a uniform approach–a MeDALL–GA2LEN–ARIA position paper. Int Arch Allergy Immunol. 2012;158(3):216–31.
5. Canonica GW, Triggiani M, Senna G. 360 degree perspective on allergic rhinitis management in Italy: a survey of GPs, pharmacists and patients. Clin Molec All. 2015;2:13–25.
6. Passalacqua G, Bousquet PJ, Carlsen KH, Kemp J, Lockey RF, Niggemann B, et al. ARIA update: systematic review of complementary and alternative medicine for rhinitis and asthma. J Allergy Clin Immunol. 2006;117(5):1054–62.
7. Canonica GW, Baena-Cagnani CE, Compalati E, Bohle B, Bonini S, Bousquet J, et al. 100 years of immunotherapy: the monaco charter. Int Arch Allergy Immunol. 2013;160:346–9.
8. Belhassen M, Demoly P, Bloch-Morot E, de Pouvourville G, Ginoux M, Chartier A, Laforest L, Serup-Hansen N, Toussi M, Van Ganse E. Costs of perennial allergic rhinitis and allergic asthma increase with severity and poor disease control. Allergy. 2016: 25.
9. Passalacqua G, Canonica GW. AIT (allergen immunotherapy): a model for the "precision medicine". Clin Mol Allergy. 2015;8(13):24.
10. Wheatley LM, Togias A. Clinical practice, allergic rhinitis. N Engl J Med. 2015;372(5):456–63.
11. Demoly P, Calderon MA, Casale T, Scadding G, Annesi-Maesano I, Braun JJ, Delaisi B, Haddad T, Malard O, Trébuchon F, Serrano E. Assessment of disease control in allergic rhinitis. Clin Trans Allergy. 2013;3:7.
12. Bousquet PJ, Combescure C, Neukirch F, Klossek JM, Méchin H, Daures JP, Bousquet J. Visual Analog Scales assess the severity of rhinitis graded according to ARIA guidelines. Allergy. 2007;62:367–72.
13. Hellings PW, Muraro A, Fokkens W, Mullol J, Bachert C, Canonica GW, Price D, Papado-poulos N, Scadding G, et al. A common language to assess allergic rhinitis control: results from a survey conducted during EAACI Congress Clin Trans. Allergy. 2015;27(5):36.
14. Demoly P, Jankowski R, Chassany O, Bessah Y, Allaert FA. Validation of a self-questionnaire for assessing the control of allergic rhinitis Clin. Exp All. 2011;41:860–8.
15. Meltzer EO, Schatz M, Nathan R, Garris C, Stanford RH, Kosinski M. Reliability, validity and responsiveness of the rhinitis control assessment test in patients with rhinitis. J All Clin Immunol. 2013;131(2):379–86.
16. Azevedo P, Correia de Sousa J, Bousquet J, Bugalho-Almeida A, Del Giacco SR, Demoly P, Giacco SR, Demoly P, et al. Control of allergic rhinitis and asthma test (CARAT): dissemination and applications in primary care. Prim Care Respir J. 2013;22(1):112–6.
17. Hellings PW, Fokkens WJ, Akdis C, Bachert C, Cingi C, Dietz de Loos D, et al. Uncontrolled allergic rhinitis and chronic rhinosinusitis: where do we stand today? Allergy. 2013;68(1):1–7.
18. Long JS, Freese J. Regression models for categorical and limited dependent variables using stata. 2nd ed. College Station: Stata Press; 2006.
19. Powers D, Xie Y. Statistical methods for categorical data analysis. Bingley: Emerald Group Publishing Limited; 2008.
20. Anderson JA. Regression and ordered categorical variables (with discussion). J Roy Stat Soc B. 1984;46:1–30.
21. Rogers WH. Quantile regression standard errors. Stata Technical Bulletin 9: 16–19. Reprinted in Stata Technical Bulletin Reprints, 1992; vol. 2, pp. 133–137.
22. Price D, Scadding G, Ryan D, Bachert C, Canonica GW, Mullol J, Klimek L, et al. The hidden burden of adult allergic rhinitis: UK healthcare resource utilization survey. Clin Trans. Allergy. 2015;5:39.
23. Canonica GW, Bousquet J, Mullol J, Scadding GK, Virchow JC. A survey of the burden of allergic rhinitis in Europe. Allergy. 2007;62(suppl. 85):17–25.

24. Bousquet J, Bousquet J, Gaugris S, Kocevar VS, Zhang Q, Yin DD, Polos PG, Bjermer L. Increased risk of asthma attacks and emergency visits among asthma patients with allergic rhinitis: a subgroup analysis of the investigation of montelukast as a partner agent for complementary therapy. Clin Exp Allergy. 2005;35(6):723–7.
25. Lombardi C, Passalacqua G, Gargioni S, Senna GE, Ciprandi A, Scordamaglia A, Canonica GW. The natural history of respiratory allergy: a follow-up study of 99 patients up to 10 years. Respir Med. 2001;95(1):9–12.
26. Grabenhenrich LB, Gough H, Reich A, Eckers N, Zepp F, Nitsche O, et al. Early-life determinants of asthma from birth to age 20 years: a German birth cohort study. J Allergy Clin Immunol. 2014;133(4):979–88.

Amelioration of patients with chronic spontaneous urticaria in treatment with vitamin D supplement

Nazila Ariaee[†], Shima Zarei[†], Mojgan Mohamadi and Farahzad Jabbari[*]

Abstract

Background: Spontaneous urticaria is a common allergic skin condition affecting 0.5–1% of individuals and may burden on health care expenditure or may be associated with remarkable morbidity.

Aim: In this study, we measured the effect of vitamin D supplementation in patients with a diagnosis of CSU. Furthermore, quality of life and cytokine changes were evaluated.

Methods: The clinical trial was conducted on 20 patients with idiopathic chronic urticaria. Vitamin D was administered orally for 8 weeks and disease activity was measured pre- and post-treatment using USS and DLQI. On the other hand expressions of IL-17, IL-10, Foxp3, and TGF-β by Real-time RT-PCR were assessed.

Results: USS questionnaire showed that severity of idiopathic urticaria after the intervention, which compared with the first day reached a significant 55% reduction. The DLQI quality of life questionnaire 2 months after treatment showed 55% improvement. Along with the significant improvement of clinical symptoms, use of vitamin D increase FOXP3 gene expression and downregulation of IL-10, TGF-B, and FOXP3, IL-17, but these changes were not statistically significant.

Limitation: These might happen due to lack of enrolled population in the investigation.

Conclusion: Vitamin D can be used along with standard medical care and it's a safe and cost-effective method for the treatment of chronic urticaria with deficiency of vitamin D.

Keywords: Spontaneous chronic urticaria, Vitamin D, T reg

Background

Chronic spontaneous urticaria (CSU) is a common allergic skin condition affecting 0.5–1% of individuals and may burden on health care expenditure or may be associated with remarkable morbidity [1]. It is characterized by urticarial itchy-wheals occurring almost daily and lasting more than 6 weeks, a remarkable proportion of the urticaria patients experience this condition for 10 years [2]. According to various recommendations; the diagnosis of the disease depends on clinical parameters, and therapeutic management still remains almost unclear.

Generally, more severe urticaria symptoms are, more difficult to treat [3].

Many of the patients with CSU, approximately 35–40% have circulating autoantibodies against the immunoglobin E (IgE) or against high-affinity receptor for IgE (FcεRI). These patients are considered to have CSU. Some studies suggest of T lymphocyte and its related subpopulations including T helper 1 (Th1), T helper 2 (Th2), T regulatory (Treg) cells particular roles in the onset and maintenance of chronic inflammatory responses in CSU [4].

There is a vivid association with the T cell subpopulation, especially Tregs and Th 17, of such patients with autoimmunity [5]. H1-antihistamines (second-generation) are recommended as first-line therapy [6]; the doses of antihistamines and choosing the most appropriate

*Correspondence: Jabbarif@mums.ac.ir

[†]Nazila Ariaee and Shima Zarei are equivalent as the first author

Allergy Research Center, Ghaem Hospital, Mashhad University of Medical Sciences, Shariati Square, Mashhad, Iran

antihistamine or other associated drugs including anti-leukotrienes, immunomodulatory, and immunosuppressives are not specified [7].

A role for vitamin D (Vit D) in allergic diseases increased attention in recent decades when the causative role for it in the treatment of the immune-mediated issue, including some autoimmune diseases, cancers, transplant rejection, had been proved [8]. Furthermore, a large number of investigations indicated vitamin D deficiency had linked with asthma, dermatitis or even allergic rhinitis [9]. It also displayed considerable functions in anti-inflammatory or immunoregulatory diseases [10].

In this study, we tried to evaluate Vit D level in sera of chronic spontaneous urticaria patients and had a treatment with Vit D supplement to assess the outcome in the alleviation of the severity of urticaria and life quality of enrolled patients. Moreover, the Tregs specific cytokines such as Transforming growth factor β (TGF-β), Interleukin 10 (IL-10), Interleukin 17 (IL-17), Forkhead box P3 (FOXP3) concentrations were compared before and after the intervention to evaluate the possible role of Vit D in Treg function and its relation to chronic idiopathic urticaria.

Methods
Patients
Chronic urticaria patients who referred to Allergy Clinic, Ghaem hospital (Mashhad University of Medical Science, Mashhad, Iran) from March 2014 to March 2015, were enrolled. The patients were visited separately by two different allergists and entirely fulfilled the criteria of idiopathic chronic urticaria [13].

All the patients should have a history of involving with urticaria at least for 6 weeks of and 4 days a week with Vit D concentration lower than 10 ng/ml were selected to study. In addition, the negative allergy skin prick test for common local aeroallergens [11], and foods allergies were checked patients with allergic rhinitis were excluded from the study. After that their CH50 and IgE level were evaluated, patients with normal CH5 and total IgE level (less than 150 IU per ml) and CH50 were selected for the study. Patients were also evaluated by autologous test to find if they have active autoantibodies, to eliminate patients with the active autoantibodies meanwhile, patients with auto immune diseases were also excluded. In addition, all patients were checked for normal hematological indices including Complete blood count, erythrocyte sedimentation rate. While they were checked for normal biochemical factors such as blood urea nitrogen, creatinine, and leaver functional tests. They were also checked for normal C-reactive protein, Antinuclear Antibody, beside that negative Hepatitis

B and *Helicobacter pylori* antigens were considered. Patients with Vit D concentration higher than 30 ng per ml were also excluded.

Patients had administrated with the highest dose of antihistamines for 3 months before adding Vit D supplement to their treatments strategy. Antihistamines were selected distinctly from patients with urticaria usually had demonstrated different responses to the various treatments so the most appropriate one had chosen for every individual. After these 3 months of treatment, our intervention was initiated, and oral Vit D was added to their conventional treatment. They have administrated a pearl of 50,000 unit every week during 8 weeks. The effects of intervention with Vit D compared with before intervention, so there was no inquiry of the control group.

Firstly, quality of life and urticaria severity were evaluated, by filling Dermatology Life Quality Index (DLQI) and Urticaria Severity Score (USS) questioners with a range of 0–30 and 0–56, respectively. Two mounts after addition of Vit D supplement to the conventional treatment as previously talked, the questioners filled again to evaluate urticaria severity and patients' quality of life and comparing with previous one.

Sample collection and gene expression
To evaluate cytokine changes, before and after intervention 8 cc brachial blood was obtained from patients and after isolating peripheral blood mononuclear cell (PBMCs), the cells were cultured in RPMI (Fermentas, Canada). The PBMCs were harvested after stimulating by Phytohaemagglutinin (PHA) when 6 h lasting. Afterward, RNA extracted and cDNA was synthesized (Fermentas, Canada). cDNA quality checked by PCR with GAPDH universal primers. The process followed by SYBR Green real-time PCR of interested genes including IL-10, IL-17, TGF-β, FOXP3, β2μ gene and its universal primers was used as internal control the sequence of primers can be seen in Table 1. All the PCR products were sequenced to clarify the accuracy of Real-time PCR amplification in Bioneer Company, South Korea.

Statistical analysis
Data analysis was carried out using the SPSS software (version 16, USA). To analyze the normal distribution of cytokines in both groups, the Kolmogorov–Smirnov test was applied. As a result of the normal distribution of data in both groups, a paired t test was applied to compare the averages before and after treatment. In the case of abnormal distribution, Mann–Whitney test and other nonparametric tests were applied. Differences were considered to be significant when $p < 0.05$.

Table 1 Designed primers for genes of interest

Name	Accession number	Product length (bp)	Sequence (5′ → 3′)
IL-10	NM_000572.2	111	Forward: TTGCTGGAGGACTTTAAGGGT Reverse: CTTGATGTCTGGGTCTTGGTT
IL-17	NM_000619.2	142	Forward: GTCAACCTGAACATCCATAACCG Reverse: ACTTTGCCTCCCAGATCACAG
FOXP3	NM_000589.2	95	Forward: ACTACTTCAAGTTCCACAACAGC Reverse: GAGTGTCCGCTGCTTCTCTG
TGFβ	NM_000660.5	192	Forward: GCAAGTGGACATCAACGGG Reverse: CGCACGCAGCAGTTCTTCTC

Results

Demography

In this investigation, 20 patients with urticaria were visited in Allergy clinic during the year of study. The mean age of the patients was (Mean ± SD) 35.6 ± 13.1 while the youngest patient was 14 and the oldest one was 57 years old. 11 (55%) of them were females and other 9 (45%) were males. The average time that patients involved with urticaria was 22.1 ± 7.6 months.

Clinical effects

According to DLQI, the quality of life of enrolled patients was changed after treatment with Vit D supplements and their quality of life was significantly increased. In this case, according to the parameters of DLQI, and based on patients' answers, patients were subdivided into 4 groups including without effect, low, moderate and intensive effects. Vit D was the dramatically inhibited impact of chronic urticaria on the quality of lives in all 4 groups. The details of DLQI outcomes can be seen in Table 2.

The severity of idiopathic urticaria in conducted patients after treatment with Vit D was statistically decreased. According to USS parameters enrolled patients were subdivided into 4 groups including very low, low, moderate, and severe. The amount of the abatement was 55% after the intervention. The details of the USS outcomes in both stages including before and after treatment with Vit D can be vividly seen in Table 3.

Cytokines assay

The results of SYBR Green Real-time PCR for TGFβ gene transcript apparently indicated that TGFβ expression was dropped out after treatment with Vit D. The outgrowth decline was not statistically significant, the mean ± SD of the TGFβ was 1.42 ± 0.43 at the first, and after the intervention, it decreased only to 0.98 ± 0.2.

The result of the assessment of IL-10 expression before and after the intervention indicated that the concentration of this cytokine was 2.7 ± 0.7 and during the treatment it decreased and achieved to 1.4 ± 0.3, the average of IL-10 was dropped out but not significantly according to paired t test in p < 0.05.

Evaluating IL-17 before and after treatment with Vit D in chronic idiopathic urticaria showed that the amount of IL-17 expression was dropped out from 2.4 ± 0.6 to 1.1 ± 0.6. Although the decline was reached to half of primer amount, this decline was not statistically significant.

Our data showed that FOXP3 was increased after treatment with Vit D and raised from 0.65 ± 0.2 to 0.77 ± 0.1 but the rise was not also significant.

Discussion

We undertook this study based on the hypothesis that vitamins and minerals effect some allergic issues [12] and the reports that proved that Iranian population had

Table 2 Quality of life Index before and after treatment with Vit D

	DLQI in CSU	N	Mean ± SD	Mean ± SD
Before treatment with Vit D	No effect	2	1	10.8 ± 1.6
	Low	9	6 ± 2	
	Moderate	7	16.1 ± 3.1	
	Severe	2	23.5 ± 0.7	
After treatment with Vit D	No effect	5	0.6 ± 0.54	0.9 ± 4.8
	Low	13	5 ± 2.7	
	Moderate	2	13.5 ± 3.6	
	Severe	0	0	

Table 3 Severity of urticaria according to USS questionnaire parameter before and after treatment with Vit D

	Urticaria severity score	N	Mean ± SD	Mean ± SD
Before treatment whit Vit D	Very low	0	0	23.5 ± 13.9
	Low	9	10.3 ± 3.1	
	Moderate	3	23.3 ± 2.5	
	Severe	8	38.4 ± 6.1	
After treatment whit Vit D	Very low	0	0	11.2 ± 9.6
	Low	13	5.1 ± 2.5	
	moderate	6	19.5 ± 2.6	
	Severe	1	39	

a profound deficiency of Vit D [13]. Meanwhile, some other studies reported the variety of gene expression and their fluctuation, and cytokine changes involved in urticaria, the furthermore presence of different T cell subsets in active lesions of patients with CSU were observed [14]. So we tried to uncover associations of Vit D with severity CSU and the possible role of T reg and Th17 related cytokines.

Previously, some authors reported symptom alleviation of urticaria after administration of vitamin D supplementation [15]. Our data also support this theory in different ways regarding improving health outcome, quality of life, and severity of the disease in a patient with CSU. In comparison with similar works that evaluate patients with urticaria, we tried to have strict inclusion criteria to have evaluation only for CSU; since it is more challenging to find a specific diagnostic strategy [16].

In this study, we revealed that FOXP3, a clinical determinant of Treg, increased in CSU patients after treating with Vit D supplement. The data were aligned with other studies focused on the phenotype or functional analysis of Tregs, they had revealed Treg which isolated from patients with autoimmune disorder reduced regulatory function comparing with healthy individual Tregs [17]. Treg devoted to aiding immune tolerance, hence their expansion is necessary for the resolution of inflammation and in preventing tissue damage or autoimmunity [18]. Tregs are usually characterized by the expression of FOXP3, which is the main transcription factor and also a master regulator of the immune suppressive activity of Treg [19]. It may be concluded that increase percentage of FOXP3 contributes to reducing the autoimmune pathogenic process of CSU. Although in our study, there was no significant rise in the concentration of FOXP3 in CSU patients before and after intervention in p > 0.05, the results were consistent with others who exhibited an increasing number of Tregs and FOXP3 expression while alleviating CSU symptoms.

Our investigation revealed that IL-17 had decreased after treatment with Vit D supplement in patients with CSU. In several skin diseases were proved previously that Treg and Th17 immune cells have to oppose immunomodulatory act in the inflammatory process [20], so we expected to have decreased in IL-17 while we had an increase in FOXP3. The opposing functions of Treg and Th17 cells have led many studies to suggest that unbalanced Th17/Treg outcome may be involved in the pathogenesis of some chronic inflammatory diseases [21]. These findings were confirmed by our experiments in which the constituent ratio of IL-17 cytokines significantly decreased. The imbalance of Th17/Treg cell subsets has been proposed to involve

in CSU pathogenesis and functional role in ameliorating patients with CSU [22, 23]. It speculated that inflammation can be subsided by the balance of Th17/Treg cell populations [24]. However, the mechanism still remains unclear. Further study may determine delicately how each cytokine interplays to exhibit the disease severity [25].

In evaluating IL-10 concentration, it was found that it had the reduction after treatment with Vit D in patients with CSU. Some studies have been previously shown levels of IL-10 significantly increased in the sera or cutaneous samples of patients with CSU, compared with the healthy population which is consistent with our data [26]. By contrast, some other studies discovered patients with CSU had lower serum levels of IL-10 compared with the healthy population [27].

IL-10 is an anti-inflammatory cytokine that secreted by some immune cells like T lymphocytes and macrophages [28]. It has inhibitory effects on mast cells and also controls proinflammatory cytokine release or their function [29]. It is not yet understood what is the specific role of IL-10 in urticaria, and still remain unclear this increase/decrease in IL-10 is a consequence of onset of CSU or compensatory response [26, 28].

Same as happened for IL-10, we had experience attenuation of TGF-B after treatment with Vit D in Patients with CSU. TGF-β has been demonstrated to have the ability to promote apoptosis of mast cells. Meanwhile, it can suppress the expression of both of the FcϵRI and IgE on mast cell surface [29]. Furthermore, it interferes with mediator release from mast cells so it may play an important role in homeostasis of mast cells [30]. Some studies illustrated that TGF-β can be a marker of mast cell degranulation and it usually rises during the active stage of urticaria. However; Anti-histamines help relieves the symptoms in some patients, some other patients do not respond sufficiently to this treatment due to the complexity of CSU pathogenesis [2]. such as TGF-β1 and IL-10 as their immunoregulatory function inhibit both Th1 and Th2 cells [31], so we expected to have dropped out of this two cytokine by amelioration of patients with CSU after treatment with Vit D.

CSU is a heterogeneous group of disorders, and it is unclear if this proportion of subjects [20] with CSU can truly represent all aspect of this disorder, so limitations of this study include the small number of subjects and lack of information about Th2 cytokines regarding cell specificity associated with altered gene expression. The single time point sampled during treatment might be beneficial to prove changing mentioned cytokines during the intervention. Furthermore, we did not have any placebo group so we may have some placebo effects.

Conclusion

In conclusion, our findings showed that Vit D supplement had a profound impact on CSU severity and patients' quality of life. Since Vit D is a cost-effective, profitable, and safe alternative that can be added to any therapeutical strategy in the management of the disease. On the other hand, due to its tremendous effects, it may apply in order to reduce other treatments like corticosteroids and immune suppressive. Moreover, the adverse side effects of conventional treatment can be avoided in this way.

Authors' contributions
NA, SZ: experimental work, preparation manuscript. MM: developed idea. FJ: visit, follow up, and evaluate health indices of the patients. All authors read and approved the final manuscript.

Acknowledgements
The authors wish to thank Mrs. Rashin Ganjali for collaboration in Real-time PCR.

Financial support
This investigation was performed under financial support of Research deputy of Mashhad University of Medical Sciences (Code: 910974).

References

1. Maurer M, Bindslev-Jensen C, Gimenez-Arnau A, Godse K, Grattan C, Hide M, et al. Chronic idiopathic urticaria (CIU) is no longer idiopathic: time for an update. Br J Dermatol. 2013;168(2):455–6.

2. Goldstein S, Weinberg JM. Recurrent and persistent urticaria: is it chronic idiopathic urticaria?: Narrative Review on Diagnosis and Management. J Dermatol Nurses Assoc. 2016;8(4):250–60.

3. Maurer M, Magerl M, Metz M, Zuberbier T. Revisions to the international guidelines on the diagnosis and therapy of chronic urticaria. JDDG J der Deutschen Dermatologischen Gesellschaft. 2013;11(10):971–8.

4. Chen W, Si S, Wang X, Liu J, Xu B, Yin M, et al. The profiles of T lymphocytes and subsets in peripheral blood of patients with chronic idiopathic urticaria. Int J Clin Exp Pathol. 2016;9(7):7428–35.

5. Negro-Alvarez J, Miralles-Lopez J. Chronic idiopathic urticaria treatment. Allergol Immunopathol. 2001;29(4):129–32.

6. Zuberbier T, Aberer W, Asero R, Bindslev-Jensen C, Brzoza Z, Canonica G, et al. The EAACI/GA2LEN/EDF/WAO Guideline for the definition, classification, diagnosis, and management of urticaria: the 2013 revision and update. Allergy. 2014;69(7):868–87.

7. Grzanka A, Machura E, Mazur B, Misiolek M, Jochem J, Kasperski J, et al. Relationship between vitamin D status and the inflammatory state in patients with chronic spontaneous urticaria. J Inflamm. 2014;11(1):1.

8. Rorie A, Goldner WS, Lyden E, Poole JA. Beneficial role for supplemental vitamin D 3 treatment in chronic urticaria: a randomized study. Ann Allergy Asthma Immunol. 2014;112(4):376–82.

9. Cheng HM, Kim S, Park G-H, Chang SE, Bang S, Won CH, et al. Low vitamin D levels are associated with atopic dermatitis, but not allergic rhinitis, asthma, or IgE sensitization, in the adult Korean population. J Allergy Clin Immunol. 2014;133(4):1048–55.

10. Mirzakhani H, Al-Garawi A, Weiss ST, Litonjua AA. Vitamin D and the development of allergic disease: how important is it? Clin Exp Allergy. 2015;45(1):114–25.

11. Oskouei YM, Hosseini RF, Ahanchian H, Jarahi L, Ariaee N, Azad FJ. Report of common aeroallergens among allergic patients in northeastern Iran. Iran J otorhinolaryngol. 2017;29(91):89.

12. Ariaee N, Farid R, Shabestari F, Shabestari M, Azad FJ. Trace elements status in sera of patients with allergic asthma. Rep Biochem Mol Biol. 2016;5(1):20–5.

13. Heshmat R, Mohammad K, Majdzadeh S, Forouzanfar M, Bahrami A, Ranjbar Omrani G. Vitamin D deficiency in Iran: A multi-center study among different urban areas. Iran J Public Health. 2008;37(suppl):72–8.

14. Holick MF, Chen TC. Vitamin D deficiency: a worldwide problem with health consequences. Am J Clin Nutr. 2008;87(4):1080S–6S.

15. Oguz Topal I, Kocaturk E, Gungor S, Durmuscan M, Sucu V, Yıldırmak S. Does replacement of vitamin D reduce the symptom scores and improve quality of life in patients with chronic urticaria? J Dermatol Treat. 2016;27(2):163–6.

16. Saini SS, Bindslev-Jensen C, Maurer M, Grob J-J, Baskan EB, Bradley MS, et al. Efficacy and safety of omalizumab in patients with chronic idiopathic/spontaneous urticaria who remain symptomatic on H 1 antihistamines: a randomized, placebo-controlled study. J Investig Dermatol. 2015;135(1):67–75.

17. Cousens LP, Najafian N, Mingozzi F, Elyaman W, Mazer B, Moise L, et al. In vitro and in vivo studies of IgG-derived Treg epitopes (Tregitopes): a promising new tool for tolerance induction and treatment of autoimmunity. J Clin Immunol. 2013;33(1):43–9.

18. Zohar Y, Wildbaum G, Novak R, Salzman AL, Thelen M, Alon R, et al. CXCL11-dependent induction of FOXP3-negative regulatory T cells suppresses autoimmune encephalomyelitis. J Clin Investig. 2014;124(5):2009–22.

19. Arshi S, Babaie D, Nabavi M, Tebianian M, Ghalehbaghi B, Jalali F, et al. Circulating level of CD4+ CD25+ FOXP3+ T cells in patients with chronic urticaria. Int J Dermatol. 2014;53(12):e561–6.

20. Kleinewietfeld M, Hafler DA, editors. The plasticity of human Treg and Th17 cells and its role in autoimmunity. Seminars in immunology. Amsterdam: Elsevier; 2013.

21. Tsur A, Hughes GC, Shoenfeld Y. Progestogens and autoimmunity. progestogens in obstetrics and gynecology. Berlin: Springer; 2015. p. 183–90.

22. Barbi J, Pardoll D, Pan F. Metabolic control of the Treg/Th17 axis. Immunol Rev. 2013;252(1):52–77.

23. Noack M, Miossec P. Th17 and regulatory T cell balance in autoimmune and inflammatory diseases. Autoimmun Rev. 2014;13(6):668–77.

24. Kimura A, Kishimoto T. IL-6: regulator of Treg/Th17 balance. Eur J Immunol. 2010;40(7):1830–5.

25. Hou F, Li Z, Ma D, Zhang W, Zhang Y, Zhang T, et al. Distribution of Th17 cells and Foxp3-expressing T cells in tumor-infiltrating lymphocytes in patients with uterine cervical cancer. Clin Chim Acta. 2012;413(23):1848–54.

26. Papadopoulos J, Karpouzis A, Tentes J, Kouskoukis C. Assessment of interleukins IL-4, IL-6, IL-8, IL-10 in acute urticaria. J Clin Med Res. 2014;6(2):133.

27. Hamad MA, Mitskevich N, Machavariani K. The Serum cytokines' network and Th1/Th2 profile balance in patients with chronic urticaria. Clin Transl Allergy. 2015;5(1):1.

28. de Kouchkovsky D, Esensten JH, Rosenthal WL, Morar MM, Bluestone JA, Jeker LT. microRNA-17–92 regulates IL-10 production by regulatory T cells and control of experimental autoimmune encephalomyelitis. J Immunol. 2013;191(4):1594–605.

29. Tavakol M, Movahedi M, Amirzargar AA, Aryan Z, Zare Bidoki A, Heidari K, et al. Association of interleukin 10 and transforming growth factor β gene polymorphisms with chronic idiopathic urticaria. Acta Dermatovenerologica Croatica. 2014;22(4):239.

30. Mohammed J, Gunderson AJ, Khong H-H, Koubek RD, Udey MC, Glick AB. TGFβ1 overexpression by keratinocytes alters skin dendritic cell homeostasis and enhances contact hypersensitivity. J Investig Dermatol. 2013;133(1):135–43.

31. Xie Y, Li X, Xu Z, Qian P, Li X, Wang Y. Effect of compound Maqin decoction on TGF-β1/Smad proteins and IL-10 and IL-17 content in lung tissue of asthmatic rats. Genet Mol Res GMR. 2016;15(3):1–7.

Role of genetic variations of *chitinase 3-like 1* in bronchial asthmatic patients

Kazuyuki Abe[1], Yutaka Nakamura[2]*, Kohei Yamauchi[1] and Makoto Maemondo[1]

Abstract

Background: Single nucleotide polymorphisms (SNPs) in *chitinase 3-like 1* (*CHI3L1*) are associated with bronchial severity and pulmonary function. CHI3L1 proteins are involved in both innate and adaptive immune responses; however, to date, the correlation of these SNPs and their age of onset of bronchial asthma has not been demonstrated.

Methods: To address the role of these genetic variations, 390 patients with well-controlled bronchial asthma and living in Japan were recruited, genotyped, and had a pulmonary function test performed on them in this study. To analyze the concentration levels of CHI3L1 protein, bronchial lavage fluids were examined.

Results: Forced expiratory volume in one second, %predicted (%FEV1), was significantly decreased in homozygotes of rs1214194 compared to heterozygotes and wild type. The age of onset of adult bronchial asthma was significantly younger in GG homozygotes of rs4950928 and AA homozygotes of rs1214194 than in the other two genotypes. The concentration of CHI3L1 protein in bronchial lavage fluid increased in both homozygotes of rs4950928 and rs1214194.

Conclusions: Our study demonstrated that the homozygotes of rs4950928 and rs1214194 of *CHI3L1* might predict an early onset of bronchial asthma and have the propensity to promote airway remodeling.

Keywords: Bronchial asthma, Single nucleotide polymorphisms, Chitinase 3-like 1

Background

Bronchial asthma is a disorder of the conducting airways that leads to variable airflow obstructions in association with airway hyperresponsiveness and a local accumulation of inflammatory cells, particularly Th2-type lymphocytes, eosinophils, and mast cells [1]. Allergens, such as those from mite and fungal exposure, up-regulate adaptive and innate immune responses, leading to the production of proinflammatory and profibrotic factors that may ultimately contribute to airway remodeling [2, 3]. Polysaccharide chitin, which is a polymer of *N*-acetylglucosamine, is found in the walls of fungi; exoskeleton of crabs, shrimp, and insects; the microfilarial sheath of parasitic nematodes; and the lining of

the digestive tracts of many insects [4–8]. Chitinases are the enzymes that digest chitin polymer, and human subjects have 2 chitinases encoded in their genome: chitotriosidase and acidic mammalian chitinase (AMCase). AMCase and the chitinase-like protein YKL-40/chitinase 3-like 1 (CHI3L1), which lacks chitinase activity, were shown to play a critical role in inflammation driven by Th2-type cells and were expressed at high levels in tissues from patients with asthma [9–11]. YKL-40/CHI3L1 are produced by a variety of cells, including neutrophils, monocytes, macrophages, chondrocytes, synovial cells, endothelial cells, and tumor cells [12, 13]. Serum [10], lung, bronchial tissues [14], and sputum [15] have been noted in patients with bronchial asthma. Moreover, single nucleotide polymorphisms (SNPs) in *CHI3L1* have been associated with a risk of bronchial asthma, bronchial asthma severity, and pulmonary function in populations of European ancestry [15]. Although it appears that YKL-40/CHI3L1 is strongly associated with both innate

*Correspondence: ICB75097@nifty.com
[2] Department of Allergy and Rheumatology, Nippon Medical School Graduate School of Medicine, 1-1-5 Sendagi, Tokyo 1138603, Japan
Full list of author information is available at the end of the article

and adaptive immune responses [16], the correlation of these SNPs and the age of onset of bronchial asthma has not been demonstrated. In the current study, we aimed to assess whether variants in the CHI3L1 rs4950928 and rs1214194 genotypes were associated with lung function, the age of onset, and the airway expression of CHI3L1 protein in Japanese adult asthmatic patients.

Methods
Study subjects
All study subjects were recruited from the Iwate Medical University Hospital. Patients aged $\geq$ 18 years were eligible if they had a diagnosis of asthma as defined by the American Thoracic Society criteria for $\geq$ 5 years and were using inhaled corticosteroid (ICS) at a stable dose for $\geq$ 1 year before screening. Well-controlled asthmatic patients who had no other medical disorders, who had smoked less than 10-pack-years, and who had not been exposed to environmental hazards were considered for the study to exclude concomitant COPD. Well-controlled asthma symptoms were defined as meeting none of the following criteria in the previous 4 weeks [17]: (1) daytime asthma symptoms showing more than twice/week, (2) any night walking due to asthma, (3) a reliever needed for symptoms more than twice/week, and (4) any activity limitation due to asthma. This study was approved by the Iwate Medical University Hospital Ethics Committee (H20-119) and registered with Clinical Trials (JMA-IIA00045 remodeling-ICS). Prospective patients were notified of our desire to include them in our study and were asked if they would be willing to participate. Upon acceptance, the subjects provided written informed consent according to the ethical protocols of our institution. Subjects were assessed for age, height, body weight, sex, age of onset, eosinophil counts, serum IgE concentration, and spirometry. The data for age of onset of bronchial asthma were self-reported. Spirometry was performed (HI-801, CHEST, Tokyo, Japan) according to the ERS/ATS Guidelines [18]. Airway methacholine responsiveness was measured using an Astograph (Jupiter 21, CHEST, Tokyo, Japan) according to the method described by Takishima et al. [19]. The examination was performed by measuring dose–response curves of respiratory resistance during continuous inhalation of methacholine at a stepwise incremental concentration. Methacholine hydrochloride in isotonic saline was gradually increased to 49, 98, 195, 390, 781, 1563, 3125, 6250, 12,500, and 25,000 µg/mL [20]. DNA was isolated from lymphocytes using standard procedures. Subjects were genotyped for rs4950928 and rs1214194 using a 7500 Fast Real-Time PCR System (Life Technologies Japan, Tokyo, Japan).

Fiberoptic bronchoscopy and specimen handling
Asthmatic patients underwent fiberoptic bronchoscopic examinations during ICS treatment. Asthmatic bronchial lavage fluids (BLF) were obtained from (i) patients harboring CC (wild type) of rs4950928; (ii) patients harboring GG (homozygous) of rs4950928; (iii) patients harboring GG (wild type) of rs1214194; and (iv) patients harboring AA (homozygous) of rs1214194. Bronchial lavage was performed by inserting a flexible fiberoptic bronchoscope (Olympus; Olympus Optical Co Ltd, Tokyo, Japan) under local anesthesia, as previously described [21]. BLF was extracted from one of the subsegmental bronchi of the left lingular division by injection of 20 mL aliquots of sterile saline pre-warmed to 36.5 °C twice and gently aspirated back into polypropylene tubes kept on ice. We obtained 20–25 mL of BLF from each asthma patient. Immediately after lavage, mucus was removed from the fluid by filtration through gauze, total and differential cell counts were performed, and the fluid was then centrifuged at $200 \times g$ for 10 min at 4 °C. The supernatant was decanted and stored at -80 °C. Ten milliliters of BLF supernatant was concentrated to 1.0 mL (tenfold) by centrifugation using Centrifugal Filter Devices (Amicon Ultra-0.5, Merck Millipore, Darmstadt, Germany). CHI3L1 levels were measured in duplicate in BLF specimens using a commercially available ELISA kit for Human Chitinase 3-like 1 Immunoassay (R&D Systems, Inc., Minneapolis, MN, USA). The mean value of the 2 duplicates was used in the statistical analyses. Duplicate samples with coefficients of variation greater than 20% were reassayed.

Statistical analysis
Statistical analyses were performed using JMP version 11 (SAS Institute Inc., Tokyo, Japan). All data were expressed as the mean $\pm$ standard error. Comparisons of the patients' characteristics between the three groups were performed using one-way ANOVA. Post hoc multiple comparisons were performed using the Tukey–Kramer test for differences among all groups. Comparisons of the total and differential cell counts, and the concentration of CHI3L1 in BLF were performed using a t-test. P values < 0.05 were considered significant.

Results
Subject demographics and enrolment
Of 390 asthmatic patients screened, 381 of rs4950928 and 368 of rs1214194 were successfully genotyped ($\geq$ 94%). We identified 270, 90, and 21 subjects that had CC wild type, CG heterozygotes, and GG homozygotes, respectively, for rs4950928 (Table 1). There were no significant differences in age at study enrolment, sex, eosinophil count status, serum IgE concentration, pulmonary

Table 1 Patient characteristics according to the rs4950928 genotype

rs4950928 genotype	CC (n = 270)	CG (n = 90)	GG (n = 21)	P value
Age, years	57.6 ± 1.0	58.5 ± 1.7	55.8 ± 3.7	NS
Height, cm	158.4 ± 0.6	159.1 ± 1.0	160.4 ± 2.1	NS
Body weight, kg	59.4 ± 0.7	60.7 ± 1.2	60.8 ± 2.7	NS
Sex, n (%)	110 men (41)	41 men (46)	12 men (57)	NS
Age of onset, years	42.5 ± 1.3	44.3 ± 2.2	31.1 ± 4.5	0.032
Eosinophil count/ μL	300.9 ± 17.4	359.5 ± 29.9	277.6 ± 65.1	NS
IgE level, IU/mL	412.1 ± 58.0	435.2 ± 77.9	565.4 ± 233.2	NS
GINA asthma severity, n (%)				
Mild	58 (21.5)	21 (23.3)	6 (28.6)	–
Moderate	105 (38.9)	33 (36.7)	12 (57.1)	–
Severe	107 (39.6)	36 (40.0)	3 (14.3)	–
Pulmonary function				
%FVC	103.3 ± 2.0	104.3 ± 3.4	103.51 ± 9.8	NS
FEV1, L	2.3 ± 0.1	2.3 ± 0.1	2.3 ± 0.2	NS
FEV1/FVC, %	72.9 ± 0.7	70.8 ± 1.2	70.2 ± 2.6	NS
%FEV1	98.9 ± 1.5	98.8 ± 2.6	95.1 ± 5.3	NS
Mild	105.8 ± 3.1	106.8 ± 5.4	91.0 ± 26.5	–
Moderate	100.0 ± 2.3	100.5 ± 4.3	103.3 ± 22.6	–
Severe	94.2 ± 2.3	92.5 ± 4.1	92.2 ± 33.1	–
Equivalent FP CFC dose (μg/ day)	382.1 ± 17.0	362.4 ± 29.3	228.0 ± 63.7	NS

Data are expressed as the mean ± standard error

GINA, Global Initiative for Asthma; FVC, forced vital capacity; FEV1, forced expiratory flow volume in one second; NS, not significant among the three groups; FP, fluticasone propionate; CFC, chlorofluorocarbon propellant

function, or receiving dose of ICS. We also identified 170, 157, and 41 subjects that had GG wild type, GA heterozygotes, and AA homozygotes, respectively, for rs1214194 (Table 2). AA homozygotes had a significantly lower forced expiratory flow volume in one second, %predicted (%FEV1) compared to other genotypes (Table 2). There were significant differences in the age of bronchial asthma onset among the three groups for rs4950928 and rs1214194 (Tables 1, 2). We next restricted the study to adult-onset bronchial asthma (excluded child-onset asthma) and compared the age of onset. The age of onset of adult bronchial asthma was significantly lower in GG homozygotes of rs4950928 (Table 3) and AA homozygotes of rs1214194 than in the other two genotypes (Table 4).

Detection of clinically relevant CHI3L1 levels in BLF supernatants

We performed a bronchoscopy and collected BLF from the two groups to confirm whether GG and AA homozygotes of rs4950928 and rs1214194, respectively, expressed

any increased CHI3L1 protein levels. Four patients who were genotyped as CC and 5 patients as GG of rs4950928 harboring wild type of rs1214194 and 6 patients who were genotyped as GG and 4 patients as AA of rs1214194 harboring wild type of rs4950928 were accepted for the BLF studies, which was performed following recommended safety procedures and was well tolerated in all subjects. There were no significant differences in total and differential cell counts between wild type and homozygous. In contrast, CHI3L1 levels in BLF were significantly increased in patients who were homozygous compared to wild type (Table 5).

Discussion

In this study, we investigated genetic variants of *CHI3L1* related to clinical characteristics in Japanese asthmatic patients. Several new findings have emerged from this study. First, we demonstrated that asthmatic patients with genetic variants of rs1214194 had a reduced %FEV1. Second, the age of onset of bronchial asthma was significantly younger in homozygotes of rs4950928 and rs1214194 than in other genotypes. When compared with restricted adult-onset asthma, the age of onset was significantly younger in homozygotes than in the wild type and heterozygotes genotypes. Third, CHI3L1 in BLF from *CHI3L1* homozygotes of GG of rs4950928 and AA of rs1214194 increased compared to the wild type in asthmatic patients. Previous population studies of genetic variation in the *CHI3L1* gene and bronchial asthma have shown an association with the promoter SNP rs4950928, intronic SNP rs1214194, and a decreased %FEV1 [15]. However, our studies demonstrated that %FEV1 was decreased in asthmatic patients harboring only homozygotes of rs1214194. One explanation for these differences may depend on medical treatment. Our prospective studies have indicated that *STAT4* TT of rs925847 and *IL13* AA of rs20541 are potential genomic biomarkers that predict lower pulmonary function. High-dose inhaled corticosteroid treatment increased the pulmonary function of patients homozygous for *IL13* AA of rs20541 but not of patients homozygous for *STAT4* TT of rs925847 [22]. Another analysis revealed an association between the homozygous *GLCCI1* rs37972 and rs37973 and the asthmatic treatment steps used with the Japanese population, showing an OR of 2.78 and 2.28, respectively, but not with pulmonary function [23]. We concluded that the recent wide use of anti-IgE and tiotropium produced a clinically meaningful reduction in the exacerbation rate and a sequential improvement in pulmonary function. Thus, decreased FEV1 was dependent on the genetic background and treatment content.

YKL-40/CHI3L1 plays a role in the pathophysiology of bronchial asthma by modulating innate and adaptive

Table 2 Patient characteristics according to the rs1214194 genotype

rs1214194 genotype	GG (n = 170)	GA (n = 157)	AA (n = 41)	P value
Age, years	57.8 ± 1.2	57.7 ± 1.3	58.4 ± 2.7	NS
Height, cm	158.8 ± 0.7	159.0 ± 0.7	157.7 ± 1.5	NS
Body weight, kg	60.5 ± 1.9	59.6 ± 1.0	59.1 ± 1.9	NS
Sex, n (%)	71 men (42)	71 men (45)	15 men (37)	NS
Age of onset, years	43.5 ± 1.6	43.2 ± 1.7	34.2 ± 3.3	0.032
Eosinophil count/μL	315.6 ± 21.7	310.6 ± 23.4	331.7 ± 46.1	NS
IgE level, IU/mL	473.7 ± 97.5	504.4 ± 101.2	235.7 ± 199.2	NS
GINA asthma severity, n (%)				
Mild	35 (20.6)	34 (21.7)	4 (9.8)	–
Moderate	70 (41.2)	61 (38.9)	18 (43.9)	–
Severe	65 (38.2)	62 (39.5)	19 (46.3)	–
Pulmonary function				
%FVC	104.0 ± 2.6	104.0 ± 2.4	97.2 ± 5.9	NS
FEV1, L	2.3 ± 0.1	2.3 ± 0.1	2.1 ± 0.2	NS
FEV1/FVC, %	72.4 ± 0.9	72.2 ± 1.0	70.9 ± 1.8	NS
%FEV1	99.6 ± 2.0	98.8 ± 1.8	87.9 ± 3.6	0.04
Mild	106.7 ± 4.3	102.7 ± 3.8	91.0 ± 11.8	–
Moderate	103.1 ± 3.0	99.3 ± 2.8	89.5 ± 5.6	–
Severe	92.0 ± 3.1	95.1 ± 3.8	85.8 ± 5.4	–
Equivalent FP CFC dose (μg/day)	325.6 ± 20.8	363.1 ± 22.3	432.1 ± 44.1	NS

Data are expressed as the mean ± standard error

GINA, Global Initiative for Asthma; FVC, forced vital capacity; FEV1, forced expiratory flow volume in one second; NS, not significant among the three groups; FP, fluticasone propionate; CFC, chlorofluorocarbon propellant

Table 3 Age of adult-onset asthma according to the rs4950928 genotype

rs4950928 genotype	CC (n = 233)	CG (n = 78)	GG (n = 18)	P value
Age of onset, years	47.6 ± 1.1	48.4 ± 1.9	35.7 ± 4.0	0.013

Data are expressed as the mean ± standard error

Table 4 Age of adult-onset asthma according to the rs1214194 genotype

rs1214194 genotype	GG (n = 148)	GA (n = 135)	AA (n = 34)	P value
Age of onset, years	48.2 ± 1.4	48.6 ± 1.5	38.9 ± 2.9	0.009

Data are expressed as the mean ± standard error

immune responses. Surprisingly, to date, the effects of genetic variation in *CHI3L1* on the age of onset of bronchial asthma have not been addressed. To clarify this issue, we compared the ages of adult-onset bronchial asthma between the genotypes for SNPs in *CHI3L1* in Japanese patients. It is generally considered that early-onset asthma included child-onset asthma and

adult-onset asthma. However, based on the remaining possibility of the prevention of bronchial asthma development via an improvement of lifestyle habit, it should be distinguished from the perspective of preventive medicine. Genotyping of *CHI3L1* could be considered significant if the development of bronchial asthma can be avoided in men who are found to have a genetic variation of *CHI3L1*, have a family history of bronchial asthma, and are notified early enough to be able to sufficiently adjust their lifestyle habits. Studies of this have added to our understanding of the importance of genetic variations by demonstrating that *CHI3L1* rs4950928 and rs1214194 genotypes play a critical role in early-onset adult asthma. Bronchial asthma should be suspected in anyone with episodic wheezing, shortness of breath, and cough, especially if more than one of the symptoms is worse at night or is precipitated by an upper airway infection; however, these symptoms are relatively nonspecific in adult individuals. Using an examination of SNPs in *CHIL3L1* might promote early detection and intervention in preventing airflow obstructions.

Increased levels of the YKL-40 protein have been found in patients with a broad spectrum of pathologies, including those with rheumatoid arthritis [13], obstructive sleep apnea syndrome [24], solid malignancies [25],

Table 5 Cell differentials and CHI3L1 levels in bronchial lavage fluid

	rs4950928		rs1214194	
	CC (n = 4)	GG (n = 5)	GG (n = 6)	AA (n = 4)
Total cell/mL ($\times 10^4$)	11.5 ± 2.7	10.2 ± 2.4	12.0 ± 2.3	13.3 ± 2.9
Eosinophils, %	1.5 ± 0.5	1.9 ± 0.5	4.0 ± 1.5	6.5 ± 1.9
Macrophages, %	81.3 ± 4.7	75.0 ± 4.2	78.3 ± 4.0	72.5 ± 4.9
Lymphocytes, %	12.5 ± 3.1	15.0 ± 2.8	13.8 ± 3.1	15.0 ± 3.8
Neutrophils, %	2.3 ± 0.9	4.6 ± 0.8	3.3 ± 1.1	5.3 ± 1.4
CHI3L1, pg/mL	140.3 ± 313.5	1144.8 ± 280.4*	179.3 ± 155.30	770.8 ± 190.2¶

Data are expressed as the mean ± standard error

* $P < 0.05$ compared with CC, ¶ $P < 0.05$ compared with GG

atherosclerosis [26], and diabetes mellitus [27, 28]. Previous asthmatic models have demonstrated that diminished antigen-induced responses in chitinase knockout mice were associated with increased eosinophil apoptosis [12]. The potential importance of YKL-40 can also be seen in rheumatoid arthritis, in which elevated serum YKL-40 levels were correlated with the severity of joint involvement [29]. As a result, these observations indicated that YKL-40 might reflect a local inflammation. To our limited knowledge, no other reports have analyzed YKL-40 in BLF, but only in serum [10], sputum [15], and bronchoalveolar lavage fluid (BALF) [30]. With respect to asthma pathophysiology, only BLF reflects chronic airway allergic inflammation and the exact concentration of chemical mediators; therefore, it is still too early to regard the concentration of YKL-40 in the sputum and BALF as a marker of whole bronchial inflammation in bronchial asthma. The aim of the present study was to determine the concentration of YKL-40 in BLF. Further investigations to compare the concentrations in serum, sputum and BLF are needed. The expression of the chitinase breast regression protein (BRP)-39, which is the murine equivalent of YKL-40, was induced by cigarette smoke exposure in a mouse model [31]. The induction by cigarette smoke is IL-1 receptor (R) 1 dependent, which is unique from BRP-39 induction in house dust mite-induced allergic inflammation, which is both IL-1R1 and IL-13 independent. In a human specimen study, YKL-40 promoted bronchial smooth muscle cell proliferation and migration. The cells expressing YKL-40 and BRP-39 in the airways were identified as bronchial epithelial cells and macrophages. Bronchial epithelial expression of YKL-40 is positively correlated with bronchial smooth muscle mass in patients with bronchial asthma [14]. This suggests that cigarette smoke-induced YKL-40 in a Th2 milieu progresses airway remodeling in asthmatic patients. We cannot deny the possibility of advancement in the airway remodeling of bronchial asthmatic patients

harboring genetic variants of rs4950928 or rs1214194 and who had an increased YKL-40 in the bronchus due to cigarette smoke. Further examinations are needed to verify the relationships between genetic background, smoking, and declined pulmonary function data.

Conclusions

In conclusion, this study demonstrated that rs4950928 and rs1214194 homozygotes of *CHI3L1* might be promising genomic biomarkers as predictors of progressing airway remodeling. Before the age of onset of bronchial asthma for patients who have these genetic variants, we need to consider the development of a preventative program that can be implemented before symptoms occur or worse.

Abbreviations
CHI3L1: chitinase 3-like 1; SNPs: single nucleotide polymorphisms; BLF: bronchial lavage fluid; FVC: forced vital capacity; FEV1: forced expiratory flow volume in one second; NS: not significant; BALF: bronchoalveolar lavage fluid; BRP-39: breast regression protein-39.

Authors' contributions
KA and YN conceived the idea and designed, were responsible for this cohort from the beginning and participated in the planning and collection of the data. KY and MM performed the data analysis. All authors have written the manuscript together. All authors read and approved the final manuscript.

Author details
[1] Division of Pulmonary Medicine, Allergy, and Rheumatology, Department of Internal Medicine, Iwate Medical University School of Medicine, 19-1 Uchimaru, Morioka 0208505, Japan. [2] Department of Allergy and Rheumatology, Nippon Medical School Graduate School of Medicine, 1-1-5 Sendagi, Tokyo 1138603, Japan.

Acknowledgements
The authors would like to acknowledge M. Niisato, T. Yamaguchi, and S. Oura (Iwate Medical University School of Medicine) for their help in performing this study. All authors thank Drs. Qutayba Hamid and James G. Martin (McGill University) for their helpful comments.

References

1. Robinson DS, Hamid Q, Ying S, Tsicopoulos A, Barkans J, Bentley AM, et al. Predominant TH2-like bronchoalveolar T-lymphocyte population in atopic asthma. N Engl J Med. 1992;326:298–304.

2. Kim HY, DeKruyff RH, Umetsu DT. The many paths to asthma: phenotype shaped by innate and adaptive immunity. Nat Immunol. 2010;11:577–84.

3. Humbles AA, Lloyd CM, McMillan SJ, Friend DS, Xanthou G, McKenna EE, et al. A critical role for eosinophils in allergic airways remodeling. Science. 2004;305:1776–9.

4. Araujo AC, Souto-Padron T, de Souza W. Cytochemical localization of carbohydrate residues in microfilariae of Wuchereria bancrofti and Brugia malayi. J Histochem Cytochem. 1993;41:571–8.

5. Debono M, Gordee RS. Antibiotics that inhibit fungal cell wall development. Annu Rev Microbiol. 1994;48:471–97.

6. Fuhrman JA, Piessens WF. Chitin synthesis and sheath morphogenesis in Brugia malayi microlariae. Mol Biochem Parasitol. 1985;17:93–104.

7. Neville AC, Parry DA, Woodhead-Galloway J. The chitin crystallite in arthropod cuticle. J Cell Sci. 1976;21:73–82.

8. Shahabuddin M, Kaslow DC. Plasmodium: parasite chitinase and its role in malaria transmission. Exp Parasitol. 1994;79:85–8.

9. Zhu Z, Zheng T, Homer RJ, Kim YK, Chen NY, Cohn L, et al. Acidic mammalian chitinase in asthmatic Th2 inflammation and IL-13 pathway activation. Science. 2004;304:1678–82.

10. Chupp GL, Lee CG, Jarjour N, Shim YM, Holm CT, He S, et al. A chitinase-like protein in the lung and circulation of patients with severe asthma. N Engl J Med. 2007;357:2016–27.

11. Lee CG, Dela Cruz CS, Ma B, Ahangari F, Zhou Y, Halaban R, et al. Chitinase-like proteins in lung injury, repair, and metastasis. Proc Am Thorac Soc. 2012;9:57–61.

12. Lee CG, Hartl D, Lee GR, Koller B, Matsuura H, Da Silva CA, et al. Role of breast regression protein 39 (BRP-39)/chitinase 3-like-1 in Th2 and IL-13-induced tissue responses and apoptosis. J Exp Med. 2009;206:1149–66.

13. Hakala BE, White C, Recklies AD. Human cartilage gp-39, a major secretory product of articular chondrocytes and synovial cells, is a mammalian member of a chitinase protein family. J Biol Chem. 1993;268:25803–10.

14. Bara I, Ozier A, Girodet PO, Carvalho G, Cattiaux J, Begueret H, et al. Role of YKL-40 in bronchial smooth muscle remodeling in asthma. Am J Respir Crit Care Med. 2012;185:715–22.

15. Gomez JL, Crisafi GM, Holm CT, Meyers DA, Hawkins GA, Bleecker ER, et al. Genetic variation in chitinase 3-like 1 (CHI3L1) contributes to asthma severity and airway expression of YKL-40. J Allergy Clin Immunol. 2015;136:51–8.

16. Reese TA, Liang HE, Tager AM, Luster AD, Van Rooijen N, Voehringer D, et al. Chitin induces accumulation in tissue of innate immune cells associated with allergy. Nature. 2007;447:92–6.

17. Global Initiative for Asthma, Global Strategy for Asthma Management and Prevention 2015. http://ginasthma.org/wp-content/uploads/2016/01/GINA_Report_2015_Aug11-1.pdf. Accessed 1 Oct 2017.

18. Miller MR, Hankinson J, Brusasco V, Burgos F, Casaburi R, Coates A, et al. Standardisation of spirometry. Eur Respir J. 2005;26:319–38.

19. Takishima T, Hida W, Sasaki H, Suzuki S, Sasaki T. Direct-writing recorder of the dose-response curves of the airway to methacholine. Clinical application. Chest. 1981;80:600–6.

20. Hoshino M, Nakamura Y. Anti-inflammatory effects of inhaled beclomethasone dipropionate in nonatopic asthmatics. Eur Respir J. 1996;9:696–702.

21. Nakamura Y, Hoshino M, Sim JJ, Ishii K, Hosaka K, Sakamoto T. Effect of the leukotriene receptor antagonist pranlukast on cellular infiltration in the bronchial mucosa of patients with asthma. Thorax. 1998;53:835–41.

22. Nakamura Y, Suzuki R, Mizuno T, Abe K, Chiba S, Horii Y, et al. Therapeutic implication of genetic variants of IL13 and STAT4 in airway remodelling with bronchial asthma. Clin Exp Allergy. 2016;46:1152–61.

23. Chiba S, Nakamura Y, Mizuno T, Abe K, Horii Y, Nagashima H, et al. Impact of the genetic variants of GLCCI1 on clinical features of asthmatic patients. Clin Respir J. 2017. https://doi.org/10.1111/crj.12647.

24. Mutlu LC, Tülübaş F, Alp R, Kaplan G, Yildiz ZD, Gürel A. Serum YKL-40 level is correlated with apnea hypopnea index in patients with obstructive sleep apnea syndrome. Eur Rev Med Pharmacol Sci. 2017;21:4161–6.

25. Johansen JS, Jensen BV, Roslind A, Nielsen D, Price PA. Serum YKL-40, a new prognostic biomarker in cancer patients? Cancer Epidemiol Biomarkers Prev. 2006;15:194–202.

26. Fach EM, Garulacan LA, Gao J, Xiao Q, Storm SM, Dubaquie YP, et al. In vitro biomarker discovery for atherosclerosis by proteomics. Mol Cell Proteomics. 2004;3:1200–10.

27. Rathcke CN, Persson F, Tarnow L, Rossing P, Vestergaard H. YKL-40, a marker of inflammation and endothelial dysfunction, is elevated in patients with type 1 diabetes and increases with levels of albuminuria. Diabetes Care. 2009;32:323–8.

28. Nielsen AR, Erikstrup C, Johansen JS, Fischer CP, Plomgaard P, Krogh-Madsen R, et al. Plasma YKL-40: a BMI-independent marker of type 2 diabetes. Diabetes. 2008;57:3078–82.

29. Garnero P, Piperno M, Gineyts E, Christgau S, Delmas PD, Vignon E. Cross sectional evaluation of biochemical markers of bone, cartilage, and synovial tissue metabolism in patients with knee osteoarthritis: relations with disease activity and joint damage. Ann Rheum Dis. 2001;60:619–26.

30. Gavala ML, Kelly EA, Esnault S, Kukreja S, Evans MD, Bertics PJ, et al. Segmental allergen challenge enhances chitinase activity and levels of CCL18 in mild atopic asthma. Clin Exp Allergy. 2013;43:187–97.

31. Nikota JK, Botelho FM, Bauer CM, Jordana M, Coyle AJ, Humbles AA, et al. Differential expression and function of breast regression protein 39 (BRP-39) in murine models of subacute cigarette smoke exposure and allergic airway inflammation. Respir Res. 2011;12:39.

Permissions

The contributors of this book come from diverse backgrounds, making this book a truly international effort. This book will bring forth new frontiers with its revolutionizing research information and detailed analysis of the nascent developments around the world.

We would like to thank all the contributing authors for lending their expertise to make the book truly unique. They have played a crucial role in the development of this book. Without their invaluable contributions this book wouldn't have been possible. They have made vital efforts to compile up to date information on the varied aspects of this subject to make this book a valuable addition to the collection of many professionals and students.

This book was conceptualized with the vision of imparting up-to-date information and advanced data in this field. To ensure the same, a matchless editorial board was set up. Every individual on the board went through rigorous rounds of assessment to prove their worth. After which they invested a large part of their time researching and compiling the most relevant data for our readers.

The editorial board has been involved in producing this book since its inception. They have spent rigorous hours researching and exploring the diverse topics which have resulted in the successful publishing of this book. They have passed on their knowledge of decades through this book. To expedite this challenging task, the publisher supported the team at every step. A small team of assistant editors was also appointed to further simplify the editing procedure and attain best results for the readers.

Apart from the editorial board, the designing team has also invested a significant amount of their time in understanding the subject and creating the most relevant covers. They scrutinized every image to scout for the most suitable representation of the subject and create an appropriate cover for the book.

The publishing team has been an ardent support to the editorial, designing and production team. Their endless efforts to recruit the best for this project, has resulted in the accomplishment of this book. They are a veteran in the field of academics and their pool of knowledge is as vast as their experience in printing. Their expertise and guidance has proved useful at every step. Their uncompromising quality standards have made this book an exceptional effort. Their encouragement from time to time has been an inspiration for everyone.

The publisher and the editorial board hope that this book will prove to be a valuable piece of knowledge for researchers, students, practitioners and scholars across the globe.

List of Contributors

Christer Janson, Fredrik Sundbom and Mary Kämpe
Department of Medical Sciences, Respiratory, Allergy and Sleep Research, Uppsala University Hospital, Uppsala University, Uppsala, Sweden

Peter Arvidsson
ALK Nordic, Kungsbacka, Sweden

Francesca Wanda Rossi, Nella Prevete, Antonio Lobasso, Filomena Napolitano, Francescopaolo Granata and Amato de Paulis
Department of Translational Medical Sciences and Center for Basic and Clinical Immunology Research (CISI), University of Naples Federico II, Via S. Pansini 5, 80131 Naples, Italy

Felice Rivellese
Department of Translational Medical Sciences and Center for Basic and Clinical Immunology Research (CISI), University of Naples Federico II, Via S. Pansini 5, 80131 Naples, Italy
Centre for Experimental Medicine and Rheumatology, William Harvey Research Institute, Barts and The London School of Medicine and Dentistry, Queen Mary University of London, London, UK

Carmine Selleri
Hematology Branch, Department of Medicine, University of Salerno, Salerno, Italy

Valerio Pravettoni, Marta Piantanida and Laura Primavesi
Clinical Allergy and Immunology Unit, Foundation IRCCS Ca' Granda, Ospedale Maggiore Policlinico, Milan, Italy

Stella Forti
Unit of Audiology, Foundation IRCCS Ca' Granda, Ospedale Maggiore Policlinico, Milan, Italy

Elide A. Pastorello
Unit of Allergology and Immunology, Niguarda Ca' Granda Hospital, Milan, Italy

Eleonora Savi and Silvia Peveri
Allergy Unit, G. Da Saliceto Hospital, AUSL Piacenza, Piacenza, Italy

Elena Makri and Cristoforo Incorvaia
Allergy/Pulmonary Rehabilitation, ICP Hospital, Via Bignami 1, 20100 Milan, Italy

Valerio Pravettoni
Department of Internal Medicine, Clinical Allergy and Immunology, IRCCS Foundation Ca' Granda Ospedale Maggiore Policlinico, Milan, Italy

Mona-Rita Yacoub, Maria Grazia Sabbadini and Giselda Colombo
Department of Allergy and Clinical Immunology, IRCCS San Raffaele Hospital, Via Olgettina 60, 20132 Milan, Italy
Vita-Salute San Raffaele University, Milan, Italy

Alvise Berti, Corrado Campochiaro, Enrico Tombetti and Giuseppe Alvise Ramirez
Vita-Salute San Raffaele University, Milan, Italy

Andrea Nico, Elisabetta Di Leo, Paola Fantini and Eustachio Nettis
Section of Allergy and Clinical Immunology, Dept. of Internal Medicine, University of Bari, Bari, Italy

Alessandra Chiappori, Laura De Ferrari, Chiara Folli, Anna Maria Riccio and Giorgio Walter Canonica
DIMI-Department of Internal Medicine, Respiratory Diseases and Allergy Clinic, University of Genoa, IRCCS AOU S.Martino-IST, Genoa, Italy

Pierluigi Mauri
Institute for Biomedical Technologies, CNR, Segrate, Milan, Italy

Carlo Lombardi
Allergy and Pneumology Departmental Unit, Fondazione Poliambulanza Hospital, Brescia, Italy

Valerie Melli and Erminia Ridolo
Department of Clinical and Experimental Medicine, University of Parma, Via Gramsci 14, Parma, Italy

Cristoforo Incorvaia
Pulmonary Rehabilitation, Centro Specialistico Gaetano Pini/CTO, Milan, Italy

Darío Antolín-Amérigo, Mercedes Rodríguez-Rodríguez, José Barbarroja-Escudero, María José Sánchez-González and Melchor Alvarez-Mon
Servicio de Enfermedades del Sistema Inmune-Alergia, Hospital Universitario Príncipe de Asturias. Departamento de Medicina y Especialidades Médicas, Universidad de Alcalá, Carretera de Alcalá-Meco s/n, 28085 Alcalá de Henares, Madrid, Spain

Luis Manso and Beatriz Huertas-Barbudo
Hospital del Sureste. Arganda del Rey, Unidad de Alergia, Madrid, Spain

Marco Caminati
Allergy Unit, Verona University and General Hospital, Verona, Italy

Belén de la Hoz Caballer
Servicio de Alergia, Hospital Universitario Ramón y Cajal, IRYCIS, Madrid, Spain

Inmaculada Cerecedo
Servicio de Alergia, Hospital Universitario Clínico San Carlos, Madrid, Spain

Alfonso Muriel
Unidad de Bioestadística Clínica, Hospital Universitario Ramón y Cajal, IRYCIS, Madrid, Spain

Mizuho Nagao, Mayumi Sugimoto and Takao Fujisawa
Allergy Center and Department of Clinical Research, Mie National Hospital, IDD, Tsu, Mie, Japan

Carl Johan Petersson and Patrik Dykiel
Thermo Fisher Scientific, Uppsala, Sweden

Magnus P. Borres
Thermo Fisher Scientific, Uppsala, Sweden
Department of Women's and Children's Health, Uppsala University, Uppsala, Sweden

Satoshi Nakayama
Thermo Fisher Scientific, Uppsala, Tokyo, Japan

Yu Kuwabara
Department of Pediatrics, Mie National Hospital, Tsu, Mie, Japan

Sawako Masuda
Department of Otorhinolaryngology, Mie National Hospital, Tsu, Mie, Japan

Marco Toscano
Clinical Chemistry and Microbiology Laboratory, IRCCS Galeazzi Orthopaedic Institute, Via R. Galeazzi 4, 20164 Milan, Italy

Lorenzo Drago
Clinical Chemistry and Microbiology Laboratory, IRCCS Galeazzi Orthopaedic Institute, Via R. Galeazzi 4, 20164 Milan, Italy
Medical Technical Sciences Laboratory, Department of Biomedical Science for Health, University of Milan, Via Mangiagalli 31, 20133 Milan, Italy

Roberta De Grandi
Medical Technical Sciences Laboratory, Department of Biomedical Science for Health, University of Milan, Via Mangiagalli 31, 20133 Milan, Italy

Gianfranco Altomare and Paolo Pigatto
Clinical Dermatology, IRCCS Galeazzi Orthopaedic Institute, Via Galeazzi 4, 20164 Milan, Italy
Department of Biomedical Science for Health, University of Milan, Milan, Italy

Oliviero Rossi
SOD Immunoallergy Caraggi University-Hospital, Largo Giovanni Alessandro Brambilla, 3, 50134 Florence, Italy

Luisa Ricciardi, Francesco Papia, Giuseppe Cataldo and Sebastiano Gangemi
Department of Clinical and Experimental Medicine, School and Division of Allergy and Clinical Immunology, University of Messina, Messina, Italy

Mario Giorgianni and Giovanna Spatari
Department of Biomedical Sciences, Dental, Morphological and Functional Investigations, University of Messina, Messina, Italy

Gian Galeazzo Riario Sforza and Androula Marinou
Division of Sub Acute Care, Sesto San Giovanni Hospital, ASST Nord Milano, Sesto San Giovanni, Italy

Letizia Lombardelli, Federica Logiodice, Ornela Kullolli, Sergio Romagnani, Enrico Maggi and Marie-Pierre Piccinni
Department of Experimental and Clinical Medicine and DENOTHE Excellence Center, University of Florence, Largo Brambilla 3, 50134 Florence, Italy

Maryse Aguerre-Girr, Ysabel Casart, Fatima-Ezzahra L'Faqihi-Olive, Valérie Duplan and Philippe Le Bouteiller
INSERM UMR1043, CNRS UMR5282, Centre de Physiopathologie Toulouse-Purpan, Université de Toulouse III, 31024 Toulouse, France

Alain Berrebi
Gynécologie-Obstétrique, Hôpital Paule de Viguier, Toulouse, France

Daniel Rukavina
Department of Physiology and Immunology, Medical Faculty, University of Rijeka, 51000 Rijeka, Croatia

Herman Haller
Department of Gynecology and Obstetrics, Medical Faculty, University of Rijeka, 51000 Rijeka, Croatia

Maria Sandra Magnoni, Fabio Arpinelli and Andrea Rizzi
Medical and Scientific Department, GlaxoSmithKline, Verona, Italy

Marco Caminati, Gianenrico Senna, Anna Rita Dama and Michele Schiappoli
Allergy Unit, Verona University and General Hospital, Piazzale Stefani 1, 37126 Verona, Italy

Germano Bettoncelli
Società Italiana di Medicina Generale, Florence, Italy

Gaetano Caramori
Dipartimento di Scienze Mediche, Sezione di Medicina Interna e Cardiorespiratoria, Centro Interdipartimentale per lo Studio delle Malattie Infiammatorie delle Vie Aeree e Patologie Fumo-Correlate (CEMICEF, formerly termed Centro), Università di Ferrara, Ferrara, Italy

Paola Lucia Minciullo
School and Division of Allergy and Clinical Immunology, Department of Clinical and Experimental Medicine, University Hospital "G. Martino", Messina, Italy

Sebastiano Gangemi
School and Division of Allergy and Clinical Immunology, Department of Clinical and Experimental Medicine, University Hospital "G. Martino", Messina, Italy
Institute of Applied Sciences and Intelligent Systems (ISASI), Messina Unit, Messina, Italy

Giovanni Paolino
Unit of Dermatology, "Sapienza" University of Rome, Rome, Italy

Maddalena Vacca and Eustachio Nettis
Section of Allergology and Clinical Immunology, Department of Internal Medicine and Infectious Diseases, University of Bari Medical School, Bari, Italy

Enrico Heffler and Nunzio Crimi
Department of Clinical and Experimental Medicine, Respiratory Medicine and Allergy, University of Catania, Catania, Italy

Massimo Landi
Pediatrician Primary Care, Turin, Italy

Silvana Quadrino
"Change" Institute, Turin, Italy
"Slow Medicine Italy", Turin, Italy

Cristoforo Incorvaia
Allergy/Pulmonary Rehabilitation, ICP Hospital, Milan, Italy

Stefano Pizzimenti
ASL-TO3, Allergy Outpatients' Clinic, "Edoardo Agnelli" Hospital, Pinerolo, TO, Italy

Sandra Vernero
"Slow Medicine Italy", Turin, Italy

Giovanni Rolla
Department of Medical Sciences, Allergy and Clinical Immunology, University of Torino, Turin, Italy

Giorgio Walter Canonica
Allergy and Respiratory Diseases Clinic, DIMI-Department of Internal Medicine, IRCCS AOU S.Martino-IST, Genoa, Italy

I. Djuric-Filipovic
Faculty of Medical Science, University of Kragujevac, Svetozara Markovica 64, 34000 Kragujevac, Serbia

Marco Caminati
Allergy Unit and Asthma Center, Verona University and General Hospital, Piazzale Stefani 1, 37126 Verona, Italy

D. Filipovic
Institution for Emergency Medical Care, Bulevar Franša Depera 5, 11000 Belgrade, Serbia

C. Salvottini
Department of Internal Medicine and Therapeutics, University of Pavia, Strada Nuova 65, Pavia, Italy

Z. Zivkovic
Children's Hospital for Lung Diseases and Tuberculosis, Medical Center "Dr. Dragiša Mišović", Belgrade, Pilota Mihajla Tepica 1, 11000 Belgrade, Serbia
Faculty of Pharmacy, University Business Academy in Novi Sad, Trg Mladenca 5, 2100, Novi Sad, Serbia

Roberto Paganelli, Claudia Petrarca and Mario Di Gioacchino
Dipartimento di Medicina e Scienze dell'invecchiamento, Università "G. d'Annunzio" of Chieti-Pescara, Via dei Vestini, 5, 66013 Chieti, Italy
Ce.S.I.-Me.T., Chieti, Italy

Matteo Bonini
Airways Division, Airways Disease Section, National Heart and Lung Institute (NHLI), Royal Brompton Hospital and Imperial College, Dovehouse Street, London SW3 6LY, UK

Nicola Scichilone
Department of Biomedicine and Internal and Specialistic Medicine (DIBIMIS), University of Palermo, Palermo, Italy

Maria Teresa Ventura
Department of Interdisciplinary Medicine, University of Bari, Policlinico, Piazza G. Cesare no 11, 70124 Bari, Italy

Marco Casciaro and Sebastiano Gangemi
School and Operative Unit of Allergy and Clinical Immunology, Department of Clinical and Experimental Medicine, University of Messina, Messina, Italy

Rosalba Buquicchio
Dermatological Clinic, Department of Biomedical Science and Human Oncology, University of Bari Medical School, Policlinico, Italy

Marcello Albanesi, Andrea Nico, Alessandro Sinisi, Lucia Giliberti, Maria Pia Rossi, Georgios Kourtis, Anna Simona Rucco, Filomena Loconte, Loredana Muolo, Marco Zurlo, Danilo Di Bona and Luigi Macchia
School and Chair of Allergology and Clinical Immunology, Department of Emergency and Organ Transplantation, University of Bari-Aldo Moro, Piazza Giulio Cesare 13, Policlinico, 70124 Bari, Italy

Margherita Rossini
Unit of Clinical Pathology, Policlinico di Bari, Piazza Giulio Cesare 13, Policlinico, 70124 Bari, Italy

Maria Filomena Caiaffa
School and Chair of Allergology and Clinical Immunology, Department of Medical and Surgical Sciences, University of Foggia, Via Luigi Pinto 1, 70100 Foggia, Italy

Jenny van Odijk
Dept of Respiratory Medicine and Allergology, Sahlgrenska Academy at Göteborg University, Göteborg, Sweden
Internal Medicine and Clinical Nutrition, Sahlgrenska Academy at Göteborg University, Göteborg, Sweden

Sigrid Sjölander, Peter Brostedt and Hillevi Englund
R and D, ImmunoDiagnostic Division, Thermo Fisher Scientific, Uppsala, Sweden

Magnus P. Borres
R and D, ImmunoDiagnostic Division, Thermo Fisher Scientific, Uppsala, Sweden

Department of Women's and Children's Health, Uppsala University, Uppsala, Sweden

Federica Gani and Laura Barrocu
Allergy Service, Azienda Ospedaliera "San Luigi Orbassano", Turin, Italy

Carlo Lombardi
Departmental Unit of Allergology and Respiratory Diseases, Fondazione Poliambulanza, Brescia, Italy

Massimo Landi
Primary Care Pediatrician, National Healthcare System, Turin, Italy

Erminia Ridolo
Experimental and Clinical Medicine, University of Parma, Parma, Italy

Massimo Bugiani
Consultant Physician of Professional Diseases Observatory, Procura della Repubblica, Turin, Italy

Giovanni Rolla
Allergology and Immunology, University of Turin, AO Mauriziano, Turin, Italy

Gianenrico Senna
Asthma Center and Allergy Unit, Verona University and General Hospital, Verona, Italy

Giovanni Passalacqua
Allergy and Respiratory Diseases, IRCCS San Martino-IST University of Genoa, Genoa, Italy

Nazila Ariaee, Shima Zarei, Mojgan Mohamadi and Farahzad Jabbari
Allergy Research Center, Ghaem Hospital, Mashhad University of Medical Sciences, Shariati Square, Mashhad, Iran

Kazuyuki Abe, Kohei Yamauchi and Makoto Maemondo
Division of Pulmonary Medicine, Allergy, and Rheumatology, Department of Internal Medicine, Iwate Medical University School of Medicine, 19-1 Uchimaru, Morioka 0208505, Japan

Yutaka Nakamura
Department of Allergy and Rheumatology, Nippon Medical School Graduate School of Medicine, 1-1-5 Sendagi, Tokyo 1138603, Japan

Index